THE Men'sHealth
BIG
BOOK
OF FOOD
& NUTRITION

Rodale books may be purchased for business or promotional use or for special sales. For information, please write to:
Special Markets Department, Rodale Inc., 733 Third Avenue, New York, NY 10017

Men's Health is a registered trademark of Rodale Inc.

Printed in the United States of America
Rodale Inc. makes every effort to use acid-free ∞, recycled paper ♻.

Book design by George Karabotsos,
design director, *Men's Health* Books and *Women's Health* Books,
with Courtney Eltringham

Photo editor: Lila Garnett

Cover, openers, and recipe photography by Charles Masters
Food styling by Jamie Kimm • Prop styling by Tiziana Agnello

Individual food photography by Thomas MacDonald and Mitch Mandel
Food styling by Melissa Reiss

Library of Congress Cataloging-in-Publication Data is on file with the publisher.

ISBN-13 978–1–60529–310–3   paperback

Distributed to the book trade by Macmillan

2 4 6 8 10 9 7 5 3   paperback

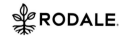
RODALE.

We inspire and enable people to improve their lives and the world around them.

Contents

Acknowledgments

Many good people helped *The Men's Health Big Book of Food & Nutrition* arrive in your hands, and I'd like to take this opportunity to thank them.

First among them are Rodale Inc. chairman and CEO Maria Rodale and the members of the Rodale family. Rodale is a truly unique publishing company and never ceases "to inspire and enable people to improve their lives and the world around them." My parents were *Organic Gardening* subscribers many decades ago, and the wisdom from those pages nurtured the gardens that fed me during my childhood. Thank you. I also praise *Men's Health* senior vice president, editor-in-chief, and brand leader David Zinczenko. DZ's Midas touch is simply phenomenal, and it's been an honor to work with him. Ditto Stephen Perrine, vice president and editor-in-chief of *Men's Health* Books, who has opened so many doors for me that I'll probably never be able to fully thank him. A sincere, heartfelt thanks for giving me so many wonderful opportunities.

The world-class brand that is *Men's Health* is a testimony to the editors, writers, copy editors, researchers, designers, photographers, illustrators, Web producers, doctors, personal trainers, advisors, nutritionists, and interns—past and present—who have worked tirelessly to create the world's best men's magazine. Thanks to all of them, and especially Matt Goulding, Adam Campbell, Paul Kita, Carolyn Kylstra, Laura Roberson, Clint Carter, and Adina Steiman for their contributions and guidance on the subject of nutrition.

The very fact that *The Men's Health Big Book of Food & Nutrition* made it into your hands is a testament to a handful of very special people: Mike Zimmerman, one of the hardest-working writers I know, who helped bring the book across the finish line when the going got tough; Senior Managing Editor Debbie McHugh, whose presence always made me feel a little bit better; Erin Williams, whose attention to details surpasses everyone's I know; nutrition number-crunchers Sara Cann, Andrew Del-Colle, and Sean Sabo; Lila Garnett, who guided the photo front; Chris Krogermeier, Brooke Myers, Liz Krenos, and Keith Biery at Rodale Books; and designers George Karabotsos, Mark Michaelson, and especially Courtney Eltringham, who created such a visually arresting book in such a short period of time. Thank you, thank you, thank you.

Last but not least: my wife, Laurel. In many ways we first bonded over food, and I look forward to cooking many meals together and tasting a multitude of flavors for years to come.

Eat wisely, America.

—*Joel Weber*

Introduction:
Indulge Your Way to a Better Body

Eating is easy.

But making smart choices about
what to eat seems harder and harder each day.
Well, that's about to change.

■

Here in 21st-century America, where we've become experts at building bridges, erecting skyscrapers, and posting cat videos to YouTube, we've also become experts at producing food. In 1920, the average American farmer could harvest 20 bushels of corn an acre. Ninety years later, his great-grandson can bag upward of 180 bushels on the same acre. Food is everywhere in America, and it's dirt cheap: 89¢ crunchy tacos, $1 cheeseburgers, and $5 footlongs. Take your pick—it's all been engineered to taste pretty darn good.

The problem with all that easy food? Humans are hardwired to feed. We're animals, after all, so when it's feeding time, our instinct is to feast mindlessly until we can feast no more, just like pigs lining up at a trough, cows entering a pasture, or chickens wandering a coop. If there's still soup in the bowl, you'll slurp it. If there's still food on a plate, you'll eat it. If there's still Coke in your Big Gulp, you'll drink it. Your gut basically just steamrolls over your brain; it'll alert you once you've chewed through the takeout and hit Styrofoam or reached an inedible wrapper. Food researchers call this phenomenon "mindless eating."

And mindless eating is exactly why so many of us carry *too much weight*—even as we're taking in *too little nutrition*.

Feeding has become so easy that since the Carter administration, Americans have added the equivalent of two extra meals to their days. We now consume 2,533 calories daily—21 percent more than we did in 1977, according to a 2010 study in the *American Journal of Clinical Nutrition*. And the results are predictable: Obesity and diabetes rates have grown as much as 50 percent since 1960.

We've given ourselves the power to produce and consume food at will. But we haven't given ourselves the information we need to manage all that power. What we've done is the equivalent of giving a brand-new Harley to a 9-year-old who's been taught to ride a 10-speed. No instructions, no training, no speed limits—just a lot of horsepower, set loose on a dangerous obstacle course. It's no wonder there are so many wrecks.

Well, here at last is the rule book, the authoritative guide to eating in the 21st century— the book they should have given all of us the first time we picked up a fork and a knife. Armed with the information within, you'll become a much smarter eater, one capable of harnessing the power of food. You'll learn to eat what you want, but in a smarter, leaner, healthier way. You'll learn to enjoy more, better, and less-expensive food. And, to quote that hairy guy from the Men's Warehouse commercials, you're going to like the way you look.

15 reasons you can't go another meal without this book.

1. You'll Eat Your Way to a Leaner Body

This is not a "diet" book. Most diet plans force you to cut calories until you're practically starving, leading you to lose not just fat but valuable muscle as well. And muscle is crucial to protecting you from injury, helping you burn fat, and developing the lean, firm shape you desire. What's more, it also keeps your metabolism—your body's internal furnace—firing. Sacrifice muscle by restricting calories, and you're priming your body to gain weight back more easily than before. That's what happens in "yo-yo dieting," and it's exactly why this book won't teach you to eat less. It will teach you to eat better.

2. You'll Enjoy Better Food

Not rabbit food. In fact, *The Big Book of Food & Nutrition* will establish some easy rules to eat by. You'll learn about E-A-T-S, the easiest nutrition plan ever, which will help you enjoy foods like, oh, steaks, burgers, ribs . . . the stuff you crave! Because humans crave protein, and protein is good—it helps us maintain muscle, enhances metabolism, and leads the assault on body fat.

64

Percentage of men who spend little or no time preparing their daily meals.

Not only does protein promote satiety by slowing down your appetite and making you feel full more quickly than either carbohydrates or fats, your body uses more energy to digest protein than it does to process carbohydrates or fat. "That means that the more protein you eat, the harder your body has to work to digest it, and the more calories you'll burn in the process," says Douglas Kalman, MS, RD, director of nutrition and research at Miami Research Associates. When a high-protein diet was compared with a high-carbohydrate diet at Arizona State University, for instance, people who ate the former burned more than twice as many calories in the hours following their meal as those eating carbs. And people who begin their days with high-protein eggs lose 65 percent more weight than those who eat a bagel with the same number of calories, according to a study in the *International Journal of Obesity*.

3. You'll Eat More and Weigh Less

It probably sounds counterintuitive: In order to weigh less, you need to eat more often. Skipping a meal creates a biological billboard that says, "We're starving here!" Your body responds by slowing your metabolism—its calorie-burning furnace—in order to hold on to its existing energy stores. If the food shortage continues, you'll begin burning muscle tissue,

which will lower your metabolic rate further. Even something as minor as rushing out the door without eating breakfast can reduce your metabolic rate by 10 percent, according Leslie Bonci, RD, MPH, director of sports nutrition at the University of Pittsburgh Medical Center. With *The Big Book of Food & Nutrition*, you'll learn to snack—smartly and often—to keep your metabolism's furnace stoked. Five small meals is a good number to strive for—breakfast, lunch, and dinner, as well as two protein-packed snacks, such as almonds or cheese—but you can even try for seven or eight. "People tend to eat around their cravings, snacking and nibbling until they've taken in 500 calories and still aren't satisfied," says D. Milton Stokes, MPH, RD. Instead of fighting your food urges, you'll just find a healthier way to satisfy them.

4. You'll Lose More Fat— Without Going "Low-Fat"

Contrary to popular belief, you actually have to eat fat in order to lose fat. But you don't have to go whole hog on a low-carb diet to see results. Swapping just a few hundred carb calories for fat calories a day—by, say, using butter instead of jam on toast or drinking milk instead of a sports drink after you work out—will help you stay fuller longer and gain fewer pounds, according to a recent study at the University of Alabama.

5. You'll Keep Your Brain Young

Rush University researchers discovered that eating certain nutrients (highlighted throughout *The Big Book of Food & Nutrition*) may keep your brain young. In a study of 3,000 people age 65 and over, scientists calculated that those who ate more than two servings of vegetables a day had a 40 percent slower rate of cognitive decline than those who ate one serving or less. Specifically, green leafy vegetables, such as collard greens, kale, romaine lettuce, and spinach, were the most effective mental medicine. The likely reason: They're all rich in folate and vitamin E, a potent compound that fights the oxidative stress and inflammation that age your brain.

6. You'll Sleep Better

In these pages, you'll discover which foods trigger the neurochemicals that induce sleepiness—and help you wake up feeling refreshed. Eating better may even lead to a more interesting night's sleep, scientists at Santa Clara University report. In their study, people who maintained healthy diets experienced more-vivid dreams, including the sexual kind, than those who regularly ate the most fast food. The researchers aren't sure how specific foods affect dreaming, but emerging research suggests that higher blood-sugar levels, which are often the result of weight gain or high carbohydrate intake, may reduce the amount of time spent in deep slumber.

7. You'll Be More Productive

If you need to stay sharp and focused for an afternoon business meeting, parking yourself at the local Starbucks will only go so far. Instead, eat foods known to enhance energy and sharpness, says Oxford University biochemist John Stanley, PhD. Choosing a combination of protein (which produces neurotransmitters, supporters of cognitive performance); minerals and vitamins like magnesium, iron, and B vitamins that help battle fatigue; and secret mind/body foods (like the Indian spice turmeric) that improve brain cell function could make the difference in your day. You'll discover a list of foods with such brain- and energy-boosting effects in the coming pages.

8. You'll Derail Diabetes

Although not an infectious disease, type 2 diabetes seems to be spreading like mono at a kissing booth. Since 1980, its prevalence in the United States has risen by 47 percent, a trend that's expected to hike northward during the next decade, as more than 1.6 million new cases will be diagnosed each year. Nearly half of American men today either have the condition or are on the verge of developing it, according to one report from the National Institutes of

47,000
The number of products in the average American grocery store.

Health. The consequences of this potential increase will be considerable: Diabetes is already the primary cause of cardiovascular disease, and can slash a man's life span by an average of 13 years. Can preventing diabetes and its complications be as simple as eating the right foods? Certain foods, especially carbohydrates, can cause blood sugar levels to spike, whereas nutrients in other foods—such as the calcium in dairy products, according to a research review in the *Journal of the American College of Nutrition*—may reduce the risk of metabolic syndrome, a precursor to diabetes. And a 2010 article in the journal *Clinical Diabetes* found that, in addition to just 30 minutes of physical activity five days a week, people at risk for diabetes should 1) cap their caloric intake from fat at 30 percent, 2) reduce their overall calorie intake, and 3) eat as many fruits, vegetables, and fiber-rich foods as possible. You'll get a better understanding of each recommendation in this book.

9. You'll Look Younger

After researchers in Australia, Indonesia, and Sweden studied the diets of 400 elderly men and women, they found that those who ate the most leafy green vegetables and beans had the fewest wrinkles. Spinach and beans—two all-stars explored in-depth in *The Big Book of Food & Nutrition*—are full of compounds that help prevent and repair damaged skin cells as you get older. Keep orange-colored foods, such as sweet potatoes, in your pantry, too. They're loaded with vitamin C, which smoothes out wrinkles by stimulating the production of collagen. A study in the *American Journal of Clinical Nutrition* found that volunteers who consumed 4 milligrams of vitamin C, about half a small sweet potato, daily for three years decreased the appearance of wrinkles by 11 percent.

10. You'll Cut Your Cancer Risk

If pharmaceutical companies were allowed to patent vegetables, we'd all need a prescription to buy tomatoes. "Tomatoes are loaded with lycopene, an important phytochemical with antioxidant properties, as well as glutamic acid, an amino acid, which work together to prevent prostate cancer," says Keith Block, MD, medical director of the Block Center for Integrative Cancer Treatment in Evanston, Illinois. You may have also heard that cooked tomato products contain the highest levels of lycopene, but only in *The Big Book of Food & Nutrition* will you learn cool tips on maximizing its effects. Example: adding a carrot, which is rich in beta-carotene, to your Bolognese will guide the lycopene to your prostate gland. USDA researchers found that when men were simultaneously given beta-carotene and lycopene supplements, more lycopene ended up in their bodies. And eating spaghetti is obviously a lot

3,000
The number of ingredients on the FDA's list of "safe" food additives.

more fun than eating pills. There are dozens of similar food combinations that have the same miraculous disease-fighting effects. You'll discover them in this book.

11. You'll Build Stronger Bones—with Beer

You probably know that a glass of milk can help cut your risk of osteoporosis by giving your body a much-needed blast of calcium and vitamin D. But another overlooked nutrient the body uses for maintaining strong bones is silicon, and to consume enough to keep your bones healthy, you may need to eat more whole grains and drink some beer, according to a report in the *American Journal of Clinical Nutrition*. Most men's consumption of silicon goes down as they grow older, and that lower consumption could help explain why a man's bones become more fragile as he ages, says Douglas Kiel, MD, the study's author. "Increasing the amount of silicon in your diet by eating more whole grains and drinking more beer could help fight the problem," he says. *The Big Book of Food & Nutrition* will fill you up with everything else that's been missing from your diet.

12. You'll Improve Your Fitness and Your Physique

Every guy in the gym knows he should consume some protein before and after a workout. Resistance training breaks down muscle, which requires a fresh infusion of amino acids to repair and rebuild it. "If you're lifting weights and you don't consume protein, it's almost counterproductive," says Jeffrey Volek, PhD, RD, a nutrition and exercise researcher at the University of Connecticut. "When you work out, your muscles are primed to respond to protein," he says, "and you have a window of opportunity to promote muscle growth." Protein also helps build enzymes that allow your body to adapt to endurance sports like running and biking. But how much protein, and when, and what kind? *The Big Book of Food & Nutrition* will help you time your meals and snacks for peak performance. Volek recommends splitting your dose of protein, eating half 30 minutes before the workout and the other half 30 minutes after. (One study, published in the *American Journal of Clinical Nutrition*, pinpointed 20 grams as the best amount of post-workout protein to maximize muscle growth.) A simple protein shake or nutrition bar is most portable and convenient. But the more time and thought you put into it, the more benefits you'll receive, because the quickest option isn't always the best one. "Whole foods provide a higher quality of the proteins, carbs, and fats your body needs," says Alan Aragon, MS. For a quick fix, pair a protein with a carbohydrate—some turkey or almond butter with a slice of bread, for instance.

20

Percentage of people who eat the recommended five servings of fruits and vegetables a day.

13. You'll Handle Stress Better

You may not be able to escape to a beachside hammock every time stress sets in, but you might find the same effect just by hitting the kitchen. Example: A piece of fruit may have caused a good deal of strife in the Garden of Eden, but here in modern times, it's actually a great chaos reducer. That's because the sugar in fruit will give you the little burst of energy that your adrenaline-charged body is craving. Any kind of fruit is fine, but reach for oranges on particularly crazy days, recommends Pam Peeke, MD, MPH, an assistant professor of medicine at the University of Maryland. Not only can the vitamin C help lower your body's production of cortisol, a stress hormone that breaks down muscle, but peeling an orange will also keep your hands and mouth busy. What's more, there might even be some truth to that old wives' tale that people who eat produce—an important element of the E-A-T-S plan—never get fat. According to Louisiana State University researchers, people who ate half a grapefruit three times a day lost 4 pounds in 12 weeks, even though they hadn't deliberately altered any other part of their diets. They also lowered their blood pressure by 6 points, enough to reduce their risk of stroke by 40 percent. The mechanism isn't clear, but the researchers speculate that grapefruit's acidity may slow your rate of digestion, helping to keep you full longer.

14. You'll Add (Happy, Healthy) Years to Your Life

Every day, you make hundreds of decisions that are pointing you toward a longer life or a shorter one. Nowhere are those decisions more clear than at the dinner table, and *The Big Book of Food & Nutrition* will help you understand just how easy healthier decisions can be. For example, when Loma Linda University researchers tracked the lifestyle habits of 34,000 Seventh-Day Adventists—a population famous for its longevity—they discovered that those who munched nuts five days a week earned an extra 2.9 years on the planet. Similarly, Italian researchers found that eating as little as one cup of raw vegetables daily can add two years to your life. (Why raw? Cooking can deplete up to 30 percent of the antioxidants in vegetables.) And as long as you're going to seriously consider eating a salad before your next meal, stop bothering with those low-fat dressings. A recent Ohio State University study showed that salads eaten with full-fat dressings help with the absorption of a carotenoid called lutein, which is found in leafy green vegetables and has been shown to benefit vision.

20

Percentage of calories in a typical fast-food meal that come just from the oil used to fry the french fries.

15. You'll Still Be at the Top of Your Game—in 2055!

More and more research indicates that, just like the body, the brain ages relative to the way it's fed and exercised. For example, did you know that 35 percent of your brain is pure fatty acids, and that you can lose fat from your brain even as you're gaining it around your belly? But eating the right kinds of fats can help your brain stay as highly functioning as the day you took your SATs. A 2008 University of Cincinnati study, for instance, found that the brain tissue of 65- to 80-year-olds contained 22 percent less docosahexaenoic acid (DHA), an important type of omega-3 fatty acid, than the brain tissue of 29- to 35-year-olds. "If you want to keep your wits about you as you age, start consuming omega-3s now," says William Harris, PhD, a nutrition researcher at the University of South Dakota. You'll find them in fatty fish like tuna and sardines and in certain nuts and seeds, like flax and walnuts, and *The Big Book of Food & Nutrition* will help you understand why the average guy isn't getting enough of them.

That's a lot of promises for one book, but it doesn't even begin to scratch the surface of the nutritional information you'll find in these pages. From simple food swaps that can strip away calories (just having two glasses of 1 percent milk instead of whole milk every day will save you more than 32,000 calories, or 9 pounds, a year), to simple ways to maximize your nutritional intake (pick a red bell pepper over a green one and get nine times as much vitamin A), *The Big Book of Food & Nutrition* is packed with essential information that will make your nutritional life healthier than ever.

Yes, eating is easy.

Now eating smart has become even easier!

459

Number of calories the average person consumes from beverages each day.

Chapter 1:
Your Most Frequently Asked Food Questions, Answered

WHY EATING EGGS WON'T GIVE YOU HIGH CHOLESTEROL, ORDERING RIB EYE WON'T ESCALATE YOUR RISK OF HEART DISEASE, AND PICKING FISH ISN'T ALWAYS THE HEALTHIEST CHOICE.

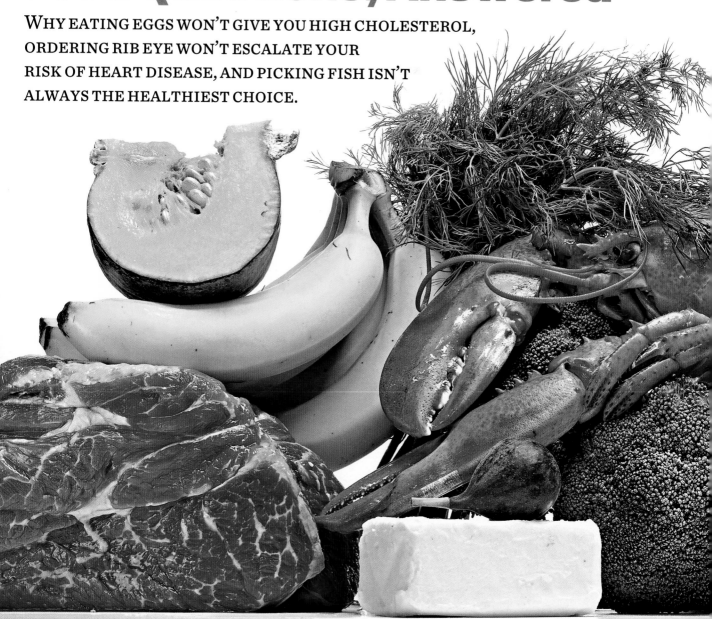

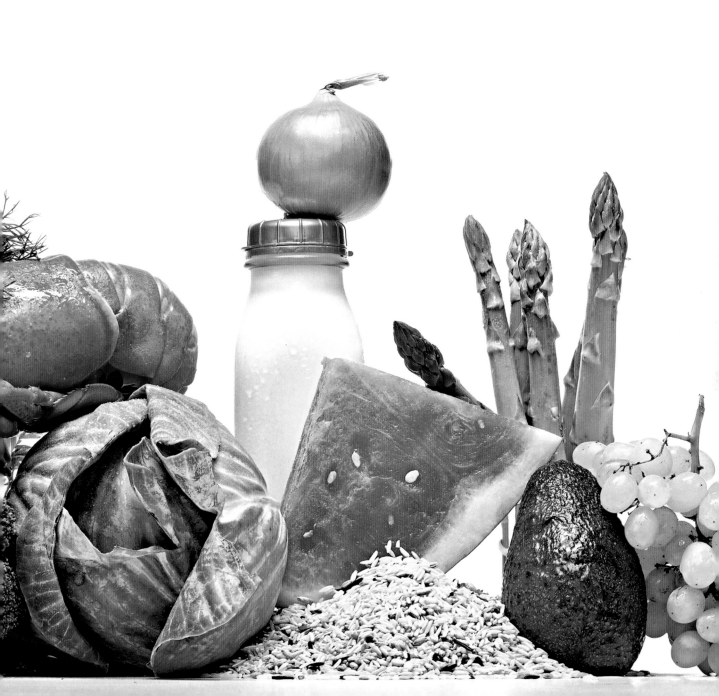

The biggest problem with food in today's society—other than our tendency to eat too much of it—is a simple lack of basic knowledge. Growing up, our primary nutritional authority was Mom. And yes, while "eat your vegetables" was a bigger household staple than the vegetables themselves, and a noble sentiment, Mom's bread pudding, buttered noodles, and candied carrots made our collective pancreases shudder.

Today, however, we're bombarded with information—from the TV, the internet, the labels plastered all over our foods, and from the self-taught trainers at the gym. We now have so much research available about food that it's difficult today to blame lack of knowledge for our lousy diet.

But let's be frank: Most of what passes for information is actually misinformation—or, in the case of those food labels, downright disinformation. What you need is authoritative information from a reliable source.

You've taken a terrific first step: picking up this book. You have not just a hunger for the best food, but you now have the best knowledge about food. Here it is.

Consider this chapter to be your official re-introduction to food, a collection of the most commonly asked questions about stuff you might think you know, or thought you might have heard, or are simply curious about. Along with the answers, you'll get tons of little-known facts, fast fixes, and smart tips for better eating. Our goal? Too much information.

Oh, who are we kidding? When it comes to smart eating, there's no such thing.

Q: Will eating fat make me fat?

A: Eating too much of anything will make you fat, but dietary fat itself doesn't have any magic weight-gain properties. However, fat does contain more calories than either carbohydrates or proteins; per gram, carbohydrates and protein provide about four calories, whereas fat yields nine calories per gram. So the more fat you eat, the more calories you consume—and downing too many calories every day will put you on the fast track to growing a big ol' potbelly. But in general we're far, far too afraid of fat. It's a fact of life and a crucial part of our anatomies. It encases our internal organs, courses through our veins, and provides a nice cushion whenever we take a load off our feet. It's even where you'd never expect it, like inside our skulls, where it provides 70 percent of the protective coating for our brains and makes up 60 percent of our gray matter. The main reason you shouldn't fear fat is that as long as you're eating the appropriate number of calories every day (more on that in a few), your body won't store it in your soft spots but rather burn it for energy. Research even shows that diets containing up to 60 percent fat are just as effective for weight loss as those in which fat provides only 20 percent of the calories. The bottom line is that fat is filling and flavorful, both of which can help keep your belly from feeling deprived. And that means that you can eat the natural fat in meat, cheese, milk, butter, avocados, nuts, and olive oil without furrowing your brow. (For a complete guide to good and bad fats, see page 46.)

Q: Is there any food out there that I should never, ever eat?

A: No, but there's one ingredient that you should avoid like the plague: trans fats. Like hotel bars on business trips, little good can come from them.

BIG FAT LIES

The US government ruled that a convenience food can claim "no trans fat" on its label if it carries less than 0.5 grams of the stuff. In other words, you could eat four servings of supermarket convenience foods that say "no trans fat" on the label and still come to close to exceeding your daily allowance of trans fats.

A completely artificial invention that studies have linked to an increased risk of heart disease and diabetes, trans fats turn the dietary fat in foods into especially hard-to-move body fat—on your belly, in your heart, and everywhere else that matters. They're created by combining vegetable oil (a liquid) with hydrogen to create "hydrogenated" or "partially hydrogenated" oil—a.k.a. trans-fatty acids. Once infused with the hydrogen, the liquid vegetable oil turns into a solid at room temperature. Historically, the food industry has loved trans fats because they are cheap and can help food stick around until cockroaches inherit the earth. Once they're inside your body, however, the enzymes that break down fat in your body can't effectively handle artificial trans fats. Trans fats are the equivalent of the hair balls women leave behind in shower drains: They clog your pipes. So check ingredient lists for trans fat or the words "hydrogenated" or "partially hydrogenated." Processed baked goods and shortenings such as margarine are two of the most common ways in which trans fats find their way into our bodies. Try not to let them pass through your lips.

Q: Do fruits pack carbs?

A: Fruits contain healthier carbs than cookies, but not all fruits are created equal. Sure, bananas, pears, and most dried fruits are good for you, but they offer relatively few nutrients for the carbs in each. When possible, opt for blackberries, raspberries, and papaya, which are loaded with fiber and powerful nutrients and carry far fewer carbs per serving. You can learn more about the fiber in fruits on page 44.

Q: Is chicken a better choice than beef?

A: It used to be. Organic, pasture-raised, skinless chicken breast is still remarkably healthy. But unless you're buying your own or eating in a restaurant that makes it a priority to source good food, your chicken probably isn't much better than most beef. Consider this: The average piece of chicken has 266 percent more fat than it did in 1971, while its protein content has dropped by a third, according to researchers at the Institute of Brain Chemistry and Human Nutrition at London Metropolitan University. That's because most of us no longer eat chickens that roam the farm eating bugs and grasses. Instead, today's chicken is actually higher in fat than yesteryear's because the birds are bred, fed, and raised in a way that promotes fat growth. Similarly, not all beef is the same. All cows are raised on grass for the first year or so of their lives, after which point, if they're headed to a conventional slaughterhouse, they'll eat an unlimited supply of corn to fatten them up as quickly as possible. A cow raised solely on grass, however, yields a completely different type of meat—in taste as well as in chemistry—because it's practically a wild animal. Grass-fed beef, as it's called, has 16 percent fewer calories than conventional beef, 27 percent less fat, 10 percent more protein, and a healthier balance of omega-3 to omega-6 fatty acids. So while chicken isn't necessarily better than beef, there are choices that can make either one dramatically better from a nutrition standpoint.

Q: Are vegetables better for you raw or cooked?

A: In general, go raw. A 2004 meta-analysis in the journal *Cancer Epidemiology* found an inverse relationship between consumption of raw vegetables and most cancers. For cooked veggies, the relationship was also present, but only in about half as many studies. The authors concluded this was likely due to heat slightly diminishing good stuff like vitamin C, beta-carotene, and enzymes.

Q: Is a glass of fruit juice equivalent to a piece of fruit?

A: No. Whole fruit is always the better option: A medium orange contains just 62 calories and 12 grams of sugar, and it has 3 grams of belly-filling fiber. By comparison, an 8-ounce glass of Minute Maid OJ has 110 calories, 24 grams of sugar, and no fiber.

What's more, so-called "juice drinks" contain not only the natural sugar from the fruit but also copious amounts of added sugars, so that they aren't as tart. (Cranberry juice, in fact, is too sour to drink when it hasn't been sweetened.) Plus, even drinks labeled 100 percent pure juice aren't necessarily made exclusively with the advertised juice. For instance, pomegranate and blueberry may get top billing, even though the ingredient list reveals that pear, apple, and grape juices are among the first four ingredients. These juices are used because they're cheap to produce and because they're supersweet, which increases the likelihood of you coming back for more. (Juice brands loaded with of-the-moment superfoods, such as açai, are especially prone to this type of trickery.) To avoid the huge sugar surge, pick single-fruit juices, pour half a glass, and fill the rest with water or seltzer—you'll barely notice the difference. But the best decision of all is to simply opt for the whole fruit.

Q: Does red meat cause cancer?

A: There's no solid evidence that it does. In a 1986 study, Japanese researchers discovered cancer developing in rats that were fed "heterocyclic amines," compounds that are generated from overcooking meat using high heat. Since then, some studies of large populations have suggested a potential link between meat and cancer.

PROTEIN POWER

Protein provides a sense of satiety—or the feeling of fullness—that can help prevent gorging, so it's important to integrate it into all of your meals and snacks. Sneaking in a little protein before your meal, such as a glass of milk, will help keep your hunger (and portion size) in check. Also, know that your sense of satiety is less adept in the evening than in the morning.

Yet no study has ever found a direct cause-and-effect relationship between red-meat consumption and cancer. As for the population studies, they're far from conclusive. They rely on broad surveys of people's eating habits and health afflictions, and those numbers are simply crunched to find trends, not causes. If you're a meat lover who's worried about the supposed risks of grilled meat, you don't need to avoid burgers and steak altogether; instead, just trim off the burned or overcooked sections of the meat before eating. Marinating is a good idea, too—and not just because it can enhance flavors. Soaking red meat in a wine- or beer-based marinade for six hours drops levels of the alleged carcinogenic compounds from grilling by up to 88 percent, according to a study from the University of Porto in Portugal. This complements a 2006 study from Kansas State University that found that cooking beef with rosemary reduced the same compounds by up to 77 percent.

60

Number of pounds of high-fructose corn syrup produced for every person in the United States each year. In 1970, that number was a half-pound per person.

Q: Do spicy foods cause heartburn?

A: No, so you can consider jalapeño peppers exonerated. A Stanford University study review shows that tobacco, alcohol, and excess body weight—not hot tamales—are the main contributors to internal combustion. "The idea that spicy foods trigger heartburn is mainly perception based

on what patients tell their doctors," says Lauren Gerson, MD, the lead study review author. That said, if you eat too much of any food right before bedtime, you're setting yourself up for heartburn; it's easier for stomach acid to creep back up your esophagus when you're lying down.

Q: Do I have to choose between losing weight and building muscle?

A: No. Building muscle can actually speed weight loss, because muscle is more metabolically active—a pound of muscle burns three times as many calories as a pound of fat. High-fiber foods that also contain protein (steel-cut Irish oatmeal contains 4 grams a serving) present a double hit to your potbelly because they make you feel full without actually filling you up.

Q: Is high-fructose corn syrup (HFCS) worse than regular sugar?

A: Sugar is sugar, and there's no evidence to show any differences between these sweeteners. Both HFCS and sucrose—better known as table sugar—contain similar amounts of fructose. For instance, the two most commonly used types of HFCS are HFCS-42 and HFCS-55, which are 42 and 55 percent fructose, respectively. Sucrose is almost chemically identical, containing 50 percent fructose.

No matter what you call it, sugar is an empty-calorie carbohydrate that will cause weight gain when consumed in excess, and you should try to limit your consumption. What makes HFCS particularly difficult on that front is that it's so cheap, it can be added to almost any food for fractions of a penny, which is why it shows up in everything from bread to ketchup to salad dressing—all foods you wouldn't necessarily expect to contain sugar. The best policy is to read the label and always opt for the product with less sugar—of any kind.

Q: Do I have to reduce my salt intake?

A: Not if your blood pressure is normal. In fact, the link between salt and blood pressure is somewhat overstated. In the 1940s, a Duke University researcher named Walter Kempner, MD, became famous for using salt restriction to treat people with high blood pressure. Later, studies confirmed that reducing salt could help reduce hypertension. Large-scale scientific reviews, however, have determined that there's no reason for people with normal blood pressure to restrict their sodium intake. (A quick clarification: Salt is a seasoning made of sodium chloride; sodium is an element that can still exist in foods marked "no salt.") Now, if you already have high blood pressure, you may be "salt sensitive." As a result, reducing the

amount of salt you eat could be helpful. That said, it's been known for the past 20 years that people with high blood pressure who don't want to lower their salt intake can simply consume more potassium-containing foods. (Deep orange and green fruits like apricot, kiwi, and cantaloupe, as well as bananas and trendy coconut water are among the top sources.) Why these foods? Because it's really the balance of the two minerals in the body that matters. In fact, Dutch researchers determined that a low potassium intake has the same impact on your blood pressure as high salt consumption does. And, as it turns out, the average guy consumes 3,100 milligrams of potassium a day—1,600 milligrams less than recommended.

Q: Does organic matter?

A: To the planet? Definitely. To your body? Sometimes. There's abundant evidence that pesticides and fertilizers have a dramatically negative impact on our environment. Pesticides have been linked to a variety of problems, from dead spots in the ocean to sexual deformities in wildlife. As to whether organic food is actually better for you from a health perspective, probably yes, but the jury's still out. In the fall of 2009, a team of British researchers, after reviewing 50 years of studies and data, concluded that organic produce offers no unique nutritional benefit. While that may be true, it's not the food

WHEN TO GO ORGANIC

The Environmental Working Group calculated that you can reduce your pesticide exposure by nearly 80 percent simply by choosing organic for the 12 fruits and vegetables shown in their tests to contain the highest levels of pesticide. They call them "The Dirty Dozen," and (starting with the worst) they are:

- peaches
- apples
- sweet bell peppers
- celery
- nectarines
- strawberries
- cherries
- kale
- lettuce
- imported grapes
- carrots
- pears

but the pesticides used on it that may be the real issue: So far studies have linked them to harming your brain, sperm, immune system, and more, and the President's Cancer Panel suggested in early 2010 that pesticides may increase our risk for certain cancers. "Exposure to pesticides can be decreased by choosing, to the extent possible, food grown without pesticides or chemical fertilizers and washing conventionally grown produce to remove residues," the report advises. Pesticides have also been linked to obesity and diabetes by the American Medical Association. To lessen your pesticide intake, choose organic whenever you're eating fruits with permeable (read: edible) skins, like apples, peaches, and berries, as well as leafy greens. These foods tend to carry the highest pesticide loads, according to the Environmental Working Group. Finally, when it comes to packaged and processed foods, "organic" does not equal "healthy." Organic sugar is still junk food.

Q: Does nuking food destroy its nutrients?

A: No. In fact, microwaves don't "nuke" food at all. "Microwave heat is really no different from ordinary heat. It just occurs faster," says Daryl Lund, PhD, a professor emeritus of food science at the University of Wisconsin. And that fast-action heat is what makes microwaves superior to conventional ovens in many circumstances, says Lund. A study in the journal *Nutrition and Food Science* found that microwaved vegetables retained up to 20 percent more vitamins than stove-cooked produce. But don't let those results lull you into thinking that all microwaved food is safe and healthy. According to the USDA's Food Safety and Inspection Service, microwaving food in plastic can leach toxic chemicals into your meal—chemicals that have been linked to both cancer and obesity. "If you wouldn't heat the container and contents in a conventional oven, don't stick it in the microwave," says Lund. Use glass or ceramic containers instead.

Q: What's best: fresh, frozen, or canned?

A: If you pluck a snap pea off its vine in July and pop it into your mouth, that's as good as it's ever going to get. But if you eat one that's been imported from Chile in mid-February, then it's lost some nutritional value in transit from the farm. (Research from Iowa State University shows that while a local Iowan apple travels only 61 miles to market, a conventional supermarket apple travels 1,726 miles.) If a supermarket's fresh produce is ever looking a little spent, consider strolling a few aisles over to the freezer section. Studies show that frozen vegetables maintain their nutrients as well as

BEST COOKING TOOL

Victorinox Forschner 8" Chef's Knife. While the market for hand-forged $300 Japanese and German chef's knives continues to spiral out of control, the best knife out there may just be this humble blade. Made by the same fine people who brought you the Swiss Army knife, this one blade can handle 90 percent of your cutting. *Cook's Illustrated*, the master of in-depth product tests, has awarded this knife their top seal of approval year after year (swissarmy.com, $40 poly handle, $144 forged).

fresh—and sometimes much better, as with that imported snap pea—because they're harvested at peak ripeness and flash-frozen within hours, a process that preserves all the valuable nutrients. The vitamin C in broccoli, for example, dipped just 10 percent when frozen at -4°F for a year, according to a 2007 study. Canned vegetables are less ideal because they often contain added sugar and excess sodium, and the preservation process can cause a loss of essential B vitamins, according to a University of California study. If you do opt for the canned route, warm the vegetables in their own liquid—it typically contains one-third of a vegetable's nutrients.

Q: If soy is so bad for men, should I not eat edamame or tofu?

A: Go ahead and eat the sushi-bar appetizers. It's true that soy has been shown in studies to lower sperm counts, but that's mainly the soy found in processed forms, such as soy cheese, soy milk, and the unpronounceable variations listed on your favorite artery-clogging processed foods. This means that eating unprocessed forms of soy, such as edamame or tofu, is perfectly fine in moderation. That's good news, because, according to Mark Messina, PhD, an adjunct associate professor at Loma Linda University, in California, an isoflavone in soy called genistein inhibits enzymes in the colon and prostate, raising the amount of vitamin D bioavailability in those tissues. "There is emerging research suggesting that vitamin D reduces cancer risk, and many people don't get enough of the vitamin," says Messina.

Q: Is brown rice really that much healthier than white rice?

A: Yes, and that's the case whenever you're comparing a whole grain to the "white" version. That goes for the rice that accompanies your Chinese takeout, the tortillas you wrap your burritos in, and the slices of bread that flank your lunch meat. Most of these products are made from grains that have had all their nutrients refined out of them. If you eat the carbs with the grain—the label will say "whole wheat"—it will be full of fiber because it's made from the entire wheat kernel: germ, bran, and endosperm. Fiber takes up room in your belly, which then sends your brain the signal that you're full. But if all the fiber is taken out (as is the case with refined carbs like white rice), fast-rising blood sugar triggers your pancreas to release a flood of insulin, the hormone that not only lowers blood sugar but also signals your body to store fat. And in about half of us, insulin tends to "overshoot," which sends blood sugar crashing. "This reinforces the binge, because it makes you crave sugar and starch again," says Valerie Berkowitz, MS, RD, the nutrition director at the Center for Balanced Health in New York City. In turn, your body craves more food—and then you eat more. And more. And more. Obviously that's bad news once you try to squeeze into your favorite Levi's. A study from Penn State University compared how much belly fat people lost when they ate whole grains instead of refined grains. The results were significant: The whole-grain eaters lost 2.4 times more fat! By avoiding refined foods, you also avoid foods that are high on the glycemic index, the scale that gauges the degree to which carbohydrates increase the level of glucose (sugar) in the blood. "If you have high glucose in the bloodstream, it causes oxidative damage, and in response to that, there's inflammation," explains Cyril W. C. Kendall, PhD, a research scientist at the University of Toronto. Dining at regular intervals, eating protein and fat at every meal, and choosing whole grains, such as whole-wheat breads and pastas, will help manage your blood sugar and thus your cravings—and your fat storage.

Q: Are eggs bad for me?

A: Once and for all: No, and stop fearing the yolk. Whole eggs contain more essential vitamins and minerals per calorie than virtually any other food, and not eating them means that you're missing out on key vitamins, nutrients, and antioxidants (egg whites provide protein but not much else). As for egg consumption and heart disease, in a recent review of dozens of scientific studies, Wake Forest University researchers found no connection. Eating eggs may even raise your HDL (good) cholesterol, according to one study in Thailand. The researchers discovered that when people ate one egg every day for 12 weeks, their HDL cholesterol rose by 48 percent, while their LDL (bad) cholesterol and triglycerides didn't budge. The only legit concern about eggs is that their yolks' fat content could impinge upon your total fat allotment for the day, according to Alan Aragon, MS. "If you're a bigger guy, six eggs per day is a safe upper range that doesn't impinge upon your total fat allotment," he says. "If you're on the smaller size, three to four eggs will still allow you to hit your macronutrient targets without going overboard on fat."

Q: Is fish always the healthiest choice?

A: It depends on the fish. Swimming with high-quality protein and omega-3 fatty acids, certain species are indeed the perfect health food. But modern aquaculture has bred some nutrients out of many fish. Take salmon. If it's labeled "wild" or "Alaskan," eat as much as you can afford. But if it's farmed (Atlantic) salmon, you're closer to eating chicken or beef from a feedlot than you might think. Most

BETTER THAN SALMON?

Just 3 ounces of mackerel contains 24 grams of protein and offers nearly twice as many brain-boosting, heart-protecting omega-3s as salmon for a quarter of the price. Rub a few fillets in minced garlic, ginger, and lime juice and bake under the broiler for 7 to 8 minutes, until the fish flakes with gentle pressure.

than you might think. Most fish farms—salmon or otherwise—use pellets made of corn and soy as feed, which negatively impacts the nutritional composition of the meat, lowering its omega-3 content. Farmed salmon can also contain up to 10 times more "persistent organic pollutants"—dioxins, PCBs, etc.—than wild salmon, according to research by environmental scientist Ronald Hites, PhD, of Indiana University. So while you're loading up on salmon to reap its health benefits, you may also be ingesting a known toxin. The prevalence of these chemicals in farmed salmon is so troubling that Hites, who has analyzed more than two tons of salmon meat, advises that farmed varieties "should be consumed at one meal or less per month." Wild Alaskan salmon, however, contains slightly less protein per ounce than skinless chicken breast—5.7 grams instead of 6.5 grams—but it also supplies a good dose of healthy fat, not to mention the cardiovascular benefit of fish oil. Learn more about navigating the fish counter on page 000.

Q: Do I have to down eight glasses of water every day?

A: You can certainly get by drinking less water—75 percent of Americans are "chronically dehydrated" and most average about four glasses a day, according to recent research—but more is definitely better. Eight glasses is a great goal, because water promotes satiety, prevents heart attacks, builds muscle, and stokes your metabolism. That last one is especially true in the morning, when your body has just spent the equivalent of a day in the office without any intake of fluids whatsoever. In fact, German scientists discovered that drinking at least 16 ounces of chilled H_2O as soon as you roll out of bed boosts metabolism by 24 percent for 90 minutes afterward, and researchers at the University of Utah in Salt Lake City have also found that volunteers who drank at least eight glasses daily had higher metabolic rates than those who sipped only four glasses. So if your glass is half full—fill it up!

Q: Are vegetarians healthier than the rest of us?

A: Most research indicates that they are, according to Marion Nestle, PhD, professor of nutrition at New York University. But is it the absence of meat, or just the fact that vegetarians eat more produce, which is linked to lower rates of cancer, obesity, and heart disease? According to the Centers for Disease Control and Prevention, 87 percent of American men don't consume the USDA's recommended five or more servings a day. Even adding just a few vegetarian foods to your diet could significantly lower your cholesterol levels, according to researchers at St.

2

Number of vegetable servings a day you need to eat to enjoy a 40 percent slower rate of cognitive decline (compared with those who eat one serving or less).

Michael's Hospital in Toronto. A month after adding several servings of vegetarian foods to their diets each day, the test subjects' LDL cholesterol levels were nearly 30 percent lower than when the trial began. But unfortunately, replacing cold cuts with celery isn't going to lead to automatic weight loss. "When people become vegetarian, they seem to simply substitute vegetarian convenience foods for those containing meat," says Allan Hackett, PhD, one of the study's authors. "And many vegetarian convenience foods are no better or are even worse, nutritionally, than their meat-containing counterparts."

Q: Do expiration dates really count?

A: They're decent guidelines, but base your final decision on a sniff test. Say you have sliced turkey with some of that slimy goo on it. Give it a whiff; if it passes, you're good to gobble. "Strong off-odors, not slime, indicate spoilage," says Brian Nummer, PhD, a food-safety professor at Utah State University. That's because that goo is produced when harmless lactobacillus bacteria start feasting on the sugar that some manufacturers add for flavor. However, if lactobacillus bacteria multiply to the point that a smell develops, there's a small chance that the bacteria responsible for foodborne illness could multiply, too. As a general rule of thumb,

you've got about a seven-day window after opening a package.

Q: How long does fresh produce retain its nutritional value?

A: For as long as it still looks appetizing. "In general, fresh-cut fruits visually spoil before any significant nutrient loss occurs," says Maria Gil, lead author of a 2006 study in the *Journal of Agriculture and Food Chemistry*. Her research concluded that after six days of refrigeration, certain fruits would lose as much as 25 percent of their vitamin C and carotenoids. (Cantaloupe and pineapple were among the fastest to deteriorate.) The same is generally true for vegetables. A 2007 meta-analysis in the *Journal of the Science of Food and Agriculture* found that the vitamin C content of fresh spinach, peas, and broccoli dropped 75, 40, and 13 percent, respectively, after being refrigerated for a week.

Q: Which vitamins should I take?

A: Whether he's an elite athlete or a desk jockey, a healthy guy with a good diet should take one low-dose multivitamin, such as Centrum, each day. Nothing more. In the most comprehensive clinical trials in the world for healthy men, low doses of vitamins and minerals have been associated

SNEAKY LEFTOVERS TIP

Sadly, the reheating process too often leaves leftover foods dry and unpalatable. Our favorite secret weapon is low-sodium chicken stock. Splash a bit on top of whatever you're reheating—pastas, meats, or vegetables—and the moisture will be reabsorbed by the food, bringing life and flavor back to the dish.

with the best results. The SU.VI.MAX French clinical trial, for instance, involved more than 10,000 healthy men and women who took either a supplement or a placebo every day for more than seven years. The men who took a daily supplement reduced their risk of heart disease, cancer, and early death. What was in the magical supplement? Only 100 mcg of selenium, 120 mg of vitamin C, 30 mg of vitamin E, 6 mg of beta-carotene, and 20 mg of zinc—roughly the daily value of a few key nutrients, in other words. Find a new multivitamin if yours doesn't have doses close to those numbers. High doses of antioxidants in pill form may actually fuel disease by not allowing our bodies to build up their own resistance to free-radical damage, essentially quashing our internal defenses.

Q: So the only thing I need to do to weigh less is eat fewer calories?

A: Or burn more off. Shedding belly fat boils down to a simple equation: Calories in - calories out = total weight loss or gain. "Calories out" is the energy your body spends keeping your heart pumping, doing daily activities, going to the gym, etc. "Calories in" is the sum of every morsel that passes between your lips. To maintain a healthy body weight, a moderately active man needs 2,400 to 2,600 calories per day. (Obviously that number can fluctuate a bit depending on your body type,

and you can use the calorie calculator at mayoclinic.com for a more accurate assessment.) But don't just watch what you eat, watch what you drink. It takes just 3,500 additional calories a week to create one pound of body fat. In other words, if you drink an extra 500 calories per day—which isn't difficult to do, considering Starbucks offers more than two dozen beverages containing at least that many—you'll earn one new pound of body fat each week.

Q: Should I always opt for the "low-fat" version?

A: No, not always. If you're trying to lose some serious weight, then sure, a lower-fat option is an easy way to save a few calories—a tub of, say, reduced-fat peanut butter indeed comes with fewer calories and a fraction less fat than the full-fat variety. But the food manufacturers have likely swapped the healthy fat in peanuts for maltodextrin, a carbohydrate used as a filler in many processed foods, so ultimately you're trading healthy fat for empty carbs and twice the sugar . . . all to spare a meager 10 calories. The difference in calories between whole and 1 percent milk, however, is significantly wider: 149 per cup versus 102. Choose whichever fits your taste. Just know that a whole-milk mustache doesn't mean you need to schedule a date for a triple-bypass surgery. A 2010 review in the *American Journal*

SNEAKY CALORIE-CUTTING TIP

Use rubs. Rather than bogging down your meat with excess calories the way sauces do, rubs infuse a dish with a variety of powerful antioxidants— potent micronutrients known to fight cancer, reduce inflammation, and even speed up metabolism. Try these:

For beef: salt and pepper, garlic salt, cayenne, cumin, pinch of cinnamon

For chicken: salt and pepper, cumin, chili powder, brown sugar

For fish: salt and pepper, smoked paprika, thyme

of Clinical Nutrition found no association between the intake of saturated fat (the kind in milk and other animal products) and the development of heart disease and stroke.

Q: What's the best strategy for snacking?

A: Every time you snack, choose a combination of three food items. Each snack should contain some protein, some fiber, and some vitamins and minerals. For example, you could pair string cheese with cherry tomatoes and grapes, yogurt with carrots and crackers, or a hard-boiled egg with a banana and trail mix. Heck, have the occasional Twinkie if you need to—just make sure you enjoy it with a glass of milk and an apple. What makes this trick work, according to its developer, nutrition counselor Karen Beerbower, RD, is that it makes you think through your snacks. And once you're more conscious of your decisions, you're no longer snacking mindlessly and emptying entire bags of Doritos in a single go. You may eat a few more calories, but you'll feel fuller longer.

Q: How bad is a day of binge eating?

A: Assuming you don't have hypertension or diabetes—in which case the extra salt and sugar are trouble—your body can deal with the occasional desertion of dietary common sense. "You'll store some of the extra fat and sugar," says Mike Roussell, PhD, a nutrition researcher at Pennsylvania State University. "And the surplus carbs and salt will make you retain water. So for the next day or two, you'll probably feel a bit bloated and may weigh a few pounds more." But at the same time, your body will compensate for the binge by releasing hormones to temporarily reduce your appetite, more or less balancing things out. A weekend-long feast, however, can cause trouble beyond Sunday. In a recent study in the *Journal of Clinical Investigation*, researchers used rats to examine the effects of palmitic acid on leptin, a hormone that helps regulate appetite. Palmitic acid is found in saturated fat, a substance often featured in your favorite weekend grub, and is known to inhibit your ability to regulate food intake when consumed in large quantities. A better reward for a week of healthy eating should be one cheat meal, not an entire weekend of them.

Q: Do certain foods require more calories to digest than they contain?

A: Nope, the "negative calorie" concept is a myth. Even celery, which is often cited as a negative-calorie food, has 18 calories in two stalks, half of them from natural sugars. Your body does burn calories to digest the food, but the total cost doesn't exceed the caloric yield.

EAT THIS BREAKFAST TOMORROW

Simmer half a can of black beans with a cup of chicken stock. Crack two eggs directly into the mixture and cook until the whites are set. Hit it with plenty of hot sauce.

Q: What's a "well-balanced" breakfast?

A: Think of your first meal of the day as the foundation of your dietary success. Eat the bulk of your daily calories—30 to 35 percent of your total intake, including snacks—in the morning, and then taper off as the day goes on, says registered dietitian Cynthia Sass. Contrary to what you see in breakfast cereal advertisements, the key is to match protein and whole grains with produce and healthy fats. If you want to get scientific about it, strive for 30 percent protein and 25 percent fat, and reserve the remaining 45 percent for carbohydrates, which includes produce. Eat eggs, peanut butter, yogurt; oatmeal, whole-wheat breads, cereals; and complementary fruits and vegetables, such as blueberries, prunes, oranges, bananas, asparagus, and spinach.

Q: Does it really make a difference if I put cream and sugar in my morning coffee?

A: Yes. Skipping a 16-calorie packet of sugar every day isn't going to shrink your waistline dramatically—you're only saving about 2 pounds' worth of calories per year. But priming your sweet tooth first thing in the morning can only lead to further cravings later in the day. If you're a sugar junkie, dial back the sweetness quotient in everything you eat—from that first cup of joe to the kind of chocolate you instinctively crave. That way it'll be harder to see what you're missing. The same goes for the cream. If eliminating both additions is too radical, try cutting one but not the other—or just gradually reducing one at a time.

Q: Do I need to take fish oil supplements?

A: Probably, but the exact amount of the two long-chain omega-3 fatty acids (EPA and DHA) you need remains open to debate. More won't hurt you, however, and according to Joseph Hibbeln, MD, one of the world's most respected sources on the link between omega-3s and depression, Americans should consume 3,700 milligrams of EPA and DHA a day (in a ratio of 2:3) to balance their current high intake of omega-6s and reap the heart- and brain-healthy benefits of these essential fatty acids—the equivalent of six high-potency fish oil capsules. The American Heart Association is more conservative: It recommends that patients with coronary heart disease get 1,000 milligrams a day.

Q: Assuming calorie content is the same, what's more likely to help me manage my weight: eating less sugar or less fat?

A: Cut out sugar over fat whenever you can. "If you have to make a choice,

3 FAST SNACKS

1. Lay a slice of Swiss cheese on a cutting board. Top with a slice of deli turkey and a spoonful of hummus or guacamole. Wrap like a jelly roll and eat.

2. Combine a can of tuna with your favorite salsa. Use Triscuits for scooping.

3. Ants on a Log: Slather celery with smooth or chunky peanut butter. Dot with raisins.

125

Calories in 12 ounces of Guinness, the best beer with the least calories. Just make sure you buy the right Guinness. Extra Stout (175 calories) will cost you an extra 300 calories a six-pack.

eat more fat, primarily because the sugar is instantly absorbed and metabolized, and it drives your blood sugar up," says Paul Lachance, PhD, a professor of food science at Rutgers University. Since sugar is more easily digested, the full feeling you get disappears faster, prompting another eating binge. That said, calories are still calories. "Whether you consume 100 extra calories of pure fat or 100 extra calories of pure sugar, it's 100 extra calories," says Kimberly Hessler, RD, research manager at the St. Louis University School of Public Health. "And an excess of calories equals weight gain."

Q: Does it matter what time of day I eat dinner?

A: For the average guy, timing matters less than total calories. "What matters most is getting your requirements over the course of the day—not at any particular points in the day," says Alan Aragon, M.S. But ideally you can consume the bulk of your calories in the first half of your day to power you through your chores. Try to keep dinner, when it's easiest to overeat if you're famished, light in calories and heavy in nutrients. Even just beginning your dinner with low-calorie, high-fiber vegetables will decrease your overall food intake by 12 percent. An old rule of thumb: Eat like a king at breakfast, a prince at lunch, and a pauper at dinner. Whatever you do, learn to listen

to your body and cut yourself off before you've stuffed yourself. "It doesn't matter when you fuel up; it's how many gallons you put in the tank," says Gary Foster, PhD, director of Temple University's Center for Obesity Research and Education.

Q: Are the skins of potatoes, apples, etc. really the best part?

A: Even a peeled apple or potato is packed with nutrition. The skins of many fruits and vegetables, however, are rich in vitamins, nutrients, and antioxidants, as well as insoluble fiber, which is what lends them a tough, chewy texture. Insoluble fiber bulks up as it absorbs liquid in your stomach, and the bulk pushes waste down and out of your system. "Think of insoluble fiber as a broom," says Tanya Zuckerbrot, RD. "Basically, it speeds up the passage of material through your digestive tract and sweeps out all the toxins in your body." But if you're planning on eating non-organic produce, make sure you remove its skin or peel before eating it—that's where the pesticides linger in surprisingly high concentrations.

Q: How much alcohol is okay for me to drink?

A: A glass or two a day. First, it really does take the edge off. University of Toronto researchers discovered that one alcoholic drink causes people's blood vessels to relax, although the effect begins to reverse with the second drink. Then there's the overwhelming research suggesting that regularly drinking a moderate amount of alcohol will help you live longer. In a study of more than 18,000 men, Harvard scientists discovered that those who had an average of two drinks every day, 5 to 7 days a week, had the lowest risk of heart attack. And according to a study in the *Journal of the American Medical Association* that analyzed the lifestyle factors of nearly 6,000 patients, consuming an alcoholic drink or two daily makes you 97 percent more likely to reach age 85. Red wine, especially pinot noir, is your best option. It contains resveratrol, an antioxidant linked to everything from cancer prevention to heart-disease protection, according to a recent review in the journal *Alcoholism: Clinical and Experimental Research*.

Q: Is diet soda really that much better for me?

A: No. Even though you'd think fewer calories is a step in the right direction, diet soda is linked even more closely to obesity than regular soda. One study revealed that people who drank at least one diet soda every day had a 23 percent greater chance of becoming overweight than those who downed one regular soda. The science isn't fully understood yet—you can read more about it in Chapter 5—but artificial sweeteners are thought to be the main culprits. Emerging research suggests that consuming sugary-tasting beverages, even if they contain no calories, may lead to a high preference for sweetness overall and that diet drinkers have an increased risk of developing type 2 diabetes and metabolic syndrome. Plus, those going no-cal with their sodas may unconsciously give themselves permission to eat a little more than they should at other times.

Q: Are all proteins created equal?

A: Not quite. While many plant foods, including nuts and beans, can provide a good dose of protein, the best sources are dairy products, eggs, meat, and fish, says Donald Layman, PhD, a professor emeritus of nutrition at the University of Illinois at Urbana-Champaign. Unlike plant-based proteins, animal protein is complete—it contains the right proportions of the essential amino acids your body can't synthesize on its own—and it's more easily accessible to our bodies. (We're able to use 94 percent of the protein in whole eggs, for instance, and some powders with whey-protein isolate and whey-protein concentrate allow our bodies to use even more than that.) It's possible to build complete protein from plant-based foods by combining legumes, nuts, and grains at one meal or over the

PROTEIN PAIRS

The proteins in vegetable products are "incomplete," meaning they don't build muscle unless eaten in combination with certain other foods. Here's an easy one: One reason that peanut butter and whole-wheat bread go so well together is that the specific amino acids absent in wheat are actually present in peanuts, according to Diane Birt, PhD, a professor at Iowa State University.

MOST UNDER-RATED BREAD

100% whole wheat English muffin: This unusual suspect may be the healthiest bread you're not using to build sandwiches. Its compact size and solid fiber count make it a perfect bookend to sliced ham and cheddar or turkey and avocado. Or use it as a healthy home to America's most famous sandwich: the cheeseburger.

course of a day. But you'll need to consume 20 to 25 percent more plant-based protein to reap the same benefits that animal-derived sources would provide, says Mark Tarnopolsky, MD, PhD, who studies exercise and nutrition at McMaster University, in Hamilton, Ontario. And beans and legumes have carbs, which means you're not getting pure protein.

Q: Is gluten bad for me?

A: Not necessarily. Removing gluten—a protein found in grains like wheat, rye, oats, and barley—from your diet doesn't offer any metabolic advantage or inherent health benefits (unless you have celiac disease, when gluten triggers an immune response that damages the lining of the small intestine). But gluten intolerance is increasingly common, and eliminating the protein will probably help you lose a few stubborn pounds, because it requires that you shelve any cookie, cake, pastry, or carb not labeled "gluten free." New Zealand researchers found that when men who were unable to lose weight stopped eating gluten, they immediately began dropping pounds. In some people, report the scientists, gluten appears to cause chronically high levels of insulin, a hormone that signals your body to store fat. Case in point: Within 3 months of adopting the diet, the study's participants had also reduced their insulin levels by 50 percent. Unfortunately, medical tests to

determine gluten intolerance are often inconclusive. If the size of your belly won't budge, the easiest way to find out if you're afflicted is to eliminate foods containing the protein for a month and monitor your weight and general health for changes.

Q: What's one nutrient deficiency that men can easily correct?

A: Magnesium. Surveys reveal that men consume about 80 percent of the recommended 400 milligrams a day, which is a serious shame, because this lightweight mineral is a tireless multi-tasker: It's involved in more than 300 bodily processes, including muscle function. Plus, a study in the *Journal of the American College of Nutrition* found that low levels of magnesium may increase your blood levels of vitamin C-reactive protein, a key marker of heart disease. "We're just barely getting by," says Dana King, MD, a professor of family medicine at the Medical University of South Carolina. "Without enough magnesium, every cell in your body has to struggle to generate energy." Fortify your diet with more magnesium-rich foods, such as halibut and navy beans.

Q: What kind of bread should I buy?

A: The bread aisle isn't as visually stimulating as, say, a sorority house, but it has about as many options. The first thing to look for is the term "whole wheat," which means the bread hasn't lost anything to refinement. (If you check the label, the first item on the list of ingredients will be whole wheat flour. Breads labeled simply "wheat bread" are usually made with about 75 percent white flour and 25 percent whole wheat flour.) Whole wheat breads are darker in color and contain a good amount of slow-digesting, belly-filling fiber. "Three to 5 grams per serving is a good mark," says Lola O'Rourke, a spokeswoman for the American Dietetic Association. Don't fall for the terms "multigrain" or "seven-grain" either. That just means more than one type of grain was used—and they may have been refined. Lastly, if it's available, opt for a thin-sliced loaf—yet another way to peel away calories.

Q: What should I look for on food labels?

A: More fiber and less sugar. That said, ideally you want to fill your cart with whole foods—the kind without labels. You'll find them around the perimeter of your supermarket, and they'll usually have much less packaging than the stuff in the middle of the store. But when you are reading a list of ingredients, think of it as the credits in a movie. The first ingredients are the main characters, whereas the latter ones play more of a supporting role . . . or just make everybody else

look a little better than they would have otherwise. The reason they're ordered this way is that, by law, manufacturers have to list them in order of their weight. If you're stumped between two products, just pick the one with fewer ingredients. It's almost always the right choice.

Q: Is stuff like turkey bacon that much better for you than the real thing?

A: Reach for the real thing. As far as calories go, the difference between the two is negligible. But while turkey is indeed a leaner meat, turkey bacon isn't made from 100 percent bird—it packs a long list of additives and extra ingredients that don't add anything of nutritional value. Both turkey bacon and bacon can give you a mouthful of sodium, but at least with the latter you'll be eating real food that makes your kitchen smell delicious.

Q: What's better for keeping me awake, a cup of coffee or an energy drink?

A: Coffee. The caffeine content in one cup of black coffee should guarantee you about 5 hours (give or take) of alertness. Even better, researchers have found that coffee is packed with antioxidants—in fact, it's the top source of these nutrients for most Americans— and studies have shown it enhances

16

Percent increase in metabolic rate of those who drank caffeinated coffee versus those who drank decaf, according to a study published in the journal *Physiology & Behavior*. Caffeine stimulates your central nervous system by increasing your heart rate and breathing.

short-term memory and helps protect against dementia and cancer. The jolt you feel from an energy drink comes mostly from sugar, which sets you up for an inevitable crash.

Q: Why is it bad for me if I eat quickly?

A: Simply put, you end up eating more. In an experiment published in the *Journal of Clinical Endocrinology & Metabolism*, 17 healthy men ate 1¼ cups of ice cream. They either scarfed it in 5 minutes or took half an hour to savor it. According to study author Alexander Kokkinos, MD, PhD, levels of fullness-causing hormones (called PYY and GLP-1), which signal the brain to stop eating, were higher among the 30-minute men. In real life, the scarfers wouldn't feel as full and could be moving on to another course. Slow down and enjoy your food, Kokkinos says: Your body is trying to tell you something, so give it a chance. Similarly, Dutch researchers have determined that people who chew food for at least 9 seconds eat much less than those who chew for only 3 seconds.

Q: Why do I want to take a nap after I eat lunch?

A: You're being drugged, but not by your food. Every day at about 2 p.m., your core body temperature drops, which triggers the release of a power-ful knockout drug/hormone called melatonin. In fact, this happens to everyone, as our brain follows a schedule set by its sleep software (known as circadian rhythms), though some people feel the effects more than others, according to Michael Breus, PhD, a clinical psychologist and sleep specialist in Scottsdale, Arizona. Squeezing in a workout at lunchtime is one surefire way to keep your energy up in the mid-afternoon.

Q: Will carrots actually help me see better?

A: Mainly they'll help prevent you from seeing worse. Orange-colored foods get their color from their high levels of beta-carotene, which your body converts into the antioxidant vitamin A. While vitamin A does a bunch of important things—from boosting your immunity to improving communication between cells—it's vital for creating the pigment in the retina responsible for vision in low-light situations. Two other nutrients you need to keep your perception sharp are the antioxidants lutein and zeaxanthin. Spinach ranks as their top source, and a study from Tufts University found that frequent spinach eaters had a 43 percent lower risk of age-related macular degeneration, which is the leading cause of blindness in America. "People with high levels of these two phytonutrients are at lower risk of both macular degeneration and

EAT YOUR VEGGIES

Only 29 percent of women and a mere 20 percent of men consume the recommended amount of produce each day. That's too bad, because a Harvard study of 110,000 men and women found that those who ate eight or more servings of fruit and vegetables a day were 30 percent less likely to have heart attack or stroke than those who ate less than 1½ servings a day.

cataracts," says Steve Pratt, MD, author of *SuperFoods Rx*.

Q: I hate vegetables. Can I just take a vitamin supplement instead?

A: There's no such thing as a magic pill you can take en lieu of vegetables, which are relatively low in calories, fat, and carbs; high in fiber; and deliver tons of other important nutrients. But if you're absolutely opposed to fresh produce, you could opt for low-sodium vegetable juice instead. "It's still the best vegetable substitute around," says Melinda Hemmelgarn, RD, a nutritionist at the University of Missouri. An 8-ounce glass of V8 is the equivalent of two servings of vegetables, and you'll also swallow some extra protection from prostate cancer, thanks to the lycopene in the tomatoes. The main catch is that you won't get as much fiber as you would if you ate the vegetables whole.

Q: What does the phrase "all natural" mean?

A: It means a food marketer is trying to make you think you're eating healthily. The USDA has no definition and imposes no regulations on the use of the term "all natural," making it essentially meaningless, because the food industry can use it almost entirely at its discretion. The one slight exception is with meat and poultry products. Regardless

of how an animal was raised—meaning it could have received hormones, antibiotics, and genetically engineered crops—the term "all natural" can only be used if, after slaughter, the meat is minimally processed and no artificial ingredients are added. The phrase "naturally raised" is slightly better than "all natural," because it means the animal didn't get juiced. The best terms of all are "organic" for produce and poultry, and "grass-fed" for meat.

Q: What happens when I skip a meal?

A: Not eating can trigger metabolism slowdown and a ravenous appetite. But it also destroys willpower, which is just as damaging. "Regulating yourself is a brain activity, and your brain runs on glucose," says Kathleen Martin Ginis, PhD, a professor of kinesiology at McMaster University in Ontario. If you skip breakfast or a healthy snack, your brain doesn't have the energy to say no to the inevitable chowfest. So skipping a meal can turn you into a glutton at night because your starving brain "just doesn't have the fuel it needs to keep you on track, monitoring your diet."

Q: If my only options are a cheeseburger, a hot dog, or a slice of pizza, what should I eat?

A: Clearly there's some room for debate about these American staples,

AVOID THE 3 P.M. ENERGY CRISIS

Eat chicken or fish for lunch. The protein isn't just vital in squashing hunger and boosting metabolism, it's also a top source of energy. University of Illinois researchers found that people who ate higher amounts of protein had higher energy and didn't feel as tired as people with proportionally higher amount of carbs in their diets.

SNEAKY POST-WORKOUT FOOD

In a test-tube study, Rutgers researchers discovered that treating human muscle cells with a compound found in spinach increased protein synthesis by 20 percent. The compound allows muscle tissue to repair itself faster, the researchers say. Add some to your turkey on whole-grain sandwich bread.

as hundreds—if not thousands—of versions exist. And, at the most basic level, each option provides a combination of protein, carbohydrates, and fat from the meat, bread, and cheese. The deciding factor, therefore, is probably the toppings; the more high-fiber vegetables you can include on each, the better. So the best option in most circumstances is probably a slice of pizza loaded with a combination of vegetables, such as bell peppers, broccoli, and mushrooms. It's not a perfect meal—the carbohydrates in the crust will likely be the refined variety—but the pile of produce certainly helps make it a healthier choice.

Q: If I eat a Quarter Pounder with Cheese, do I instantly weigh a quarter of a pound more?

A: The fact of the matter is that, according to McDonald's, its Quarter Pounder with Cheese weighs 198 grams, or 0.43 pounds, so you'll actually weigh closer to half a pound more—and that's before the fries and soda you probably ordered! So even though matter may disappear down your gullet, because of some basic laws of physics, it can't just disappear from the face of the planet. The same is true if you run a caloric surplus over a prolonged period of time; if they're not burned, calories add up. But the opposite hypothetical scenario is also true: If an active, average-size adult male eats only three Quarter

Pounders with Cheese every day and nothing else, he'll net only 1,600 calories and may find himself losing weight.

Q: Will blueberries really boost my brainpower?

A: In general, dietary polyphenols—not just the ones from berries—have multiple protective and health-promoting effects. In this particular case of defending against cognitive decline, there's evidence suggesting that it's a good idea to maintain a regular intake of a variety of fruits and vegetables. But labeling just blueberries as some sort of "superfood" is too narrow a perspective.

Q: If I eat before I work out, should I still eat afterward?

A: Yes. But don't think you have to rush to scarf down one of those expensive muscle shakes the minute you step out of the shower. The idea of eating a fast-acting recovery meal or shake as soon as possible after training is rooted in research on endurance athletes. One study focused on athletes who trained to glycogen depletion through a 2½-hour combination of intensive cycling and sprinting. On top of that, they were training after an overnight fast—and no preworkout meal. Under those circumstances, a quickly absorbed meal or shake would be smart. But hopefully your body isn't running on empty, so try a meal that balances carbs and protein, like a meat-packed deli sandwich, within an hour after your workout.

Q: Are white cheeses better than yellow cheeses?

A: In general, yes, selecting paler cheeses is a good rule of thumb if you're trying to lose weight. But no matter which type you prefer, cheese is a calorie-dense food. An ounce of cheese—which doesn't take up much space, as it's about the equivalent of four dice—is about 100 calories, more than twice as much as you'll find in the same serving of salmon. Cheddar, for instance, contains 113 calories; colby, 110; gouda, 100; brie, 94. As you can also tell from those numbers, yellower cheeses tend to have higher calorie counts than white cheeses, because of their higher fat concentrations. That ounce of cheddar or colby, for instance,

contains 9 grams of fat, whereas gouda or brie contain 8 grams each. "My recommendation is to eat the types that suit your personal taste, because, for the most part, cheese is cheese," says Alan Aragon, MS. "But calorie-dense foods add up quickly, so moderate your intake throughout the week."

Q: Why are processed foods so bad for me?

A: This depends on how you define "processed," and it depends on the food. Take whey-protein powder: It's processed via multiple steps, yet it's one of the most nutrient-dense constituents of milk. On the other hand, if most of the carbohydrates in your diet are from table sugar or corn syrup (instead of, say, cereal and fruit), then you can end up displacing the intake of more nutrient-dense foods and potentially incur deficiencies in essential vitamins and minerals.

■

SMART FOOD

Garlic: Researchers in Pakistan found that rats fed a puree of garlic and water performed better on a memory test than rats that weren't fed the mixture. That's because garlic increases the brain's levels of serotonin, which has been shown to enhance memory function.

Chapter 2:
So You're Thinking About Going on a Diet ....

WHAT WORKS, WHAT DOESN'T, AND WHY STANDARD
DIET ADVICE SIMPLY DOESN'T APPLY ANYMORE.

Here's

something that may surprise you: Every single one of the tens of thousands of diet plans available today will actually work. Sort of. Kind of. For a little while.

You see, every diet works to a certain degree, because every diet you go on forces you to monitor the food you eat, and that alone helps cut down on your calorie intake. Who cares if some of those schemes sound a little wacky—grapefruit diets, leek soup diets, cottage cheese diets, and even cookie diets! Who cares if the natural act of eating becomes an exercise in algebra as you try to calculate your calorie intake and phases and ratios and points and all the other bizarre mathematical formulas out there? The good news for the nearly 76 million Americans who are on a diet of some kind at this very moment is that, in the short term, every single one of them will work.

ORDER IT TO GO

Eating out is a caloric field day—often unintentionally. Some facts to think about:

We tend to eat more when served more.
Students at Cornell were given access to an all-you-can-eat buffet and told to go to town. Researchers took note of how much each ate; the following week, they served the same students portions of equal size, 25 percent bigger, or 50 percent bigger. Those with 25 percent more food ate 164 more calories, and those with 50 percent more food ate 221 extra calories.

We're lousy guessers.
A 2006 study published in the *American Journal of Public Health* found that consumers given an obviously high-calorie restaurant meal still underestimated the caloric load by an average of 600 calories.

Divide and conquer:
Every time you order a full-size dinner entrée, ask the server to deliver a to-go box with your food and stash half for home. The food is easier to divide before you start eating, and you won't have to fight the temptation of a half-eaten manicotti sticking in your face. The bonus benefit? Two meals for the price of one.

And the bad news? In the long term, almost every single one of them is going to fail. In fact, the number-one predictor of future weight gain is whether or not you're on a diet today. The more diets you try, the more likely it is that you'll be even heavier a year from now.

You see, "diet" really is a four-letter word. Here are the common problems with most diets, and why, sometimes, you'd be better off washing your mouth out with soap.

Most diets set you up for binge eating.

A study published in the *International Journal of Obesity* found that 91 percent of people on a diet experience food cravings—94 percent if they involve calorie restriction. Another recent study, in the journal *Psychology and Health*, found that when it comes to exercising our willpower, well, we have only so much willpower to give. That's why trying to break several bad habits at once (like overeating and not exercising) can be overwhelming: You drain your capacity for what researchers call "self-regulation," says study author Kathleen Martin Ginis, PhD, a professor of kinesiology at McMaster University in Ontario.

Even worse, our ability to control ourselves wanes after we exert self-control, according to researchers at Florida State University. The reason? Self-control is fueled by blood sugar. So the more you resist your food cravings, the less power you have over them. (Think of *The Sopranos'* New York capo, Johnny Sack, who took out a hit on a fellow mobster who made fun of his wife's weight—until he discovered candy wrappers hidden under her pillow. She was bingeing, even though— or in fact, because—she was always on a diet.) So unless you're ready to exert Gandhi-on-a-fast, Lance-Armstrong-on-a-bike, John-McCain-in-Hanoi levels of courage and self-discipline, you can forget about any restrictive diet working over the long haul.

Most diets just aren't realistic.

You're starting a new diet plan, and you're all psyched up and ready to go: You're going to fire up the stove every night and cook the healthy, low-cal dinners in your new diet book. Or you're going to eat only the pre-packed, nutritionally correct, perfectly balanced frozen dinners you've got lining your freezer. Or you're having all your meals delivered directly to your door by Abs-on-Wheels. Terrific!

But what if you never make it home in time?

Americans spend 4.2 billion hours sitting in traffic each year. Not surprisingly, the average man eats about 32 meals a year behind the wheel of his car—that's a whole month's worth of dinners spent looking at brake lights and bumpers instead of friends and family. And that's before the birthday parties, bar mitzvahs, and weddings, before the Thanksgivings and the Christmases and the Passovers, before the business dinners and the executive lunches and the power breakfasts.

Now, if most diet plans included drive-through burgers, rubber chicken, and holiday ham, that wouldn't be a problem. But diet programs are usually constructed for fantasyland, and you live in the real world. Long commutes, hungry kids, and time crunches are a reality, and unless you're a billionaire Zen master with a preternatural command of your family, your wallet, and your belly, there will be plenty of times when you're a) not in control of what's for dinner or b) needing to fuel up cheap and fast.

So let's say it's 8 p.m., the family's starving, and you're only halfway home from Grandma Rose's house. A McDonald's burger and fries isn't part of your fancy diet plan, but it's what's available, and ya gotta eat. So you either resist the craving (see above for the success rate on that plan), or you give in. Either way: *bam*, dead diet.

Of course, there are ways to get around this situation, as long as you're not trying to "diet." In fact, you could get a McDouble (with extra cheese!) off the Mickey D's Dollar Menu and add a Fruit 'N Yogurt Parfait, and if you wash it down with a bottle of water, you're looking at only 570 calories—about ¼ of what you should eat in a day. But if your fancy diet doesn't make allowances for fast-food cheeseburgers, you're in trouble. (And the only diet

plan that does belongs to that crazy guy from *Super Size Me* who tried to kill himself with french fries.) When it comes to dieting, the road to heavy is paved with good intentions.

Most diets are just quick fixes.

So your buddy, the guy who hasn't seen his feet in a decade, the one who pulled a cannonball in your pool last summer and you had to re-pour all the concrete, he's on a diet. And he looks amazing! He lost 25 pounds by eating nothing but salted grapefruit peels and foods that start with the letter R. At last, a diet that works! You gotta try it, right?

Well, hold on a minute. A recent study in the *New England Journal of Medicine* found that, as we said earlier, all diets lead to weight loss if they include a calorie deficit. And that's how fad diets typically work: by restricting one kind of food or letting you eat only one kind of food. It doesn't matter whether the diet advocates or bans carbs or fats or sodium or meat or cheese or, heck, salted grapefruit peels. This finding has been echoed in other studies in the journal *Diabetes Care,* the *American Journal of Clinical Nutrition*, and the journal *Archives of Internal Medicine*. Typically, people on diets lose 5 to 10 percent of their starting weight in the first six months. But according to researchers at UCLA, most people gain back that weight, and then some, in a year.

97

Amount of additional calories in today's average restaurant hamburger compared with 1977 portions. Amount of additional calories if you have fries with that? 165.

WEIGHT-LOSS SABOTEUR #1: YOUR SPOUSE

Researchers at the University of Minnesota found that men and women usually gain 6 to 8 pounds in the first 2 years of marriage. "Once you're married, that need to impress is gone," says Edward Abramson, PhD, author of *Marriage Made Me Fat.* "You may go to the gym less often, go out for meals or to parties more frequently, and develop new rituals, such as sitting on the couch with your spouse and snacking."

Fix your head:
Regain that need to impress. Imagine what losing excess weight could do for your sex life. As for that bowl of junk food with your wife, Abramson says, ask yourself: Why am I eating? Boredom? Habit? Better yet, ask her to stop bringing those binge foods into the house.

Fix your routine:
Establish healthful rituals. Instead of *Access Hollywood* after dinner, take regular walks. Exercise suppresses appetite. Cool down with Italian ice (120 calories per cup) instead of ice cream (290 calories per cup).

Just how gimmicky are all the different diet strategies? Let's take a look.

DIET TYPE: The Specific-Ratio Diet
EXEMPLAR: The Zone
Many popular diets focus on getting you to eat a perfectly harmonious mix of certain foods in a specific ratio—carbs vs. fats vs. proteins, or acidic foods vs. alkaline foods. This philosophy, expounded by the Zone and others, is based on the idea that balancing your body's hormones or pH level is the key to weight loss. To accomplish this goal, the Zone, for instance, prescribes that every meal has to have a specific ratio of carbs, protein, and fat. (In the Zone, it's 40 percent carbs, 30 percent protein, and 30 percent fat.) You eat low-fat proteins at every meal; focus on good fats, like the monounsaturated fat in olive oils, almonds, and avocados and the omega-3 fatty acids in fish; limit carb intake to whole grains and some fruits; and avoid processed foods. So far so good, right? Not quite. You're also supposed to avoid juice, beer, and sweets, as well as restrict saturated fat from red meat and egg yolks. Steak and eggs with a Bloody Mary? Forget about it: Dieting isn't supposed to be fun, remember?

But according to a recent study in the *Journal of the American Medical Association*, counting all those carbs, proteins, and fats—and making sure they're proportioned correctly for each meal—does little more than make you hyperaware of the foods you're eating, which can help you cut calories and lose weight. It'd be a whole lot easier if you just focused on eating foods with proven health benefits, such as heart-healthy olive oil, cholesterol-busting oats, and protein-and-fiber-rich black beans.

Worse, many of these diets are so complicated that you can only follow them successfully by purchasing the diet guru's food products. And those products aren't necessarily the foundation of a healthy eating plan: Three types of Zone meal-replacement bars had to be recalled by their manufacturer, Abbott Labs, back in February 2009; turns out their preferred peanut paste was made by the same scandal-ridden peanut-processing plant that caused an outbreak of salmonella. (Atkins Nutritionals also recalled some of its processed food offerings.) Yummy ingredients in Zone bars include calcium phosphate, d-alpha-tocopheryl acetate, zinc oxide (that's the stuff you rub on diaper rash), and sodium molybdate. A well-balanced diet? Depends on your definition.
Bottom line: There are easier ways to lose weight and stay healthy.

DIET TYPE: Low-Carbohydrate Diets
EXEMPLAR: Atkins
When you sit back and think about strategies such as the Atkins diet, they're really quite extreme. From the get-go, you'll restrict your diet to only proteins and fats and eliminate almost

all carbohydrates. With Atkins specifically, you'll get just 20 grams a day, which means no bread or pasta, but also no fruits, vegetables, or juice. After a few weeks, you'll increase your carbohydrate intake to 25 grams a day, and each week thereafter nudge it up by a mere 5 grams at a time. Now, nobody is perfect, but aside from wanting to enjoy a cookie every now and again, going without fruits and vegetables—the very foods that study after study say are the key to health and longevity—seems counterproductive.

The emphasis on protein is indeed on the right track, though. A recent study in the *American Journal of Clinical Nutrition* found that while calorie deficit is the main factor in weight loss, those who got 30 percent of their daily calories from protein felt more satiated than those who ate less protein, leading them to consume 441 fewer calories a day and lose 5 pounds over the course of 2 weeks. But the Atkins diet and other imitators take this idea to the extreme, because, in reality, it's just a calorie-restriction diet in camouflage. Of course you're going to lose weight if you severely restrict an entire nutrient group! You're dramatically decreasing the amount of calories you're putting into your body. But fruits and vegetables also enhance feelings of fullness because of their naturally high water and fiber content and provide your body with healthy fiber, folate, and other heart-protecting, brain-boosting, libido-lifting, mood-enhancing, essential vitamins and nutrients. Cut those and

you're also losing out on a whole spectrum of wonderful tastes, smells, and textures that your body craves—which leads to the bigger problem with this approach to eating: It's not sustainable. Restricting foods will only make you crave them more, and you may end up bingeing instead.

Bottom line: You might lose weight in the beginning, but keeping it off will be another story.

DIET TYPE: Point-System Diets
EXEMPLAR: Weight Watchers
A strategy such as Weight Watchers assigns every food a point value based on its calories, fat, and fiber content per serving. Fiber decreases the point value assigned to a particular food, whereas fat and calories increase the point value. Your job is to stay under a certain number of points every day. You can choose a high-carb or high-protein plan.

Now, diets like these deserve credit for helping people realize how many calories they're putting into their bodies. And the new "Points Plus" system is better than its predecessor because it rewards consumption of whole foods, some of which previously had the same point values as processed foods. But while keeping a food diary is a great exercise for those who want to lose weight, ultimately it is just that, an exercise. Counting calories is not something you want to do for the rest of your life. Food is meant to be savored, not suffered over. (And again, complicated = unrealistic. Weight Watchers even has

70

Percentage of kids who turn to their parents for information on nutrition and healthy eating, according to the American Dietetic Association.

its own line of frozen meals for folks who can't handle the math.)

Lastly, there's a serious flaw to the logic of these point-counting plans: What's to stop you from eating all your allotted points in one sitting and then starving yourself for the rest of the day? That's certainly not healthy and, even worse, will cause your body's metabolism to slow.

Bottom line: It is nearly impossible to sustain a diet based on counting calories alone.

DIET TYPE: Cleansing or Phase Diets
EXEMPLAR: Just About Every Diet!
Some of these approaches have month-long "jump start" periods where you'll eat as few as 1,200 calories a day, divided between three meals and a snack. Or you'll start with a phase in which you eat little else besides lean meats or vegetables or foods containing certain kinds of fats. Eventually you'll add another 400 calories or so, or a new group of foods, and if you successfully endure that stage, you'll add in a few more. You'll usually drink a lot of water

(often flavoring it to keep things interesting), eat slowly, and perform "mindful" eating exercises designed to explore your relationship with food.

But any kind of diet that causes you to focus on one or two food groups and eschew others isn't sustainable. Sure, it's cool to lose a lot of weight superfast, which is what happens when you radically restrict calories. (And by the way, it's restricted calories, not the magic foods, that causes rapid weight loss at the start.) But wouldn't it be cooler to lose weight more slowly and keep it off for a really long time?

Bottom line: Being "mindful" of your meals is a step in the right direction, but starving yourself for a month just sets you up for rebound weight gain. Better to have your weight head slowly downward than to have it drop off the table, only to bounce back up and hit you in the gut.

Okay, so diets don't work. What's a man to do?

Quite frankly, he's supposed to eat like a man. Check out the next chapter to discover how.

WEIGHT-LOSS SABOTEUR #2: LATE NIGHT TV

Not getting enough deep, non-REM sleep inhibits production of growth hormone, which might lead to premature middle-age symptoms—abdominal obesity, reduced muscle mass and strength, and diminished exercise capacity. You become Homer Simpson.

Fix your head:
"Mentally disengage yourself before you hit the sack," says Jim Karas, author of *The Business Plan for Your Body*. Lay off the TV, don't bring work to bed, and especially don't bring food to bed.

Fix your routine:
Exercise in the morning or afternoon, says Eric Nofzinger, MD, director of sleep neuroimaging research at the Western Psychiatric Institute. Evening workouts may leave you too stimulated to sleep. Establish a ritual that signals your body that the day is over 30 minutes before bedtime—turn off the computer, read, or stretch, says Karas.

Don't Diet, Do This

8 EASY STEPS TO A HEALTHIER BODY

By now you should be convinced that all those magical diets that have come and gone are not worth your time. In fact, they can undermine your weight-loss efforts. Better to eat more of the right foods than to starve yourself into putting on weight. Doing right by your body doesn't have to be difficult. Start by cherry-picking one or two of the following tips to start today, and add another couple every week until they become second nature.

1. **Stay hydrated.** If you are dehydrated, you may be burning up to 2 percent fewer calories, according to University of Utah researchers. Drink water.

2. **Make the water ice cold.** German researchers found that drinking 6 cups of cold water a day (48 ounces) can raise resting metabolism by about 50 calories a day—enough to shed 5 pounds a year. The increase may come from the energy it takes to heat that cool water to body temperature.

3. **Eat the heat.** Capsaicin, the compound that gives chili peppers their burn, can also fire up your metabolism. Eating about 1 tablespoon of chopped red or green chilies boosts the body's production of heat and the activity of your sympathetic nervous system, according to a study in the *Journal of Nutritional Science and Vitaminology*.

4. **Get more sleep.** A 2009 study in the *American Journal of Public Health* and other studies show that people who get enough sleep to feel rested have healthier diets and less abdominal fat.

5. **Fight fat with fiber.** Research shows that some fiber can rev your fat burn by 30 percent. And numerous studies suggest that people who eat the most fiber gain the least weight. Aim for 25 grams a day, easy to reach if you eat one serving of beans and three each of fruits and vegetables daily.

6. **Stand up when you're on the phone.** Make a habit of standing every time you talk on the phone. Missouri University researchers discovered that inactivity (of 4 hours or more) causes a near shutdown of an enzyme that controls fat and cholesterol metabolism.

7. **Drink coffee or tea.** Caffeine is a central nervous system stimulant, so your daily java jolts can rev your metabolism 5 to 8 percent—that's 98 to 174 calories a day. A cup of brewed tea can raise your metabolism by 12 percent, according to one Japanese study. Researchers believe the antioxidant catechins in tea provide the boost.

8. **Don't cut the cheese.** If you're laboring under the myth that milk, cheese, and other dairy foods are unhealthy, you're wrong—dead wrong. Dairy foods are packed with calcium, which boosts metabolism. Unfortunately, most men don't consume the recommended daily amounts. So add milk, yogurt, and cheese back into your life. Bonus benefit: Research shows that consuming calcium through dairy foods may also reduce fat absorption from other foods.

Chapter 3:
E-A-T-S, the Best Nutrition Plan Ever

THE UNBELIEVABLY SIMPLE STRATEGY FOR EATING ALL THE FOODS YOU LOVE AND STAYING LEAN, FIT, AND HEALTHY FOR LIFE!

Y

ou are on a diet. You may not actually think you're on a diet, my friend, but you are. Whether you eat nachos and mozzarella sticks or tofu and bean sprouts, whatever you put into your mouth on a regular basis is—literally—your diet. And while many of us think of diets as something we "go on" or "go off," typical diets— by which we mean the Atkins/Zone/Fat Smash variety—are more like interludes. The stuff you eat when you're not consciously following one of those programs? That's your diet.

WEIGHT-LOSS SABOTEUR #3: STRESS

Stress will spike levels of the hormone cortisol, which tells your body to store fat. That can cause a double-whammy: "Unfortunately, some people appease their anxiety by reaching for fatty foods," says Elissa Epel, PhD, an assistant professor of psychiatry at the University of California at San Francisco. Eating boosts insulin levels; combining that with cortisol leads to greater fat deposits. To break the stress/belly connection:

Fix your head:
First, identify the type of stress you're under. Is it temporary, like a bar exam, or more permanent, like your job? Short-term stress will pass. Long-term stress may require a permanent solution, like a new job.

Fix your routine:
Make healthy eating effortless. Buy snacks that won't send insulin levels soaring: high-fiber energy bars or single-serving bags of almonds or cashews. Fifteen minutes of explosive activity—hitting a speed bag or jumping rope—can alleviate anxieties after work.

So in case you haven't been paying attention to what you've been eating, let's investigate the average American man's diet. According to research by the Centers for Disease Control and Prevention, men eat about 2,618 calories daily—15 percent from protein, 35 percent from fat, and 50 percent from carbohydrates. In fact, the average American man's food intake over the last 30 years has grown by 500 calories a day, nearly 80 percent of which can be attributed to additional carbohydrates. We also know that Americans typically eat half as many fruits and vegetables as the government recommends, which means that most of these additional carbohydrate calories are coming from sugars and starches, a.k.a. "simple" carbohydrates. That's not totally surprising, considering foods made from sugars and starches are so cheap and so omnipresent: Sodas, chips, sweets, pizzas, fries, bagels, donuts, pastries, and other "packaged" and "processed" foods beg for constant attention everywhere—from grocery stores to gas stations. (You can even buy candy bars online at Staples!)

The problem is, when your "diet" is all about convenience foods like these, your body goes on a never-ending roller-coaster ride. That's because one of the main end products of digestion is glucose, or blood sugar. When you eat a balanced diet, your body digests its food slowly—protein, fiber, and fat take a while to work their way through your system, and so your body gets slow, steady doses of glucose, which it uses for all sorts of bodily activities, from growing hair to thinking big thoughts to keeping your heart pounding to fending off attacking hordes of Visigoths. But simple sugars and starches are digested very rapidly, and if you eat a lot of them, they flood your bloodstream with large amounts of glucose all at once—levels that your body never evolved to handle. Too much sugar in the blood causes all kinds of havoc—that's what diabetes is, basically—and so, to prevent the stuff that too much blood sugar can cause, like, oh, blindness and death, your endocrine system has to work overtime pumping out the hormone insulin, which helps to clean the sugar out of your bloodstream. Unfortunately, the only thing your body can do with excess sugar is to store it as flab.

A flood of sugar—and the resulting flood of insulin—is the top of the roller coaster. Once all the blood sugar is stored away in your belly, guess what? You're hungry again, because your blood sugar has dipped. That's the bottom of the roller coaster, and off you go, at that point, to look for more food. It's a never-ending cycle of hunger and fat storage, and it helps to explain why overweight people always seem to feel hungry—because they are!

In a nutshell, you can think of that typical American diet combination— 15 percent protein, 35 percent fat, and 50 percent carbs—as a shortcut to obesity, diabetes, heart disease, and the rest of the health complications plaguing modern Americans.

But there's nothing complicated at work here. Simply cutting down on those sugar-rush incidents throughout the day will curb your hunger, give you long-burning energy, and keep fat storage to a minimum—all of which will lead to big changes in your body. Eating is easy, remember? In fact, it's so easy that smart food choices can be boiled down to a four-letter acronym: E-A-T-S.

E-A-T-S is the simplest nutrition plan ever (don't call it a "diet!"), and it's designed to help you swap empty-calorie fare for healthy, filling, nutritious food.

E = Eliminate Added Sugars

The Challenge

For our ancient ancestors, who lived in a world with few ready-to-eat snacks, foods that provided sweetness—think apples, berries, dates, etc.—were nature's version of fast food. They required relatively little work to grow and harvest (compared to, say, making a loaf of bread from a field of wheat or hunting down a mammoth and dragging its carcass back to the cave). They were also packed with essential nutrients, which is why we evolved to crave sweet things.

That instinctual preference for sweetness and the instant energy that it provides remain to this day, but

nature's ingenious nutrient-delivery scheme went to hell in a handbasket when modern food manufacturers figured out how to produce less-perishable sweets via processing—things like candy bars and soda pop, for instance. Then they realized that if we liked sweet-tasting things, we could be inspired to buy more food if EVERYTHING became sweet-tasting, and so food marketers began adding sugar, especially high-fructose corn syrup, to everything—beverages, cereal, ketchup, bread, peanut butter, salad dressing, and the hundreds of other products with far-off expiration dates that now fill our lives (even the coating of aspirin tablets).

The problem with all that sugar is probably obvious to you by now. Not only do high doses of sugar and starch send our blood sugar soaring and set it up for an inevitable nose-dive, but research from the University of California at San Francisco shows that fructose—a natural sugar, but one that's now found everywhere—can trick your brain into craving more food, even when you're already full, by dulling your response to leptin, the "I've had enough" hormone. "Sweetened foods tend to make us overeat," says David Levitsky, PhD, a professor of psychology and nutritional sciences at Cornell University. "And that threatens the energy balance in our bodies."

According to a USDA survey, the average American eats 82 grams of

300+

Amount of calories you consume if you munch on a couple of Olive Garden's bread sticks or Red Lobster's Cheddar Bay Biscuits before your "real" meal arrives. A basket of chips at the Mexican joint? Around 500 calories, which can easily double the impact of an entrée.

2,000

Number of extra weekly calories consumed if you drink 2 regular beers a night.

added sugars daily. That's nearly 20 teaspoons a day, contributing an empty 317 calories. The researchers report that 91 percent of these added sugars can be attributed to the intake of regular soda (33 percent), baked goods and breakfast cereals (23 percent), candy (16 percent), fruit drinks (10 percent), and sweetened milk products, such as flavored yogurt (9 percent).

The Solution

Check out this simple four-word US dietary guideline, circa 1980: "Avoid too much sugar." Easy, right? So why don't we all follow it?

In part because dietary advice has gotten too complicated. By 2005, that simple governmental guideline had morphed into a 25-word tongue twister, as Marion Nestle points out in her book *What to Eat*: "Choose and prepare foods and beverages with little added sugars or caloric sweeteners, such as amounts suggested by the USDA Food Guide and the DASH [Dietary Approaches to Stop Hypertension] Eating Plan."

Blah? Blah.

Stick to the 1980 approach. Avoid foods that contain added sugar and you'll eliminate most junk food, reduce your overall calorie intake, and instantly make your diet healthier. And you'll feel better indulging in the occasional candy bar, cupcake, or chocolate shake knowing that you're ingesting sugar when YOU choose to and not because some manipulative food manufacturer snuck it into your Caesar salad dressing.

A= Add Quality Proteins

The Challenge

Much of the protein in the average American's diet comes not from beef or chicken, as you might expect, but from soy. *That can't apply to me*, you might think. *I don't eat a lot of tofu*. Perhaps not, but you do eat far more soy than you think: Foods that claim they're "high in protein," like cereals, energy bars, and the like usually contain soy. Most vegetable oils and "fortified flours" are made from soy, which means most baked and fried foods are as well. And soy can be found added into everything from canned tuna to bean soup.

Problem is, soy protein isn't a "complete" protein like you get from meat, dairy, or fish, so it doesn't contain all the amino acids your body needs to build and maintain muscle. Soy also contains two naturally occurring chemicals, genistein and daidzein, which mimic the effects of estrogen and counteract testosterone, the essential muscle-maintaining hormone.

To make matters worse, a diet high in soy—combined with a lack of exercise—has the same effect on the animals we eat as it does on us. Today's chicken, as established earlier, has just 63 percent as much protein (in other words, only 63 percent as much muscle per body weight) as chickens our families ate in the early seventies. Instead of roaming the land in search of grubs and seeds, they instead live their lives in cages, where they choke down feed made of soy and corn.

Not only do we need better protein, we also need more of it. The USDA recommends a daily intake of 56 grams, yet most adult men would benefit from eating more than that, according to Donald Layman, PhD, a professor emeritus of nutrition at the University of Illinois at Urbana-Champaign.

The Solution

Nutrition scientists have done a lot of research since *Rocky*, so fortunately you don't need to resort to chugging raw eggs. But you still need to think big. The benefits of a diet that's higher in protein will extend beyond muscles, too: Protein dulls hunger and can help prevent obesity, diabetes, and heart disease. A good rule of thumb is to eat 1 gram of protein per pound of your desired body weight. (If you want to weigh 175 pounds, in other words, eat 175 grams.) Concentrate on dairy; eggs; meats such as fish and poultry; and cuts of beef with the word "loin" in them, like sirloin.

T= Trade Starch for Produce & Whole Grains

The Challenge

Starches are the main carbs in white bread, pasta, and white rice. They're quickly and easily absorbed by the body, and because they're simply long chains of sugar molecules, consuming too much of them will cause your blood sugar to spike, setting you up for the whole rebound hunger problem outlined earlier in this chapter.

The easiest fix in the world? Eat whole fruits and vegetables instead. (Remember the line "No one ever got fat from eating produce"?) Most produce contains a lot of fiber, tons of vitamins and minerals, few calories, and very little starch. And eating produce is like winning the gold medal in curling or hammer toss—you can be a champion easily, because nobody's doing it! In fact, one-third of America's daily vegetable intake comes from just two sources: iceberg lettuce and potatoes. When you consider that most potatoes are fried, either as french fries or potato chips, Americans are barely eating any fresh vegetables at all. (And by the way, potatoes are about the starchiest vegetables around; eating a baked potato isn't that much different than eating a few slices of bread.) Even with fruit, we rarely challenge our taste buds. Half of the typical consumer's daily servings come from just a handful of sources: bananas, apples, oranges, and grapes.

The Solution

A good goal is to limit yourself to three or four servings of starch a day, on average. Consider one serving to be about 20 grams of carbohydrates—equal to about one slice of bread, one cup of hot or cold cereal, half of a large potato, or ½ cup cooked pasta or rice. By reducing your starch intake while also eliminating foods with added

WEIGHT-LOSS SABOTEUR #4: YOUR FRIENDS

Friends can make or break a diet or workout plan, whether it's unconscious scarfing of nachos during the game or the lure of happy hour. Worse, some guys will deliberately try to sabotage their buddy's diet just for sport. Want a cookie?

Fix your head:
Admit you need support. "Let people know how to help you, and many will," says Beth Kitchin, an assistant professor of nutritional sciences at the University of Alabama at Birmingham.

Fix your routine:
Eat a protein bar before meeting friends, so you'll feel fuller. Drink a glass of water for every glass of booze. A time-tested strategy: Recruit a friend to diet or work out with you. Having someone to answer to is the best enforcement plan.

WEIGHT-LOSS SABOTEUR #5: YOUR ROUTINE

Like Pavlov's dog, we all have food triggers that make us want to eat—for instance, the link between late-night TV and snacking. Food psychologists call these habits "eating scripts" and "they are the icebergs of our diets," says Brian Wansink, PhD, director of the Cornell University Food and Brand Lab.

Fix your head:
Recognize your triggers and rescript your behavior. Experiment until you find new patterns you can live with. Some people have success with an interception strategy: It's fine to grab a doughnut at the weekly staff meeting, but only after you first have a piece of fruit or a stick of gum and then reassess how much you still crave the doughnut.

Fix your routine:
Brown-bag a healthy lunch. Eliminate as many distractions as you can so you concentrate on your food. If you want to eat at your desk or in the car, fine—but turn off the computer or radio when you do so. Chances are you'll eat less when you pay full attention to the ingestion process.

sugars, you'll better control your blood sugar and be less likely to experience intense carb cravings—the kind that send you looking for quick hunger fixes in the first place.

Swapping those empty calories for fiber-rich produce and whole grains will do a world of good, because unlike sugar and starches, fiber stays intact until it nears the end of your digestive system. And people who add fiber to their diets lose more weight than those who don't, according to a review published in the journal *Nutrition*. Fiber requires extra chewing and slows the absorption of nutrients in your gut, so your body is tricked into thinking you've eaten enough, says review author Joanne Slavin, PhD, RD, a nutrition professor at the University of Minnesota. And some fibers may also stimulate cholecystokinin (CCK), an appetite-suppressing hormone in the gut.

One good goal to strive for is to triple your current intake of fruits and vegetables, says David Katz, MD, an associate professor of public health at Yale University. "Five servings is the minimum recommendation for a healthy diet. I aim for 12 to 15 servings myself," he says. Include them with every meal, and always eat them first. Not only will you consume more of them by making them a priority, you will also wind up getting fewer calories from other foods—and the fiber content will again help you sidestep those nasty swings in blood sugar that lead to hunger.

And if you're really ambitious, try new types of fruits and vegetables whenever you have the opportunity. In a 2006 study at Colorado State University, researchers found that people who ate higher amounts of produce from a smaller selection saw no meaningful health benefits. A group that ate the widest variety of fruits and vegetables experienced the most DNA protection.

S = Stop Fearing Natural Fat

The Challenge

Yes, it's bad for you to regularly eat fat—but only one type (man-made transaturated fats), and not the kind you've long been led to believe were unhealthy (natural saturated fats). "The health scare surrounding saturated fat and cholesterol was overblown," says Walter Willett, MD, chairman of the department of nutrition at Harvard University. Indeed, it has been the food industry's attempts to capitalize on our fear of fat that's lead in part to our growing, well, fat!

For example, every "health-conscious" American switched from butter to margarine in the 1970s and 80s. But butter is made from natural saturated fat, which, yes, the US government had urged people to cut down on. Margarine, on the other hand, is made from trans fats, which could be marketed as a healthier option. But as more and more research was conducted, it soon became clear that saturated fat wasn't the danger some had once believed and that trans fats were being linked directly to high cholesterol, heart disease, stroke, and diabetes. What are trans fats, exactly? They're vegetable-based—usually soy-based—oils that have been infused with hydrogen (i.e., "hydrogenated") to make them solid at room temperature. (Think Crisco.) That hydrogenation also allows them to retain their semisolid form once they enter your body. Imagine what that does to your arteries . . .

Today, nutrition researchers urge us to embrace fat—including fat from meat and dairy—and to focus on getting heart-healthy mono- and poly-unsaturated fats, from sources like nuts, olive oil, and avocados. Simply swapping one fat for another may be all you need: While mono- and polyunsaturated fats are not associated with noticeable weight gain, say Harvard researchers,

for every 1 percent increase in the percentage of calories you consume from trans fat, you gain 2.3 pounds.

The Solution

Eat healthy fats whenever they exist naturally in foods, as they do in meat, avocados, nuts, milk, and cheese. Fat gives food flavor and provides a filling sensation, which will help prevent you from overeating. Good fats also make all the other healthy foods you eat even healthier. That's because many essential vitamins, like A, D, and E, are fat-soluble—meaning they're activated and absorbed best when eaten with fat. So stop torturing yourself with low-fat or no-fat garbage. Opt for the whole-fat or reduced-fat versions instead and then monitor your calorie consumption. Research even shows that diets containing as much as 60 percent fat are just as effective for weight loss as those that are low in fat.

192

Extra calories at each meal consumed by people who drink alcohol beforehand. Researchers in the Netherlands gave people a premeal treatment of booze, food, water, or nothing. Those who had the booze spent more time eating, began feeling full later in the meal, and consumed more. Hold off and order a health-friendly glass of red wine with your entrée.

Unlock the Power of Food

WHAT YOU EAT FUELS YOUR BODY—AND YOU CAN
OPTIMIZE YOUR PERFORMANCE BY FINE-TUNING YOUR KNOWLEDGE
OF CARBS, FAT, AND PROTEIN.

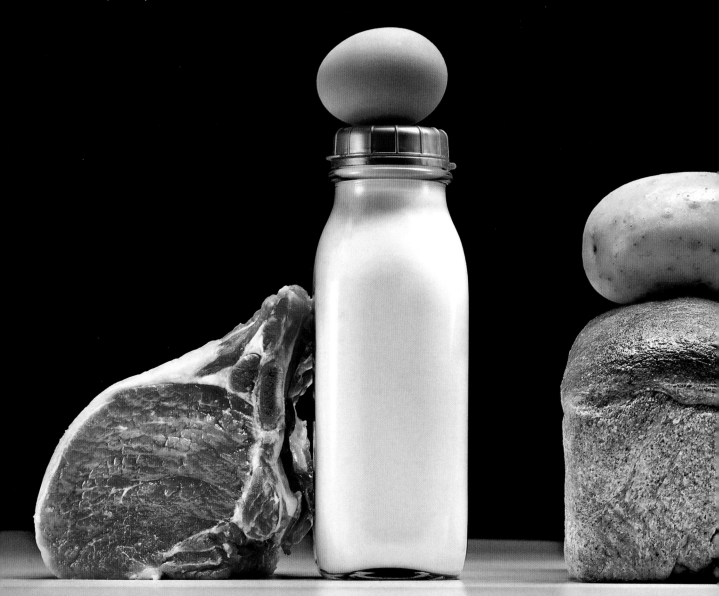

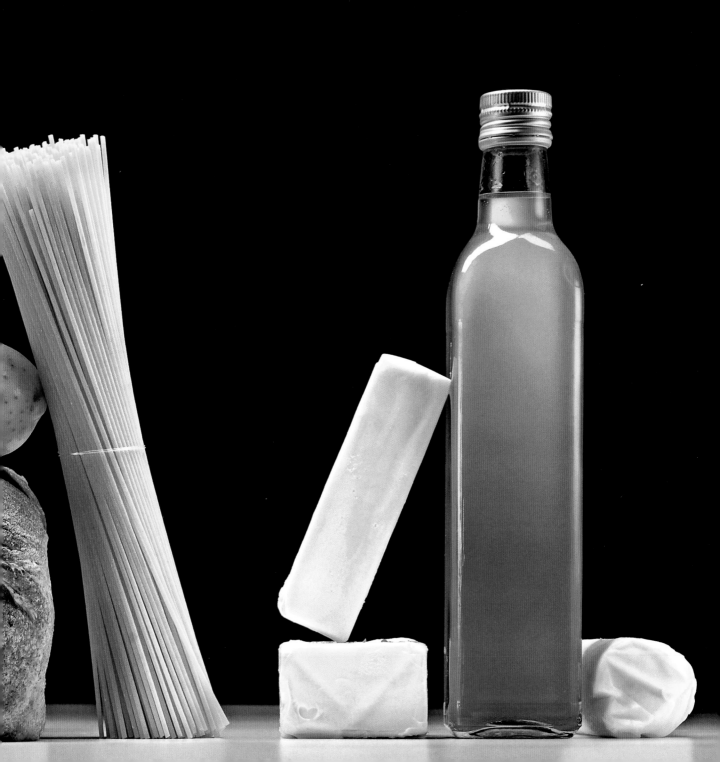

Food is power.

The power to lose weight. The power to build muscle. The power to feel energized. The power to beat disease. And the power to live a longer, healthier life.

But food can also cause you to gain weight, lose muscle, feel sluggish, and succumb to disease and disability. How are these divergent paths all possible? And, for that matter, what exactly is food, anyway?

Food is made of carbohydrates, fats, and/or proteins. Each "macronutrient," as these calorie-providing blocks are called, supplies the raw materials that your body uses for energy.

Each macronutrient's energy content varies slightly—proteins and carbohydrates contain about 4 calories per gram whereas fats contain about 9 calories per gram. This inherent energy is in the form of chemical bonds, which your body can't harness until it breaks them apart. Your organs do the real work here by slicing and dicing the three macronutrients into smaller, manageable molecules that are capable of entering the bloodstream and circulating throughout the body.

Eating may be easy, but digesting what you eat is an extremely demanding process. Depending on your age, genes, and diet, 10 to 15 percent of the calories your body uses daily are burned just by the process of digesting your meals. Eat 1,000 calories at a restaurant and your body will actually net somewhere between 850 and 900 calories—it needs the difference to process the meal. Scientists call the energy our bodies use to break down our meals the "thermic effect of food," or TEF, which is the calorie-burning effect of digesting, using, and storing food energy.

Fat has the lowest thermic effect of the three macronutrients. Protein, on the other hand, has the highest thermic effect. When Arizona State University researchers compared the benefits of a high-protein diet with those of a high-carbohydrate diet, they found that people who ate a high-protein diet burned more than twice as many calories in the hours after their meals as those eating primarily carbs. This is also why protein is said to "burn hot."

Not surprisingly, one way you can kickstart your metabolism—your body's internal calorie-burning furnace—is to eat protein with every meal. Having a total of five or six meals a day can yield a similar effect, too, as long as you control your portions and don't consume too many extra calories. You can also boost your metabolism by increasing your level of activity through exercise, which can account for as much as 15 percent of your total caloric usage. Technically this is called exercise-activity thermogenesis (EAT), and weight lifting and interval training are the most effective for enhancing your metabolism. But the most significant source of your daily burn happens when you do nothing at all. Your basal metabolic rate (BMR) is simply the cost of your body doing business: keeping your heart beating, your lungs breathing, even your cells dividing. You can make this process more efficient in a big way—provided you make an effort at improving your diet and exercise habits.

This brings us back to the food you eat throughout the day. Your body not only uses the macronutrients derived from your meals for fuel, but also to repair cells and build new muscle. So to better understand why food is truly power—and how you can harness that power to achieve the body you want—let's take a closer look at the science of carbohydrates, fat, and protein. A lot of diet books try to group them into "good" or "bad" categories, but as you'll see it's not as simple as that. In fact, you may be surprised at what you learn.

CHECK YOUR BLOOD FATS

A study at the University of California at Davis offered evidence to explain how cutting down on carbs may trigger weight loss. Researchers there found that keeping carbs to less than 40 percent of your total daily calories actually deactivates a gene that produces triglycerides—the blood fats that collect as body fats.

Carbohydrates:
The Fast-Acting Fuel Your Body Craves

Carbohydrates, which are sugars and starches, are especially prevalent in grains, fruits, and vegetables, and they provide crucial, fast-acting energy to feed your brain, muscles, and metabolism. And when they're consumed in their natural state, they can also contain loads of minerals, vitamins, and fiber. In fact, carbohydrates are generally your body's main (and preferred) source of fuel. There are two types—simple and complex—and your body uses each of them fairly differently.

Simple Carbohydrates

Ultimately, simple carbohydrates are nothing more than sugar. While there are many types of sugar (see "How Sugar Hides" on page 45 for a list of aliases), the two main ones that we consume are called glucose and fructose. These are known as single sugars, and they combine with each other to create double sugars, such as sucrose, which you know as table sugar. Whether you're eating an apple or drinking a soda, most sweet-tasting foods, from strawberries to Starburst, contain a combination of glucose and fructose.

Glucose

Your body and brain's main energy source, glucose is the "sugar" in blood sugar. And because it's already in the form your body needs, it's quickly absorbed into your blood. As a result, glucose is the type of carbohydrate that raises blood sugar the most quickly. The higher a food's number on the glycemic index (GI), the greater the impact it has on your blood sugar. In limited amounts, glucose can be stored in muscles and in the liver as glycogen—chains of glucose. During exertion, glycogen gets released into the bloodstream so that your muscles can fuel their work. When glycogen is depleted, muscles become fatigued. However, if you overeat carbohydrates—and don't burn off all those extra sugar calories through exercise—your glycogen levels can fill to capacity. When that happens, your body starts converting the excess glucose in the bloodstream

A FILLING FEELING

When Harvard University researchers analyzed the diets of more than 27,000 people over 8 years, they discovered that those who ate whole grains daily weighed an average of 2.5 pounds less than those who ate only refined-grain foods.

into body fat—the rainy-day slush fund your body will tap for energy in the event that a plague of locusts destroys your field of wheat before harvest.

Fructose

Unlike glucose, fructose—which is naturally found in fruit but is also added to processed foods—doesn't spike blood sugar. That's because to use fructose, your body must first send it from your intestines to your liver. From there, your body converts it to glucose and stores it. However, if your liver's glucose stores are already full, then the fructose is converted to body fat. So consuming extra fructose, now found in thousands of packaged foods, can lead to a rounder belly, because that's the place your body can most efficiently store excess calories, whether the calories come from carbs, fats, or proteins.

Complex Carbohydrates

Any carbohydrate that's composed of more than two sugar molecules is considered complex.

Starch

This is the stored form of glucose as found in plant foods. There's an abundance of starch in grains, legumes, and root vegetables, such as potatoes. Essentially, starch is a bunch of glucose molecules that are held together by a weak chemical bond—meaning it breaks down easily once you eat it, leaving you with pure glucose. If eaten without fat or fiber, which slow glucose's absorption, starch will quickly raise blood sugar.

Fiber

The structural material in the leaves, stems, and roots of plants, fiber is a bundle of sugar molecules as well. But unlike starch, it has no effect on blood sugar. That's because human digestive enzymes can't break the bonds that hold those bundles together, so fiber—a.k.a. "a nondigestible carbohydrate"—stays intact until it nears the end of your digestive system and binds with other foods to escort calories out of the body.

This is true for insoluble fiber as well as soluble fiber. Insoluble fiber, or roughage, is the kind found in wheat bran, nuts, and many vegetables. It has a thicker and rougher structure and won't dissolve in water, so it passes through your digestive tract and increases stool bulk. Soluble fiber, the kind found in oats, beans, barley, and some fruits, dissolves in water to form a gel-like material in your digestive tract. This slows the absorption of sugar into your bloodstream and removes cholesterol.

And what's the best part about either type? People who add fiber to their diets lose more weight than those who don't, according to a review published in the journal *Nutrition*. Review author Joanne Slavin, PhD, RD, says that fiber requires extra chewing and slows the absorption of nutrients in your gut, so your belly feels full even though you haven't stuffed yourself.

HOW SUGAR HIDES

Scanning a product's ingredients list to see if it contains sugar is smart, but you may need to expand your vocabulary. Here are 20 aliases that the sweet stuff goes by—none of which include the word sugar.

- barley malt
- brown rice syrup
- corn syrup
- dextrose
- evaporated cane juice invert syrup
- fructose
- fruit juice
- galactose
- glucose
- granular fruit grape juice concentrate
- high-fructose corn syrup
- honey
- lactose
- maltodextrin
- maple syrup
- molasses
- organic cane juice
- sorghum
- sucrose
- turbinado

Fat: The Stealthy Health Secret You've Overlooked

SURVIVAL INSTINCT

After you eat a meal, your small intestine breaks the fat molecules down into glycerol and fatty acids, which end up in your bloodstream. Fatty acids circulate through your entire body and are absorbed into fat cells, where they're assembled into fat molecules and stored for the next famine. Excess glucose from carbohydrates are also concentrated into fat molecules and absorbed by fat cells. And if the famine doesn't come, you grow wider.

While no macronutrient is an outright villain, dietary fat has been maligned as one for decades. But some of the healthiest foods we eat—including omega-3 fatty acids and monounsaturated fatty acids—are out-and-out fats. And our bodies desperately need fat to perform metabolic functions that range from the fairly basic (healing scrapes) to the extremely complicated (keeping brain cells firing). Thankfully, fat tends to taste pretty good, and it keeps your belly feeling full—which is one reason why a little fat can go a long way.

Plus, including healthy fats in your diet will make all the other healthy foods you eat even healthier. That's because many essential vitamins such as A, D, and E are fat-soluble; they are activated and absorbed best when eaten with fat. Carrots, broccoli, and peas are all loaded with vitamin A, but you won't get all the value from them unless you pair them with a healthy fat such as olive oil. As a good dietary rule of thumb, shoot for half a gram of fat daily for every pound of your desired body weight. Research shows that diets containing upward of 50 percent fat are just as effective for weight loss as those that are lower in fat. But not all fats are created equal, and the quality of the fats you eat have an enormous impact on your health.

The differences between fats are molecular, and the chemistry of fat can make your head spin. The short explanation is that the three fatty acids—monounsaturated, polyunsaturated, and saturated—are the foundations of fat. They're long chains of linked carbon atoms that attract hydrogen. Chains with less hydrogen mean the fat is "unsaturated," whereas those with more hydrogen are more "saturated." Every fat you eat actually contains at least a little of each type, but the fat ratios always vary.

Monounsaturated Fatty Acids

Fatty acids with the least amount of hydrogen are called monounsaturated. This is the main kind of "good" fat, and you'll find it in nuts, olives, avocados, and olive and canola oils. Because of their chemical structure, monounsaturated fatty acids are liquid at room temperature, solid when refrigerated, and they turn rancid when left exposed to the elements.

Why are they so good? Because monounsaturated fatty acids—"MUFAs," as they're sometimes called—do double duty on the health front, reducing bad cholesterol levels and hunger levels. They help your body burn fat, too. In one interesting study, people who ate a meal high in MUFAs burned more fat in the ensuing five hours than after a meal rich in saturated fats. Palmitoleic acid, cis-vaccenic acid, and oleic acid are the three main types, the latter of which shows up in the greatest percentages in American diets.

Oleic acid
Recent research from the University of California, Irvine, has found that this particular fat functions to bolster memory, and it also helps reduce appetite and promote weight loss. While your body can make oleic acid on its own—it's also known as omega-9 fatty acid—the most popular and most concentrated source is olive oil. Indeed, more than 70 percent of olive oil's fats come from oleic acid. It shows up in other surprising places, too, including dark chocolate and steak.

Polyunsaturated Fatty Acids
This category of fats contains both "good" fats and "bad" fats. Polyunsaturated fats are more chemically stable than monounsaturated fats and tend to remain liquid whether at a hot or cold temperature.

Omega-3 fatty acids
As you've probably heard by now, omega-3 fatty acids boost brain function, protect against coronary heart disease, fight inflammation, and may even erase wrinkles. There are different types of omega-3s. The three main ones are eicosapentaenoic acid, docosahexaenoic acid, and alpha-linolenic acid, known respectively as EPA, DHA, and ALA. EPA and DHA, the omega-3 fatty acids that are most easily used by your body, come mainly from plankton and are found in the most significant amounts among cold-water fish, which carry extra fat for insulation. ALA is obtained from terrestrial plants. But for ALA to provide any health benefits, your liver must convert it into EPA and DHA, according to Bruce Holub, PhD, a professor of nutritional sciences at the University of Guelph in Ontario. The estimated average efficiency of conversion is only around 10 percent to 15 percent, he says, which means you need to eat a fair amount of plant foods to glean an equivalent amount of EPA and DHA contained in a relatively small amount of fish.

Omega-6 fatty acids
When food manufacturers first realized that omega-6s—prevalent in

CLEAR YOUR PANTRY
The typical American eats 27.6 times more soybean oil than olive oil, and much of that comes from generic bottles labeled as "vegetable oil." Ban this oil from your life—it's the main reason why our omega-6 to omega-3 ratios are so out of whack—and replace it with canola oil, which has a near-perfect 2:1 ratio of the two omegas, as well as olive oil.

polyunsaturated seed oils such as vegetable, corn, and soybean oils—didn't go rancid as quickly as omega-3s, they cleared shelves to make room for products containing them . . . and then they quickly started adding shelving. Our pantries have never recovered, and neither have our waistlines, because omega-6s compete with omega-3s for space in our cell membranes. While our ancestors ate a ratio of omega-6s to omega-3s of approximately 1:1, our "Western" diet, characterized by high intakes of corn-fed meat, sugar, and refined carbohydrates, has a ratio of about 20:1. And, according to a 2008 review of studies by the Center for Genetics, Nutrition and Health, a high intake of omega-6 fats relative to omega-3 fats increases inflammation, which may increase your risk of heart disease, diabetes, and cancer. Omega-6s are still essential for your health, but it's important to achieve a proper balance with omega-3s.

Conjugated linoleic acid

CLA is a polyunsaturated fatty acid mixture commonly found in beef that's been shown to offer protection against cardiovascular disease and diabetes. It can also help you lose weight, according to a meta-analysis in the *American Journal of Clinical Nutrition*. The researchers found that consuming just 3.2 grams of CLA a day can strip 12 pounds off your body in the course of a year. Grass-fed beef— from cows that have been raised in

pastures and fed a natural diet—has two to three times more CLA than beef from cows raised in concentrated animal-feeding operations (CAFOs) and fed a diet of corn.

Transaturated fatty acids

The term "trans" refers to the fact that the fats are transformed from liquid polyunsaturated fats (usually soybean oil) to solid fats by adding hydrogen in a pressure-cooker–like environment. Completely man-made trans fats—like those in margarine— are not only worse for your heart than other fats, but they're also a prime culprit for weight gain, according to Harvard Medical School researchers. For every 1 percent increase in the percentage of calories you consume from trans fats, you gain 2.3 pounds. Even worse, foods that are "free of trans fats" can still contain up to 0.5 grams of trans fat per serving—and those 0.5 grams add up quickly. If the label reads "hydrogenated" or "partially hydrogenated," the food contains trans fats—and is worth avoiding.

Saturated Fatty Acids

Saturated fat—the kind found in a T-bone or a slab of butter—is solid at room temperature and turns to liquid when heated. "Butter melts in hot weather, but you have to cook steaks and pork chops to melt their fat. This tells you that meat has more saturated fatty acids than butter," writes Marion Nestle in *What to Eat*.

KNOW YOUR OMEGAS

The essential fatty acids omega-3 and omega-6 are polyunsaturated fats that your body needs but cannot manufacture itself. The former comes from certain leaves, the latter from seeds. Your body can make omega-9, a monounsaturated fatty acid also known as oleic acid, but it's good to consume foods with it, which is why you hear experts raving about its main source, olive oil.

But admit it: If you were to scan the nutritional information on the label and see a high amount of saturated fat, you'd consider that food to be bad news, right? Well, not so fast. In fact, a 2010 review of 21 studies, published in the *American Journal of Clinical Nutrition,* found no conclusive evidence that dietary saturated fat is associated with an increased risk of coronary heart disease, stroke, or cardiovascular disease. (Yes, you read that correctly!) According to a review in the *European Journal of Nutrition,* a diet high in fat from dairy products such as butter may even raise levels of HDL (good) cholesterol while having no effect on levels of potentially harmful LDL (bad) cholesterol.

What's more, it turns out there are more than 13 types of saturated fatty acids—some of which are actually good for your heart. Humans consume three types of them predominantly: stearic acid, palmitic acid, and lauric acid. This trio comprises almost 95 percent of the saturated fat in a hunk of prime rib or a slice of bacon, and nearly 70 percent of that in butter and whole milk.

Here's a quick look at some of the major forms of saturated fats.

Palmitic acid

Palmitic acid is a saturated fat that shows up everywhere. Meat and dairy products contain it, but it also shows up in coconut and palm oil (hence the name). While palmitic is known to raise total cholesterol as well as LDL (bad) cholesterol, it also raises HDL (good) cholesterol just as much, if not more. This overall effect lowers your risk of heart disease, because increasing both actually reduces the proportion of the bad kind of cholesterol in your blood to the good. Indeed, numerous studies have reported that this HDL/LDL ratio is a better predictor of future heart disease than LDL alone.

Stearic acid

It's well-established that stearic acid has no effect on cholesterol levels. In fact, stearic acid—which is found in high amounts in cocoa as well as in animal fats—is converted to oleic acid, the heart-healthy monounsaturated fat, in your liver. As a result, scientists generally regard this saturated fatty acid as either benign or potentially beneficial to your health.

Lauric acid

A recent analysis of 60 studies published in the *American Journal of Clinical Nutrition* reports that even though lauric acid raises LDL (bad) cholesterol, it boosts HDL (good) cholesterol even more. As with palmitic acid, this means that it may decrease your risk of cardiovascular disease.

Myristic acid

We had to include this because there's no way around it: This saturated fat is bad news. Fortunately it makes up only about 3 percent of the saturated fat in sirloin steak and only about 14 percent of the saturated fat in butterfat.

ANTI-SOCIAL GREASE?

In one study of crime rates in five countries, a rising ratio of omega-6 correlated with an increase in homicide rates.

Protein:
The Superfuel
Your Muscles Need

Made of amino acids, proteins are the nutritional building blocks for lean muscle mass. Stressing a muscle—by, say, raising and lowering a dumbbell—causes microscopic tears in the muscle fibers. When amino acids reach a muscle's cells, they help repair damaged muscle fibers and make new, stronger ones in a process called protein synthesis. This process can't happen, of course, unless you've got amino acids coursing through your body. There are 22 different kinds, 13 of which we produce ourselves. The other nine, called essential amino acids, must come from the food you eat. The best kinds of protein—namely meat, dairy, and eggs—provide all nine and have a high "biological value," your body can easily use them. Other foods may contain a fair amount of protein, but they're considered "incomplete" sources, because they contain fewer than nine amino acids. Your body can form complete proteins by combining incomplete ones—this happens whenever you combine legumes, nuts, and grains—but you'll need to consume as much as a quarter more plant-based foods to get all the benefits provided by animal protein.

Beyond just building muscle—which helps raise your metabolism and increase your daily calorie burn—protein helps keep you slim in another way, as well: it requires a lot of calories to digest. And of the three macronutrients, protein will make you feel full the fastest. Here's a closer look at the most common types of protein.

Whey protein

Three essential amino acids—leucine, isoleucine, and valine—are called "branched-chain amino acids," and they're the very best amino acids you can get, because they act quickly and your body uses them so efficiently. Whey protein happens to be 10 percent leucine (other animal-based proteins have as little as 5 percent), and it behaves almost like a hormone in your body. "It's more than a building block

TRIM YOUR BELLY

In a Danish study, researchers put 65 subjects on a low-protein diet, a high-protein diet, or no diet. While the low-protein dieters lost an average of 11 pounds, the high-protein dieters lost an average of 20 pounds. But even more amazingly, the high-protein dieters lost twice as much abdominal fat. One reason may be that a high-protein diet helps your body control its levels of cortisol, a stress hormone that directs fat toward the belly.

of protein—it actually activates protein synthesis," says Jeffrey Volek, PhD, RD, a nutrition and exercise researcher at the University of Connecticut. Found in dairy products and supplements, it's also known as a "fast protein" because it's quickly broken down into amino acids and appears in your bloodstream 15 minutes after you consume it, which makes it a very good protein to consume after your workout.

Casein protein

Casein, another dairy protein also sold in supplement form, digests slower and provides a slower-absorbing but more sustained source of amino acids. It's ideal for providing your body with a steady supply of smaller amounts of protein for a longer period of time—such as between meals or while you sleep. Whey and casein are ideally consumed together.

Egg protein

Your body can use 94 percent of the protein in a whole egg, making it, like whey and casein, an excellent source of high-quality protein. In fact, a recent review of more than 25 published studies on protein concluded that egg protein may help boost muscle strength and development more than other proteins do because of its high concentrations of leucine. And egg protein is also good for keeping you from getting hungry over a sustained period of time.

Soy protein

Besides not contributing to protein synthesis as much as other proteins, soy presents a number of other nutritional weaknesses as well. The researchers of a 2005 study in the *Journal of Nutrition* compared soy with casein and concluded that "the biological value of soy protein must be considered inferior to that of casein protein in humans."

And though it's promoted as a health food—especially for the heart—soy protein is anything but. In 2006, a study review in the American Heart Association journal *Circulation* cast doubt on the long-held notion that eating soy daily can lower LDL (bad) cholesterol. In fact, research now suggests that you'd have to eat the equivalent of 2 pounds of tofu every day to lower your LDL cholesterol a measly 3 percent. Soy's isoflavones have also been shown to raise estrogen levels in men and to negatively impact thyroid function when consumed in high amounts. And a 2008 Harvard study found a strong association between men's consumption of soy foods and decreased sperm counts.

And while Asian diets are often considered "healthier," contrary to popular belief, Asians don't consume huge amounts of soy protein: Studies say the average daily intake is around 10 grams in China and about 8 grams in Japan. Many Americans get north of 20 grams because soy is so abundant and inexpensive.

PROTECTING THE BUSYBODY MACRO-NUTRIENT

Muscle isn't the only thing protein is good for. Protein provides the framework of all tissue—from filaments to tendons to organs. Enzymes, hormones, and antibodies are also proteins. In short, protein plays many underappreciated roles, and your body is constantly draining its protein reserves for other uses—making said hormones, for instance. The result is less protein for muscle building. To counteract this problem, you need to "build and store new proteins faster than your body breaks down old proteins," says Michael Houston, PhD, a professor of nutrition at Virginia Tech University.

Chapter 5: Stop Swallowing Food-Label Lies!

YOUR WEIGHT ISN'T ENTIRELY YOUR FAULT—AND THAT'S EXACTLY WHAT THE FOLKS ENGINEERING YOUR FOOD DON'T WANT YOU TO KNOW. FIND OUT HOW YOU CAN BITE BACK.

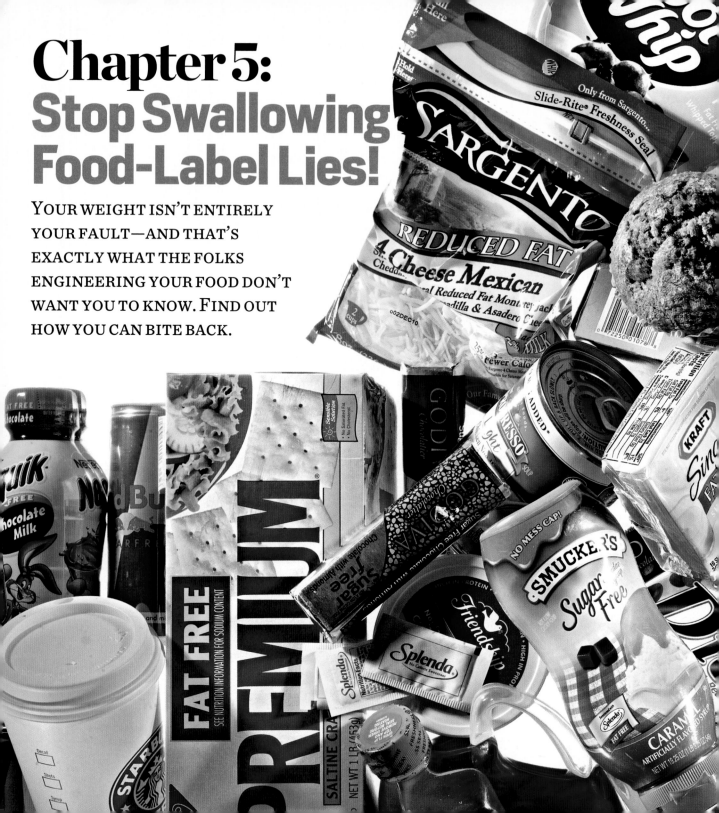

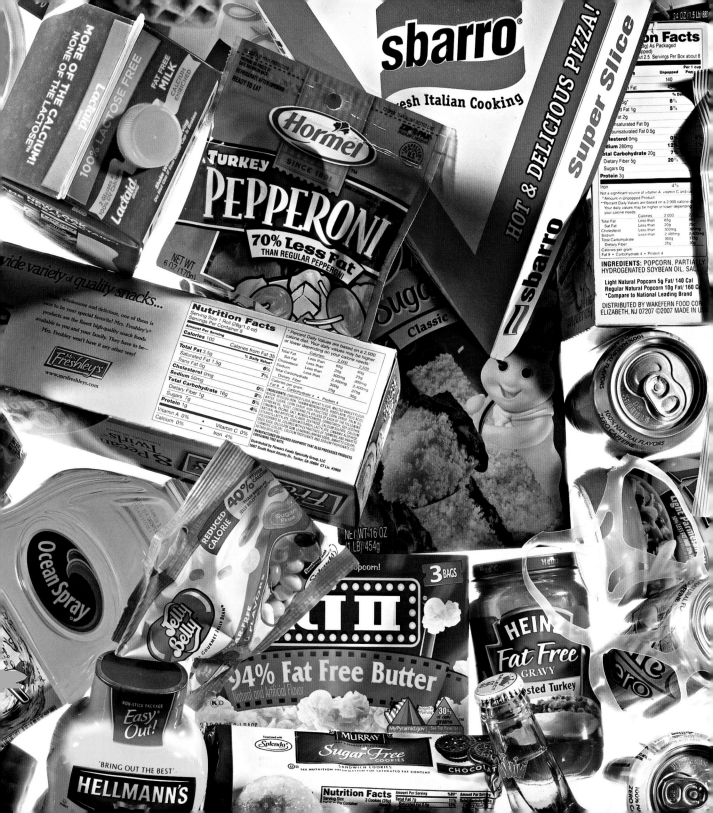

Sugar. Fat. Salt.

Combine large doses of any of these with a seemingly innocent and healthy vehicle—be it chicken breast, potatoes, salad greens, or coffee—and you can create a savory offering similar to those on the vast majority of American restaurant menus and in the thousands of packages on your supermarket shelves. That's because the folks engineering your food know that these hidden health hazards will make any meal, snack, or treat more delicious, flavorful, and satisfying. And, if they're successful, you're likely to buy more of their food. They're also fond of adjusting proportions to create so-called "low-fat" or "reduced-sodium" products.

But compare the nutrition labels and you might discover some sleight of hand. If a food manufacturer removes a product's sodium, for instance, it typically has to boost the sugar content to keep the taste desirable, according to Joanne L. Slavin, a nutrition professor at the University of Minnesota. So any way you look at it, the equation is simple and designed to make you fail:

MORE SUGAR + MORE FAT + MORE SALT = LESS NUTRITION

It's time to pull back the curtain and expose the food industry's tactics. Educate yourself and you can fight back—with your wallet.

Food labels lie when they make you think that . . .

1. "Fat-Free" Is Good for You

People hawking packaged foods equate deception with good business. Consider the labels on products such as Mike and Ike and Good & Plenty candies, where you'll find a somewhat surprising claim: "fat-free." They're not lying—these empty-calorie junk foods are almost 100 percent sugar and processed carbs. But food manufacturers clearly hope that you'll equate fat-free with healthy or nonfattening. Problem is, fat-free snacks that are loaded with sugar are digested rapidly, sending your blood sugar soaring; as soon as it drops again, you'll crave more "fat-free" empty calories. Fat-free

half-and-half is equally dubious. By definition, a half-and-half dairy product is 50 percent milk and 50 percent cream. Cream, of course, is pretty much all fat. Technically, fat-free half-and-half can't exist. So what is it exactly? Skim milk—to which a thickening agent and an artificial cream flavor have been added. You may be disappointed in the payoff: One tablespoon of Land O'Lakes traditional half-and-half contains just 20 calories; its fat-free version has 10.

Food labels lie when they make you think that . . .

2. Cherry-Picked Stats Are Meaningful

On the front of a box of crackers, marketers will often use a claim like "33% Less Fat Than the Original!" When you compare the nutritional labels, you'll see that the math is accurate. For example, the original version of the product might contain 3 grams of fat per serving (per four crackers), while the reduced-fat version has 2 grams (per five crackers). So statistically, yes, it's a 33 percent difference. But is it meaningful? After all, when was the last time you ate just five crackers? And, if you continue to study the nutrition content, you'll probably notice that the reduced-fat crackers have 33 percent more carbs than the original. In other words, when they removed 1 gram of fat, they had to replace it with 3 grams of refined flour and sugar to keep the crackers palatable. And you'd better believe that "33% More

Unhealthy "Health" Food #1
PRETZELS

The upside: One ounce has just 110 calories.

The downside: These twisted low-fat snacks have one of the highest glycemic indexes of any food. In fact, they rank above ice cream and jelly beans in their ability to raise blood sugar.

The healthy alternative: Nuts. Almonds, walnuts, cashews, pistachios, or peanuts (or a party mix of them all) will fill you faster and pack more nutrition.

Carbs Than the Original" isn't going to help any crackers fly off the shelves.

Food labels lie when they make you think that . . .

3. "Healthy" Beverages Are Actually Healthy

Through ingenious marketing, beverage companies have managed to pass off everything from sweetened green tea to vitamin-enhanced waters as good for you. Skip these drinks nine times out of ten in favor of a cool, refreshing glass of zero-calorie water. The beverage aisle is almost like the Wild West of nutritional claims. On behalf of *Men's Health*, ChromaDex laboratories recently analyzed 14 different bottled green teas for their levels of disease-fighting antioxidants called catechins. While Honest Tea's Green Tea with Honey topped the charts with an impressive 215 milligrams of total catechins, some products weren't even in the game. For instance, Republic of Tea's Pomegranate Green Tea had only 8 milligrams, and Ito En Teas' Tea Lemongrass Green had just 28 milligrams, despite implying on its label that the product is packed with antioxidants. The rainbow-colored rows of "enhanced" waters have a different dirty little secret. The crutch of every bottle of Vitaminwater, for instance, is a host of B vitamins. Everything that goes in after that—zinc, chromium, vitamins A, C, or E, etc.—hinges on whether said beverage is trying to provide "focus," "sync," "balance," or any number of

elusive and unsubstantiated health claims. The problem is that this scant collection of nutrients isn't worth the stiff sugar tariff that Vitaminwater charges: 32.5 grams—8 teaspoons' worth—stuffed into each bottle. Pop a daily multivitamin instead.

Food labels lie when they make you think that . . .

4. Your Breakfast Is Low in Sugar

Flavored yogurt seems like an ideal breakfast or snack for a man on the go—after all, it's a protein-packed dairy product paired with antioxidant-laden fruits in one convenient little cup. Unfortunately, the sugar content of these seemingly healthy products is sky-high, especially in the fruit-on-the-bottom varieties. The fruit itself is swimming in so much thick syrup that high-fructose corn syrup and other such sweeteners often must be listed in the ingredients before the fruit itself. A similar dilemma presents itself with flavored instant oatmeal. Some brands even proudly display the American Heart Association (AHA) check mark on their products' boxes. However, the fine print next to the logo will simply read that the cereal meets AHA's "food criteria for saturated fat and cholesterol." In other words, it could have as much sugar as Fruit Loops and still get this particular AHA logo! And sugar, a low-quality refined carbohydrate, is the last thing you want for breakfast. Not only can spikes in blood sugar wreck your short-term memory, according to a study in the *European Journal of Clinical Nutrition*, but Australian researchers have found that people whose diets were high in carbohydrates had a lower metabolism than those who ate proportionally more protein. Opt for non-flavored products whenever possible and simply add healthy toppings yourself.

Food labels lie when they make you think that . . .

5. "Heart-Healthy" Foods Are Always Good for Our Hearts

Why is the AHA logo on some products but absent from others, even when both meet the guidelines? Companies pay big money for the right to use most logos, because they know that consumers equate them with credibility. The NASCAR-ification of our foods means that even cornflakes can sport a "diabetes-friendly" logo on the box's side panel—never mind that Australian researchers have shown that cornflakes raise blood glucose faster and to a greater extent than straight table sugar.

Food labels lie when they make you think that . . .

6. Food Containers Are Safe

An estimated 93 percent of Americans have bisphenol A (BPA), a synthetic chemical found in plastic and used in the lining of aluminum cans, circulating in their bodies. To date, studies have linked the chemical to diabetes; obesity; mood disorders; lower sperm counts; heart disease; an increase risk of breast, prostate, and testicular cancers; and more. BPA enters our bodies by leaching into food. A recent study by the Environmental Working Group found that one in 10 cans of food, and one in three cans of infant formula, contained BPA levels more than 200 times the government's recommended level of exposure to industrial chemicals. Canned chicken soup, infant formula, and ravioli had BPA levels of the highest concern, with beans and tuna close behind. Unfortunately, jarred foods aren't much better, thanks to the plastic lining in their lids. A recent study by Health Canada tested glass-jarred baby food and found BPA in 84 percent of the samples. Acidic foods are among the worst (tomatoes, citrus, sodas, and beer), because they increase the rate of leaching. What to do? Opt for products that have minimal contact with plastic and BPA whenever possible by buying fresh or frozen produce, beer and soda in glass bottles, and foods in BPA-free cans by companies such as Eden Organic.

Food labels lie when they make you think that . . .

7. Calorie Counts Are Accurate

That's because in order to make sure you're getting at least as much as you pay for, the FDA is more likely to penalize a food manufacturer for overstating the net weight of a product than understating it. As a result, manufacturers

Unhealthy "Health" Food #2

CALIFORNIA ROLL

The upside:
The seaweed it's wrapped in contains essential nutrients, such as iodine, selenium, calcium, and omega-3 fats.

The downside:
It's basically a Japanese sugar cube. That's because its two other major components are white rice and imitation crab, both of which are packed with fast-digesting carbohydrates and almost no protein.

The healthy alternative: Real sushi made with tuna or salmon. These varieties have fewer bad carbohydrates, while providing a hefty helping of high-quality protein. Better yet, skip the rice, too, by ordering sashimi.

often either "generously" package more food than the stated net weight or make servings heavier than the stated serving-size weight. Do some investigative work yourself the next time you come home from the grocery store. Get out an ordinary food scale and check a few products' actual net weights and serving-size weights. If anything is heavier than the package says, that means you could be eating more calories than you thought you were.

Food labels lie when they make you think that . . .

8. Fruit Juice Is Full of Fruit

The claim "100 percent juice" deserves a big asterisk. Some juices, such as apple, grape, and pear, are cheap, abundant, and loaded with sugar. Others—blueberry, açai, and pomegranate, for instance—are more expensive, higher-quality nectars. So what do beverage companies do? Like drug dealers, they cut the good stuff with the cheap stuff. It's still 100 percent juice, but in reality it's nothing more than a blend of inexpensive sucrose-loaded fillers tinged with a mere splash of what you really want. Moreover, many juice "cocktails" contain as little as 20 percent real juice; sugar pads the rest. Take Ocean Spray's stable of hybrid "juices," most of which have sugar loads close to 85 percent. They'll use cane or beet sugar on the ingredients list to make it sound more appetizing, but as far as your body's concerned, sugar is sugar.

You're better off thinking of these juices as non-carbonated soft drinks or sugar-laden aperitifs.

Food labels lie when they make you think that . . .

9. All Milk Is Equal

If you're a scrupulous consumer, you've no doubt noticed the two competing messages on some milk containers. One says "from cows not treated with rbST" while the other reads "no significant difference has been shown between milk derived from rbST-treated and non-rbST-treated cows." You're not the only one who finds the pairing contradictory and *udderly*—ahem—confusing. The first claim comes from legitimate fears about the carcinogenic effects of the hormone rbST, or recombinant bovine somatotropin (also known as rBGH, recombinant bovine growth hormone), which dairy farmers give cows to increase their milk output by 10 to 25 percent. The main concern with rbST is that the cows produce milk with higher-than-normal levels of the insulin-like growth factor IGF-1. A series of studies at the Channing Laboratory in Boston show that high levels of IGF-1 increase the risk of several cancers, including breast, prostate, and colorectal. In the study, those with the highest levels of the hormone were four times as likely to develop cancer. Other studies contradict the findings, however, and the biotech that developed the hormone (Monsanto, which has since sold it) successfully lobbied for the confusing qualification.

5 Rules for Healthier Ordering

Sit-down restaurants might seem like a better option than fast-food establishments, but oftentimes that's not the case. A menu analysis of 24 national chains revealed that the average entrée at a sit-down restaurant contains 867 calories, compared with 522 calories in the average fast-food entrée. A cheeseburger from Outback Steakhouse is roughly five times the size and packs up to six times the calories as a 300-calorie cheeseburger from McDonald's. And that's before appetizers, sides, and desserts—selections that can easily double your total caloric intake. Regardless of where you place an order, these easy guidelines can help you make healthier choices.

1. Skip the Supersize

The average "value" meal contains 1,200 calories. Compared with the normal meal, that's 73 percent more empty calories for 17 percent more money. What seems like a bargain for you is really nothing more than a hefty profit for a large-scale food supplier trying to move its inventory.

2. Say "No Thanks"

Servers love to upsell by asking you questions like "do you want chips and a soda with that?" Why? Because the technique really works. A 2005 study published in the *Journal of Retailing and Consumer Services* found that you're more likely to add unwanted calories to your meal when the server verbally prompts you.

3. Stop Splurging

A 2008 study in the *International Food Research Journal* found that people are less likely to make healthy restaurant choices when they feel that they're dining out for a "special occasion." But eating out always feels special. Limit yourself to a once- or twice-a-week splurge—your wallet and waistline will reap equal rewards.

4. Order the Small

If you order soup, for instance, ask for a cup instead of a bowl. If you finish your cup and want more, ask for a second serving. No one will ever stop you from ordering seconds. Recognize your order as the business transaction that it is and, like any good businessperson, start small.

5. Eat "Real" Food

You'd think that Chicken McNuggets would contain mostly bread and chicken, but there are another 25 or so ingredients. Burger King's Chicken Fries? Thirty-five ingredients. Wendy's Frosty? Fifteen. Rule of thumb: The fewer the ingredients, the better the food.

Unhealthy "Health" Food #3

FAT-FREE SALAD DRESSING

The upside: Cutting out the fat reduces the calories that a dressing contains.

The downside: First, when you remove fat, you have to add sugar to provide flavor. But perhaps more important is that the removal of fat reduces your body's ability to absorb many of the vitamins found in a salad's vegetables. Ohio State University researchers discovered that people who ate a salad dressing that contained fat absorbed 15 times more beta-carotene and five times more lutein—both powerful antioxidants—than when they downed a salad topped with fat-free dressing.

The healthy alternative: Choose a full-fat dressing that's made with either olive oil or canola oil and has less than 2 g carbs per serving.

The good news is that many big players—Starbucks, Kroger, and Wal-Mart among them—have essentially resolved the conflict for you and decided to sell only hormone-free milk.

Food labels lie when they make you think that . . .

10. All Food Additives Are Safe

Researchers at the University of Southampton in the UK found that artificial food coloring and sodium benzoate preservatives are directly linked to increased hyperactivity in children. The additives included Yellow #5, Yellow #6, Red #40, and sodium benzoate, which are commonly found in packaged foods in the United States, but the researchers don't know if it's a combination of the chemicals or if there's a single one that's the primary culprit. You can find Red #40, Yellow #5, and Yellow #6 in Lucky Charms, for example, and sodium benzoate in products such as diet sodas, pickles, and jellies.

Food labels lie when they make you think that . . .

11. Artificial Sweeteners Are Better for You

Although diet soda is essentially calorie-free, its sweeteners may cause you to unintentionally consume extra calories. Researchers at Purdue University fed the artificial sweetener saccharin to a group of rats and found that, compared with those eating

sugar-sweetened foods, the saccharin rats gained more weight. The rush of sugar with no calories may trigger a desire for calorie-containing energy, according to one theory. That discovery parallels the findings of researchers at the University of Texas Health Science Center. After crunching the numbers collected from 622 people over a span of eight years, they learned that a daily can of diet soda amounted to a 41 percent jump in the risk of obesity. In other words, drinking diet soda doesn't really do your body any favors. True, it's a step up from regular soda—albeit a very small one—but for every can you guzzle, a genuinely healthy beverage remains untapped.

Food labels lie when they make you think that . . .

12. Lean Cuts of Meat Are Healthier

Leaner cuts of meat, by definition, are less juicy. To counteract this dried-out effect, some manufacturers "enhance" turkey, chicken, and beef products by pumping them full of a liquid solution that contains water, salt, and other nutrients that help preserve it. This practice can dramatically boost the meat's sodium level. For example, a 4-ounce serving of Shady Brook Farms' Fresh Boneless Turkey Breast Tenderloin that's enhanced by a 6 percent solution contains 55 milligrams of sodium. But the same-size serving of Jennie-O's

Turkey Breast Tenderloin Roast Turkey, which is enhanced by up to 30 percent, packs 840 milligrams—more than one-third of your recommended daily value for sodium!

Food labels lie when they make you think that . . .

13. Meat Is Actually Meat

The most common type of salami is called Genoa salami, and you can find it at sandwich shops across the country. Made from slaughterhouse leftovers—some pig, some cow—the scraps are collected via "advanced meat recovery," a mechanical process that strips the last remaining bits of muscle off the bone so that nothing is wasted. It's then processed using lactic acid, the waste product produced by bacteria in the meat. It both gives the salami its tangy flavor and cures it as well, making it an inhospitable place for other bacteria to grow. Add in a bunch of salt and spices—for a total of 15 ingredients in all—and you've got salami. What's worse than where it comes from, however, is what it can do to you. Emerging research is linking processed lunchmeats with certain lung diseases, the thinking being that they may help trigger harmful free radicals.

Food labels lie when they make you think that . . .

14. Your Food Is from a Kitchen, Not a Lab

A milkshake is a pretty straightforward concoction, right? Well, forget about a young man wearing a paper hat and a toothy grin blending ice cream, milk, and a little syrup in a metal container right in front of you. Today many shakes can't be made with fewer than 30 ingredients. One particular shake at Baskin-Robbins requires a full 50—almost 10 times more ingredients than the shakes made in ice cream parlors of yore—and delivers 1,690 calories and 46 grams of saturated fat! The ingredient list reads as if the world exhausted its supply of real food and handed the craft of culinary creation to chemists. Various types of sugar appear seven times. Partially hydrogenated oil, the source of trans fat, shows up three times. Then there's a smattering of flavoring agents such as artificial butter flavor, vanillin, and salt, and behind that comes the cabal of emulsifiers, thickeners, colors, and preservatives; industrial items such as carrageenan, polysorbate 80, annatto, potassium sorbate, sorbitan monostearate; and so forth. As a general rule, if you can't envision it in its natural state, then you probably shouldn't eat it.

REDUCED-FAT PEANUT BUTTER

The upside:
Even the reduced-fat versions pack a substantial quantity of heart-healthy monounsaturated fat.

The downside:
Many commercial brands are sweetened with "icing sugar"— the same finely ground sugar used to decorate cupcakes. In fact, each tablespoon of Skippy contains half a teaspoon of the sweet stuff. Reduced-fat versions are the worst of all, because they contain less healthy fat and even more icing sugar.

The healthy alternative: An all-natural, full-fat peanut butter—such as Crazy Richard's or Teddy's—that contains no added sugar.

What They Hide

CREEPY FOOD FACTS POPULAR RESTAURANTS DON'T WANT YOU TO KNOW

Long John Silver's

In response to public outcry, most fast-food restaurants have switched to trans-fat-free cooking oils. But Long John Silver's still fries everything in artery-clogging trans fats. Their 2 Fish Plank Combo packs 12.5 grams of the stuff—more than five times what the American Heart Association recommends you eat in an entire day! If you're held hostage and forced to eat at LJS, avoid anything on the menu that's fried.

Cold Stone Creamery

Every drink in its regular line of shakes contains at least 1,000 calories, 92 grams of sugar, and 1.5 grams of trans fat. Order a larger size and you'll get up to 2,010 calories and 4 grams of trans fat!

Dunkin' Donuts

Its muffins are worse than its dough-nuts. Even the reduced-fat blueberry muffin still has 430 calories—more than all but three doughnuts on the menu.

KFC

Partially hydrogenated oils appear 36 times on its menu's ingredients list, yet its Web site boasts that KFC chicken contains zero grams of trans fat per serving. Technically their nondisclosure, while inaccurate, isn't illegal: The FDA says that if a product contains less than 0.5 grams of trans fat per serving, the product's label can state that it's "trans fat-free." Still, there are better choices in the fast-food world.

The Cheesecake Factory

This franchise won't disclose its nutritional information. According to their Web site, the restaurants are "known for their generous portion sizes and, consequently, we have always encouraged 'sharing' at the table." Until the facts are fully disclosed, assume the worst.

IHOP

IHOP can squeeze extra calories into anything. Let's say you just wanted to sample some of IHOP's appetizers before your meal comes. It's a bit of an indulgence, but you're being good—you ordered the Herb-Roasted Chicken. But eat the whole appetizer and you've scarfed down 1,380 calories. The chicken? Another 1,280!

T.G.I. Friday's

Yet another dodger. A T.G.I. Friday's rep has even been quoted as saying, "We don't provide nutritional information unless required by law." Does that frighten anybody else?

Applebee's

In 2008, E.W. Scripps news service sent a number of dishes on the restaurant's vaunted Weight Watchers menu, taken from eight different locations, to a lab to be analyzed. Results found that certain "healthy" entrées packed double the calories and up to eight times the fat that Applebee's claims they do.

Ruby Tuesday

The average RT burger delivers an appalling 1,045 calories. But you won't do yourself any favors swapping in the healthy-sounding Chicken & Broccoli Pasta. It packs 200 calories more than the average burger!

Sbarro

How many calories does a single slice of the chain restaurant's stuffed pepperoni pizza contain? You won't find any of the company's nutritional information on its Web site, because that particular page has been "under construction" for more than 30 months (as of press time). The frightening truth, thanks to a New York City law that requires calorie counts to be displayed prominently on menu boards: 960 calories.

Starbucks

Most of its lattes pack more sugar than a two-scoop ice cream sundae. For example, a no-whip grande Gingersnap Latte packs 34 grams of the sweet stuff, a no-whip grande Cinnamon Dolce Latte offers 38 grams, and the healthy-sounding grande Earl Grey Tea Latte includes 31 grams. And cutting back from 2 percent milk to skim doesn't help, either—in fact, the fat-free versions are even sweeter.

Subway

Jared knows what he's talking about: Most of the offerings are actually quite healthy, nutritious, and relatively low-calorie. But even though you may eat less fat and sodium than at, say, McDonald's, you still might not down fewer calories at Subway than at your average fast-food joint. A 2007 study at Cornell University found that when shown two 1,000-calorie dishes, people underestimate the energy load by about 159 calories in food they consider healthy. The researchers also found that when people eat at "healthy" restaurants, they tend to order 131 percent more calories in side items than they do at known "unhealthy" restaurants. That's because people give themselves permission to overorder when they think they're eating healthy. The easiest solution? Order the sandwich but skip the chips, soda, and cookies.

Uno Chicago Grill

Unless you typically split your burger, multiply the nutrition information listed on Uno's Web site by two. Uno lists its stats as one "serving" of each dish, but if you look at the top right corner of the page, you'll see that burgers are considered to be two servings—a fact that doubles the already sizeable calories and fat grams. (Half a "Bring Home the Bacon Burger" contains 520 calories and 38 grams of fat!) Keep your calculator handy. The rest of the menu requires more multiplication, sometimes quadrupling the initial listings.

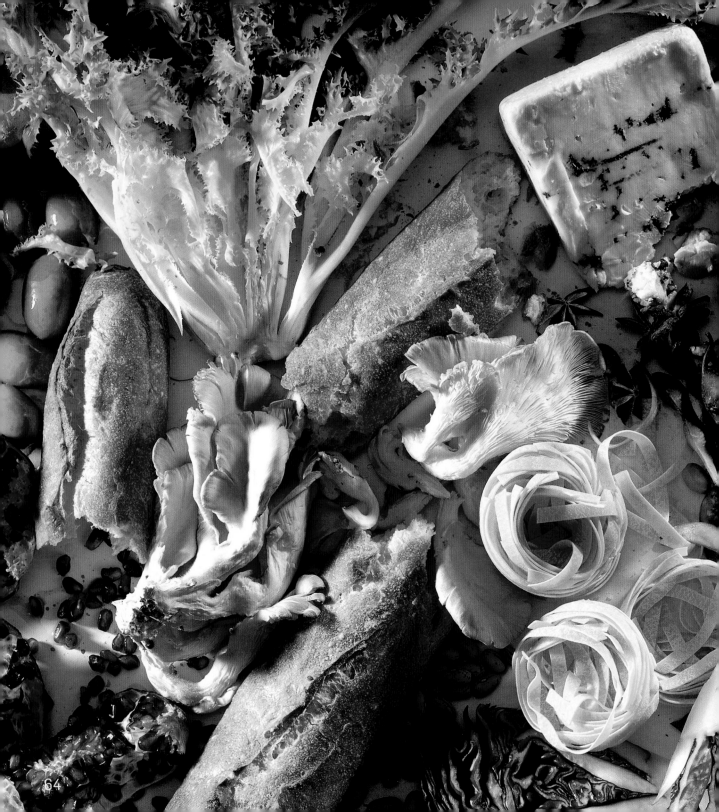

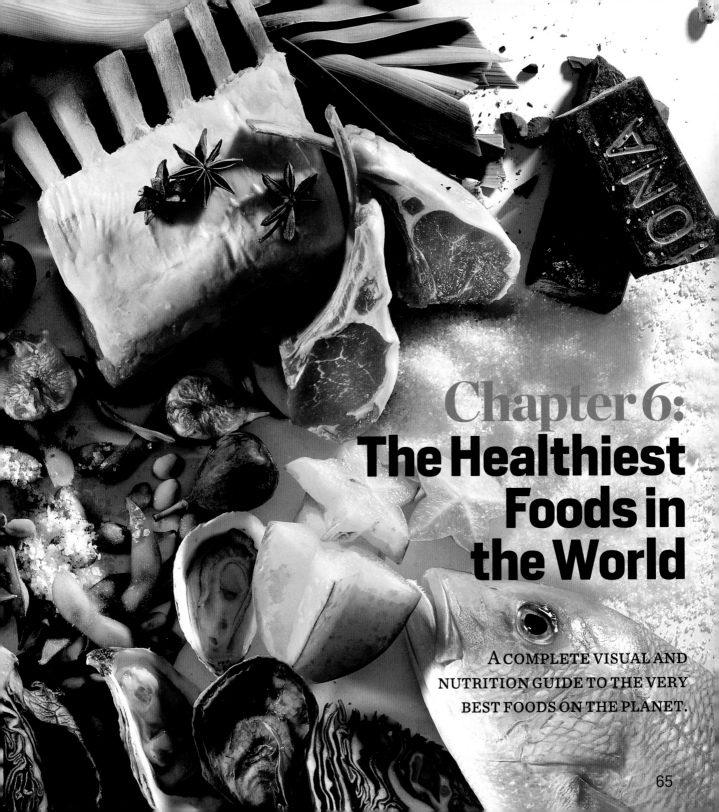

Chapter 6:
The Healthiest Foods in the World

A COMPLETE VISUAL AND
NUTRITION GUIDE TO THE VERY
BEST FOODS ON THE PLANET.

If you remember

just one fact from this big book of facts about food, remember this one: Food that can go bad is good for you. Food that can't go bad is bad for you.

As you'll read later in this book, there are more than 3,000 compounds used in today's food manufacturing, chemicals and additives that make packaged foods more stable, more transportable, more resistant to spoilage, and often, more like consumer products and less like real food.

As a result, we get "food" that can sit on a grocery store shelf for months without going bad. But that's not real food. Instead, it's what author Michael Pollen calls "food-like substances," things that you can put into your mouth, chew and swallow, but which provide hundreds of unneeded, empty calories and, often, absolutely no nutritional value. And the more food-like substances you eat, the less real food, and the less real nutrition, you're giving your body.

Unfortunately, too many of us get so confused by all these food-like substances that we go on diets, trying to reduce our calorie intake (often by substituting things like "meal replacement bars," for real food). And that's just about the worse thing you can do. Subbing in fake foods, or skipping meals altogether, is a great way to grind your metabolism to a halt. When your body goes without real food, it switches to starvation mode, storing calories rather than burning them. Fake food=real fat.

Think of this chapter, then, as your reintroduction to food. If you find it here, it's probably good for you. (It'll also spoil, so shop wisely.)

This chapter is one massive international culinary bazaar: a thoroughly researched encyclopedia of delicious whole foods with thousands of cool food facts across the entire dietary spectrum. You'll discover what they look like, why they're so good (and where the occasional nutritional pitfalls are), and what they mean to your overall eating plan.

You'll certainly find your favorites, but as you dig deeper, you'll also find dozens of new ideas for what to eat. If anything, this chapter—the heart of *The Big Book of Food & Nutrition*—is all the proof you need that healthy foods are not boring and bland. Good eats come from all over the world in all shapes, sizes, tastes, and textures.

Best of all: The terrific whole foods featured in this chapter are used to create the recipes in the following chapter. So if you love, say, steamed clams (page 178), we've also got a killer clam chowder recipe with all the taste and none of the weight gain (page 271).

Read on, eat up, enjoy.

If you want to remake your diet, here's a great place to start. Of course you know vegetables are a vital part of any healthy diet. But the ones in this section are no-brainers because you can find them in any supermarket. That fact alone is more proof of how easy it really is to eat better.

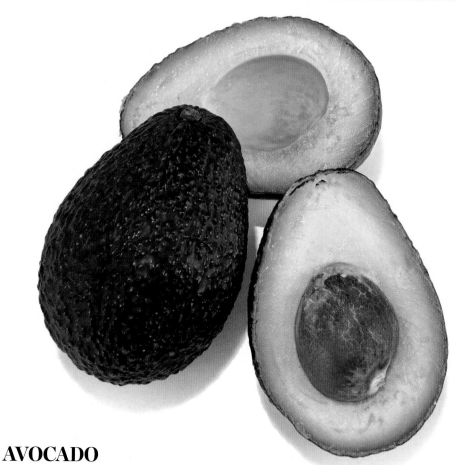

AVOCADO

Okay, avocadoes are technically fruit, but we prepare and eat them more like vegetables. Let's just call them a superfood. More than half the calories in each creamy green fruit comes from one of the world's healthiest fats, monounsaturates. Numerous studies have shown that monounsaturated fats both improve your cholesterol profile and decrease the amount of triglycerides in your blood. And with 10 grams of fiber per cup, they're a true craving-buster.

SERVING SIZE	1 cup, sliced (146 g)		
Calories/Fiber	Calories: 234		Fiber: 10 g
Macronutrients	Protein: 3 g	Fat: 21 g	Carbs: 12 g
Vitamins/Minerals	Vitamin K: 38%	Folate: 30%	Vitamin C: 24%

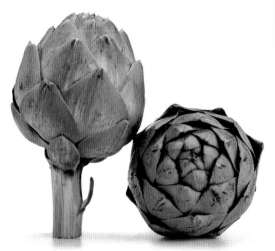

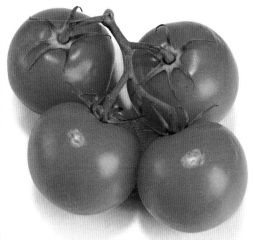

ARTICHOKE

USDA scientists found that artichokes have more antioxidants than any other vegetable they tested. This fiber-rich plant also contains healthy doses of bone-building magnesium and potassium. Besides that, artichokes are among the tastiest and most versatile vegetables in the produce aisle. Place the entire artichoke in a pot with an inch of water, cover, and steam for 20 to 25 minutes, until the base can be pierced easily with the tip of a knife. Serve the meaty petals with a bit of mayo spiked with lemon juice and chopped garlic. Slice the heart and toss it with pasta, or pile it onto a grilled-chicken sandwich.

1 medium (128 g)		
Calories: 60	Fiber: 7 g	
Protein: 4 g	Fat: 0 g	Carbs: 13 g
Vitamin C: 25%	Magnesium: 13%	Potassium: 10%

TOMATOES

Lycopene, the phytochemical that makes tomatoes red, is a prostate protector and helps eliminate skin-aging free radicals caused by ultraviolet rays. Cooking tomatoes (which, like avocadoes, are technically a fruit) helps concentrate their lycopene levels, so tomato sauce, tomato paste, and even ketchup pack on the protection. The extended heat of summer brings out the best in a tomato. Because winter hothouse and equatorial tomatoes are picked early and ripen in transit, the most nutritious tomatoes are locally grown. Try heirloom varieties like the meaty Cherokee Purple and Red Brandywine.

1 large (3" diameter, 182 g)		
Calories: 33	Fiber: 2 g	
Protein: 2 g	Fat: 0 g	Carbs: 7 g
Vitamin C: 39%	Vitamin A: 30%	Vitamin K: 18%

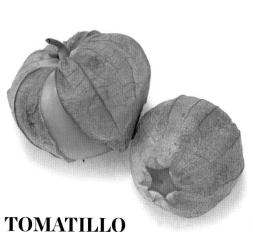

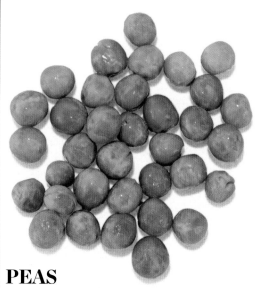

TOMATILLO

Tomatillos look like small green tomatoes with papery husks. After peeling off the husk, you can eat tomatillos raw or cooked, and they taste like a cross between a tomato and a tart strawberry. One cup of chopped tomatillos has just 42 calories and is packed with vitamin C and vitamin K. Plus, tomatillos contain lutein and zeaxanthin—carotenoids that may boost eye health. As a salsa: Roast a pound of husked tomatillos, one seeded jalapeño, and one halved onion in a 450°F oven for 20 minutes. Puree with the juice of one lime, then season. Eat with grilled chicken.

PEAS

Peas are one of the easiest ways to add a fiber-and-vitamin turbo boost to your diet. They're packed with protein, as well—8 grams in a 1-cup serving. These little guys are great on their own but versatile enough to be an effortless addition to vegetable medleys, soups, stews, or stir-frys.

SERVING SIZE	½ cup, chopped or diced (66 g)			1 cup (145 g)		
Calories/Fiber	Calories: 21		Fiber: 1 g	Calories: 117		Fiber: 7 g
Macronutrients	Protein: 1 g	Fat: 1 g	Carbs: 4 g	Protein: 8 g	Fat: 1 g	Carbs: 21 g
Vitamins/Minerals	Potassium: 20%	Vitamin C: 13%	Vitamin K: 8%	Vitamin C: 97%	Vitamin K: 45%	Manganese: 30%

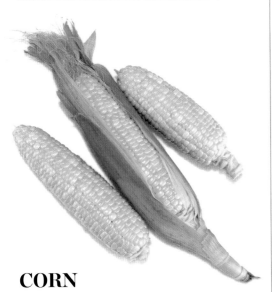

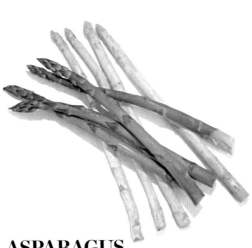

GROW FRESH MUSCLE

Researchers at the University of Georgia discovered that ginger supplements might reduce muscle soreness, allowing you to improve your range of motion—and potentially pack on more muscle. A change was noticed within 11 days using 2 grams of ground ginger each day.

CORN

When Columbus accidentally discovered America, he was not looking for a New World but rather a better route for bringing prized spices from the Orient back to Europe. However, he discovered something even more valuable: corn. Carrots get all the press as eyesight food, but corn is loaded with lutein, which can help slow macular degeneration.

ASPARAGUS

Asparagus is loaded with bone-protecting vitamin K, and it's rich in folate, which may help ward off heart disease and reduce your risk of obesity. "It's a nutritious alternative to starches as a side with fish or poultry," says Milton Stokes, MPH, RD, a spokesman for the American Dietetic Association. Toss a bunch with olive oil, cracked pepper, and Parmesan cheese. Roast for 10 minutes in a 400°F oven or on a medium-high grill. Finish with a squeeze of lemon. Or cook bite-size pieces in a screaming-hot wok with soy sauce, fresh ginger, garlic, and sesame seeds.

1 cup, raw (154 g)		
Calories: 132	Fiber: 4 g	
Protein: 5 g	Fat: 2 g	Carbs: 29 g
Thiamin: 21%	Folate: 18%	Vitamin C: 17%

1 cup, raw (134 g)		
Calories: 27	Fiber: 3 g	
Protein: 3 g	Fat: 0 g	Carbs: 5 g
Vitamin K: 70%	Vitamin A: 20%	Folate: 17%

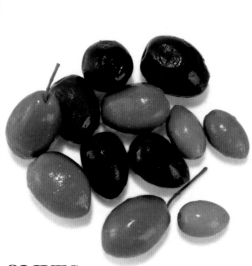

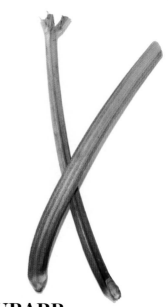

OLIVES

Three-quarters of the fats in olives are the benevolent monounsaturated kind. Foods rich in healthy fats help reduce inflammation, a catalyst for migraines. One study found that the anti-inflammatory compounds in olive oil suppress the same pain pathway as ibuprofen. Dirty martinis aren't really the answer, but black olives are a tasty addition to pizzas and quesadillas.

RHUBARB

Rhubarb is low in calories, and it's a good source of fiber, vitamin C, and vitamin K. Bonus: Most cooking methods increase its antioxidant levels. Try it on top of oatmeal or yogurt: Simmer 3 cups chopped rhubarb with 1/3 cup brown sugar, 1 teaspoon grated orange peel, and a splash of water until tender, about 15 minutes.

SERVING SIZE	1 oz, pickled (28 g)			1 cup, diced (122 g)		
Calories/Fiber	Calories: 41		Fiber: 1 g	Calories: 26		Fiber: 2 g
Macronutrients	Protein: 0 g	Fat: 4 g	Carbs: 1 g	Protein: 1 g	Fat: 0 g	Carbs: 6 g
Vitamins/Minerals				Vitamin K: 45%	Vitamin C: 16%	

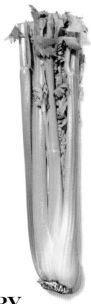

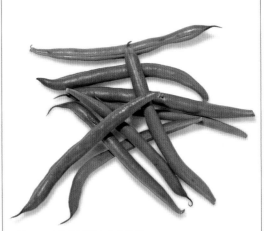

GREEN BEAN

They're easy to find frozen, and are just fine that way, but when the weather is warm, buy 'em fresh at the farmer's market. Good beans have vibrant, smooth surfaces. The best are thin, young, and velvety, and snap when gently bent. Refrigerate unwashed in an unsealed bag for up to 1 week. Green beans pack 4 grams of fiber per cup for practically no calories.

CELERY

Eating celery is almost the same as chewing water. Only iceberg lettuce contains more H_2O ... by a whopping 0.2 percent. And although your belly will hardly notice a cup of celery's 16 calories—the vegetable claims one of the lowest calorie counts of all foods—you'll still net more than a third of your daily vitamin K recommendation as well as sizeable amounts of vitamin A, fiber, folate, and potassium. It's also thought that celery's phytochemicals, called phthalides, may relax muscle tissue in artery walls, increase blood flow, and thereby help lower blood pressure.

1 cup, chopped (101 g)		
Calories: 16		Fiber: 1.6 g
Protein: .7 g	Fat: .17 g	Carbs: 3 g
Vitamin K: 37%	Vitamin A: 9%	

1 cup (110 g)		
Calories: 34		Fiber: 4 g
Protein: 2 g	Fat: 0 g	Carbs: 8 g
Vitamin C: 30%	Vitamin K: 20%	

Mushrooms

Yes, mushrooms are fungi. If you find that skeevy (an actual medical term), all we can say is try a grilled portobello just once and you will return from the dark side craving more. Use this section to fulfill all your fungal food fantasies.

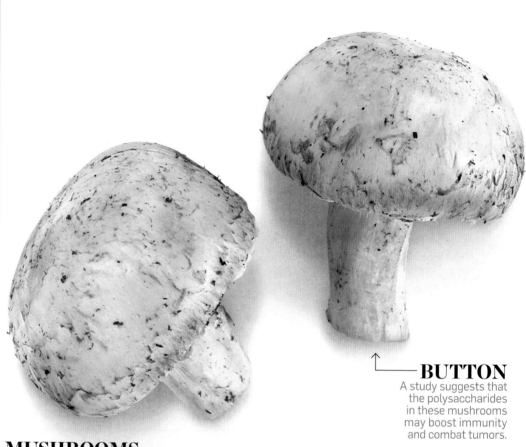

BUTTON
A study suggests that the polysaccharides in these mushrooms may boost immunity and combat tumors.

MUSHROOMS

Wild mushrooms (reiki, shiitake, maitake, portobello, lobster) are rich in the antioxidant ergothioneine, which protects cells from abnormal growth and replication. In short, they reduce the risk of cancer. Even better: Cooking them in red wine, which contains the antioxidant resveratrol, magnifies their immunity-boosting power.

SERVING SIZE	1 cup, pieces (70 g)		
Calories/Fiber	Calories: 15		Fiber: 1 g
Macronutrients	Protein: 2 g	Fat: 0 g	Carbs: 2 g
Vitamins/Minerals	Riboflavin: 17%	Selenium: 9%	

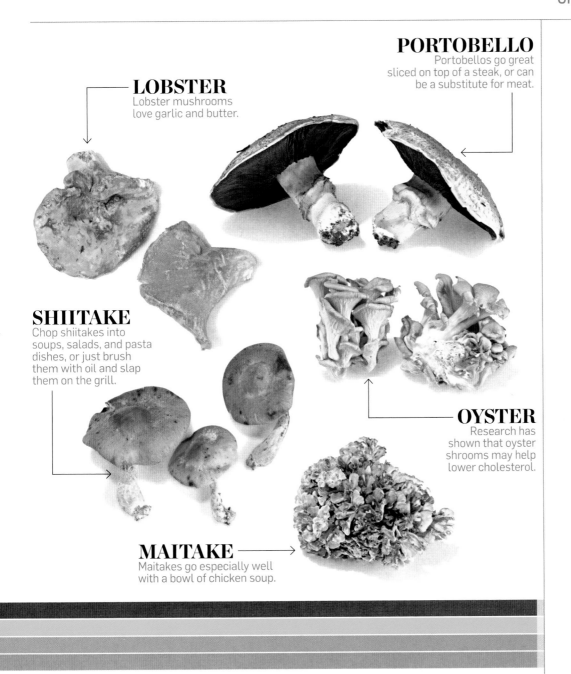

LOBSTER
Lobster mushrooms love garlic and butter.

PORTOBELLO
Portobellos go great sliced on top of a steak, or can be a substitute for meat.

SHIITAKE
Chop shiitakes into soups, salads, and pasta dishes, or just brush them with oil and slap them on the grill.

OYSTER
Research has shown that oyster shrooms may help lower cholesterol.

MAITAKE
Maitakes go especially well with a bowl of chicken soup.

Root Vegetables

Root vegetables sometimes take potshots for being a high-carb food, but get real: Eating sweet potatoes isn't like eating a scoop of confectioner's sugar. Roots deliver so much nutritional payoff in potassium and vitamins B_6 and C that to exclude them from a varied diet would be as senseless as excluding any other vegetables.

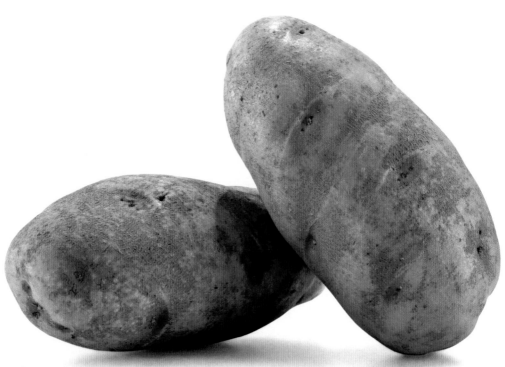

POTATOES

Though all too often a vehicle for dangerous quantities of cheese, butter, and sour cream, the potato packs blood pressure–lowering potassium and immunity-boosting vitamin C. In fact, a potato contains nearly twice as much vitamin C as a tomato and just 15 percent less potassium than a banana! Baking or boiling reduces its nutritional content, so remember to go easy on the toppings and eat the skin—that's where the most fiber lives.

SERVING SIZE	1 cup (150 g)		
Calories/Fiber	Calories: 104		Fiber: 4 g
Macronutrients	Protein: 2 g	Fat: 0 g	Carbs: 26 g
Vitamins/Minerals	Vitamin C: 50%	Potassium: 18%	Vitamin B₆: 16%

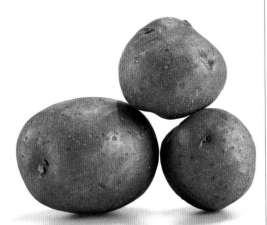

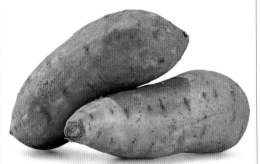

BABY RED POTATOES

This smaller, waxy variety of potato contains slightly less fiber and vitamin C than regular potatoes. They hold their shape after cooking better than regular potatoes, too, so they're ideal for potato salad.

YAMS

If you've brought home one of these tubers, which are mostly grown in Africa, Asia, and the Caribbean, it was probably the dirtiest-looking vegetable in the grocery store. They're actually quite rare stateside and are often misidentified as sweet potatoes.

1 cup (150 g)			
Calories: 104		Fiber: 2 g	
Protein: 2 g	Fat: 0 g		Carbs: 24 g
Vitamin B₆: 28%	Vitamin C: 22%		Potassium: 20%

1 cup (150 g)		
Calories: 177		Fiber: 6 g
Protein: 2 g	Fat: 0 g	Carbs: 42 g
Vitamin C: 43%	Potassium: 35%	

Root Vegetables |

SAVE THE GREENS

Although sweet-potato leaves are typically discarded, they're one of the world's richest sources of disease-fighting antioxidants, according to a report from the University of Arkansas. In all, they're packed with at least 15 different types of healthy compounds that help fight diabetes, heart disease, bacterial infections, and cancer. Beet leaves aren't too far behind, as they're also packed with vitamins, minerals, and antioxidants. Sauté either with onions and garlic.

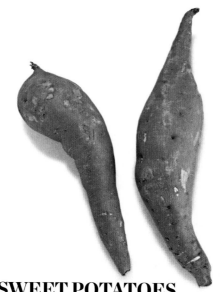

SWEET POTATOES

Eating this orange-colored native American root, which is smaller and sweeter than a yam and also less starchy, may help your skin look younger. Its beta-carotene builds up in your skin and may help defend against sun damage, according to European researchers, and just half its vitamin C content is enough to decrease the appearance of wrinkles by 11 percent if consumed daily for 3 years, according to a study in the *American Journal of Clinical Nutrition*. Sweet potatoes also contain glutathione, an antioxidant that can enhance nutrient metabolism and your immune system.

JICAMA

While this Central American root—pronounced *he-kuh-muh*—looks like a potato or turnip, it's actually quite juicy and even slightly sweet. High in fiber and vitamin C, you can slice it and eat it raw, or boil it like a potato, till soft.

SERVING SIZE	1 cup (133 g)			1 cup (120 g)		
Calories/Fiber	Calories: 114		Fiber: 4 g	Calories: 46		Fiber: 6 g
Macronutrients	Protein: 2 g	Fat: 0 g	Carbs: 27 g	Protein: 1 g	Fat: 0 g	Carbs: 11 g
Vitamins/Minerals	Vitamin A: 377%	Maganese: 17%	Potassium: 13%	Vitamin C: 40%	Potassium: 5%	

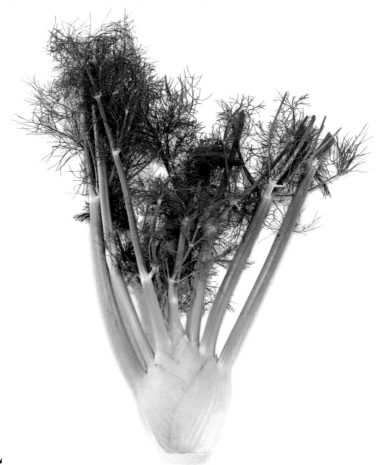

FENNEL

You might know fennel best as the little seeds speckling your Italian sausage, but from those seeds sprout something better: crunchy, sweet bulbs. Fennel packs vitamin C, fiber, and a unique mix of antioxidants, including anethole, a phytonutrient shown to reduce inflammation and cancer risk. Even better, its mellow licorice flavor may help increase bloodflow to the penis, according to a report by the Smell and Taste Treatment and Research Foundation.

1 cup (87 g)		
Calories: 27		Fiber: 3 g
Protein: 1 g	Fat: 0 g	Carbs: 6 g
Vitamin C: 17%	Potassium: 10%	

Root Vegetables

EAT COLORFUL CARROTS

Heirloom varieties of carrots, available in kaleidoscopic colors, are sweeter than the ubiquitous orange type. Yellow ones heap eye-healthy lutein, while red and purple add cancer-fighting lycopene.

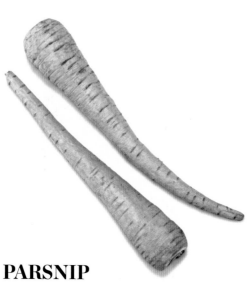

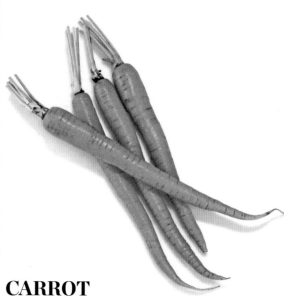

PARSNIP

As nutritious as a sweet potato, the humble parsnip is a below-the-radar root vegetable ideal for soups, stews, and roasting. It could be mistaken for an albino carrot at first glance, but it tastes sweeter, contains more vitamins and minerals, and is actually more closely related to parsley, whose mature root it resembles.

CARROT

Men who consume more beta-carotene—the very reason carrots are orange—can significantly delay cognitive aging, according to Harvard researchers. Carrots' extremely high dose of vitamin A is also good for your eyes and skin. In fact, National Cancer Institute researchers found that people with the highest intake of carotenoids—the pigments that occur naturally in carrots—were six times less likely to develop skin cancer than those with the lowest intakes.

SERVING SIZE	1 cup (133 g)			1 cup (128 g)		
Calories/Fiber	Calories: 100		Fiber: 7 g	Calories: 52		Fiber: 4 g
Macronutrients	Protein: 2 g	Fat: 0 g	Carbs: 24 g	Protein: 1 g	Fat: 0 g	Carbs: 12 g
Vitamins/Minerals	Vitamin C: 38%	Vitamin K: 37%		Vitamin A: 428%	Vitamin K: 21%	

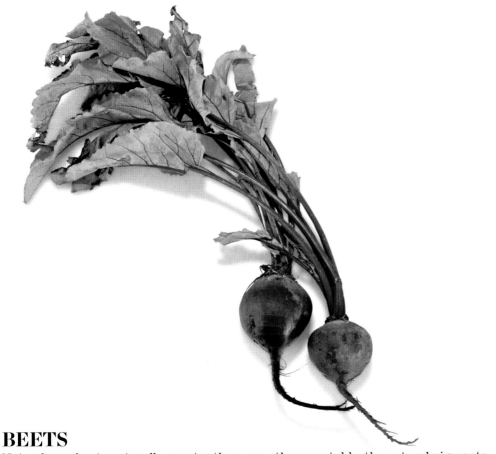

BEETS

Not only are beets naturally sweeter than any other vegetable, the natural pigments that give them their color—betacyanins—have been potent cancer fighters in laboratory mice. Plus they're one of the best sources of both folate and betaine, two nutrients that work together to lower your blood levels of homocysteine, an inflammatory compound that can damage your arteries and increase your risk of heart disease. Beet juice also contains nitrate, which may also help lower blood pressure, according to a 2008 study in the journal *Hypertension*.

1 cup (136 g)		
Calories: 58		Fiber: 4 g
Protein: 2 g	Fat: 0 g	Carbs: 13 g
Folate: 37%	Manganese: 22%	

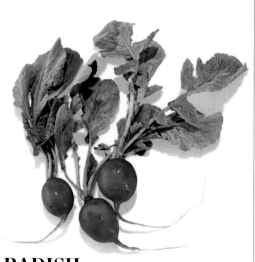

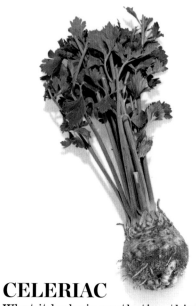

RADISH

While often sliced and used as a garnish in salads or tacos, these small-and-spicy orbs make a great snack eaten whole. Both appearance and nutritional benefits vary among the many varieties (the daikon, for instance, looks like a long, white cylinder), but in general all radishes share an abundance of vitamin C and help facilitate the digestive process.

CELERIAC

What it lacks in aesthetics, this lumpy winter root vegetable makes up with a pleasant, celerylike flavor. Also known as celery root, celeriac is loaded with bone-building vitamin K, and it's high in fiber, potassium, magnesium, and vitamin B_6. Substitute a few cups of cooked celeriac in your mashed potatoes to add a hint of earthy sweetness and reduce the dish's glycemic load, or toss julienned strips with mayo, Dijon mustard, lemon juice, and capers for a quick salad. But no matter how you use it, peel the gnarly exterior off first.

SERVING SIZE	1 cup (116 g)			1 cup (156 g)		
Calories/Fiber	Calories: 19		Fiber: 2 g	Calories: 66		Fiber: 3 g
Macronutrients	Protein: 1 g	Fat: 0 g	Carbs: 4 g	Protein: 2 g	Fat: 0 g	Carbs: 14 g
Vitamins/Minerals	Vitamin C: 29%	Folate: 7%		Vitamin K: 80%	Vitamin C: 21%	Vitamin B_6: 13%

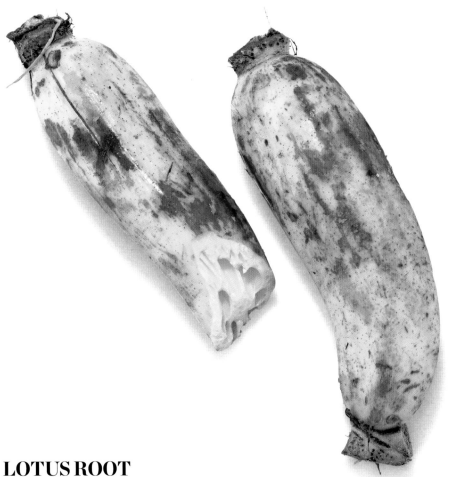

THE TOP 10 HUNGER-FIGHTING FOODS

High-satiety foods can help you feel fuller, longer. When Australian researchers fed equal portions of 38 foods to study participants, the following foods proved to have the most stick-to-your-ribs power. Incorporate them into your diet to block binges and keep hunger at bay:

- Potatoes
- Fish
- Oatmeal
- Oranges
- Apples
- Whole-wheat pasta
- Steak
- Baked beans
- Grapes
- Popcorn

LOTUS ROOT

Commonly used in Asian cooking, this root has a texture akin to a raw potato's and a flavor similar to that of a coconut. It's loaded with vitamin C, fiber, and potassium, as well as two minerals beneficial to bone health—copper and manganese. Try it as a substitute for potato chips: Peel and slice it into disks, and then rub with olive oil. Microwave for 7 to 10 minutes until crisp.

10 slices (2½" diameter, 81 g)		
Calories: 60		Fiber: 4 g
Protein: 2 g	Fat: 0 g	Carbs: 14 g
Vitamin C: 59%	Potassium: 13%	

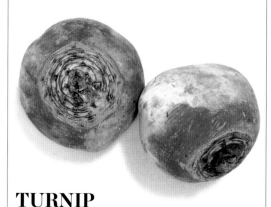

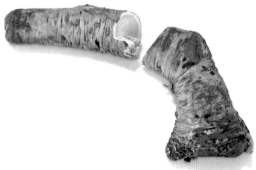

TURNIP

The calories in these white-and-purple orbs come mostly from natural sugars, but fortunately, turnips are also a good source of the mineral manganese, which helps regulate blood sugar. Eat raw or add to a roasted vegetable medley, and keep the greens—they're an excellent source of lutein and zeaxanthin, two antioxidants that protect your eyes like chemical sunglasses.

HORSERADISH

When cut or grated, this root releases a biting aroma and sharp taste that ratchets up the kick in a range of foods— it's a low-calorie, flavor-enhancing shortcut. Horseradish also contains high levels of glucosinolates, a compound that may help prevent cancer cells from forming, according to a 2009 review of studies published in *Food Science and Technology*. Mix peeled, finely grated horseradish into a half-cup of sour cream for an instant sauce for grilled fish or beef tenderloin, stir a spoonful into mashed potatoes, or try a teaspoon in a Bloody Mary.

SERVING SIZE	1 cup (130 g)			1 Tbsp (25 g)		
Calories/Fiber	Calories: 36		Fiber: 2 g	Calories: 7		Fiber: 0 g
Macronutrients	Protein: 1 g	Fat: 0 g	Carbs: 8 g	Protein: 0 g	Fat: 0 g	Carbs: 2 g
Vitamins/Minerals	Vitamin C: 46%	Manganese: 9%		Vitamin C: 6%		

SUNCHOKES

Also called Jerusalem artichokes, these vegetables look like gnarled potatoes and have a nutty, slightly sweet taste. They contain fructooligosaccharides—sweet fibers that promote gut health and may help boost immunity. Roast them instead of potatoes to lower your glycemic load.

Per 1-cup serving:
109 calories, 3 g protein, 26 g carbs, 2 g fiber, 0 g fat, and RDIs of 28 % iron, 20 % thiamin, and 18 % potassium

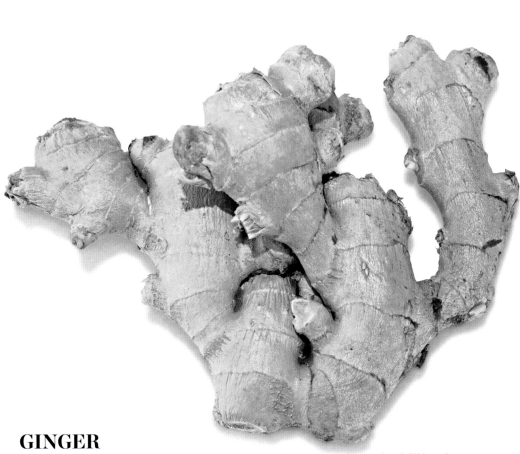

GINGER

Though it's actually a rhizome, not a root, ginger—a piquant addition to so many Asian dishes—has a fresh, sweet-tasting flavor. Beyond its role in aiding digestion, ginger may also have cancer-fighting capabilities. That's because it contains 6-gingerol, a nutrient that has been shown to stop the growth of colon-cancer cells, according to researchers at the University of Tennessee.

¼ cup (24 g)			
Calories: 19		Fiber: 0 g	
Protein: 0 g	Fat: 0 g	Carbs: 4 g	
Magnesium: 3%	Potassium: 3%		

There are some true nutritional all-stars in this section. And when Mom said, "Eat your vegetables," she was talking about a lot of these (brussels sprouts, baby!). But aside from the nutrition info you see in here, cruciferous vegetables such as broccoli contain proven anticancer compounds, including indole-3 and sulforaphanes.

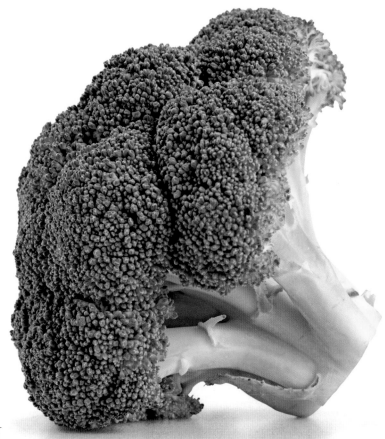

BROCCOLI

A single stalk of this cruciferous all-star packs 3 grams of protein—about as much as an ounce of chicken breast. Eat a cup and you'll get a hearty dose of calcium, as well as manganese, potassium, phosphorus, magnesium, and iron. And that's in addition to its high concentration of vitamins, including A, C, and K, not to mention the phytonutrient sulforaphane. "Broccoli may also help reduce excess estrogen levels in the body, thanks to its indole 3-carbinol content," celebrity trainer Gunnar Petersen says.

SERVING SIZE	1 cup, chopped (91 g)		
Calories/Fiber	Calories: 31		Fiber: 2 g
Macronutrients	Protein: 3 g	Fat: 0 g	Carbs: 6 g
Vitamins/Minerals	Vitamin C: 135%	Vitamin K: 116%	Vitamin A: 11%

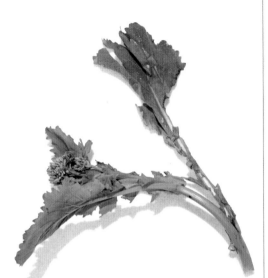

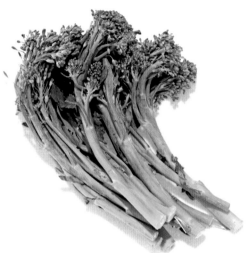

BROCCOLI RABE

Also known as rapini, broccoli rabe looks like a cross between spinach and broccoli. Like spinach, it has long, stiff stalks and dark, tender leaves; like, broccoli, it produces florets. It packs vitamins A, C, and K, folate, and as much protein as spinach.

BROCCOLINI

A hybrid of broccoli and Chinese kale, this veggie has a peppery sweet edge that isn't overly bitter—and just four stalks boost immunity with 65 percent of your day's vitamin C.

PAIR BROCCOLI WITH TOMATOES

New research shows that this combo prevents prostate cancer, but no one is sure why. In a recent study, John W. Erdman Jr., PhD, of the University of Illinois, proved that the combination shrunk prostate-cancer tumors in rats and that nothing but the extreme measure of castration could actually be a more effective alternative treatment. (What more motivation do you need to embrace this one-two punch?) "We know that tomato powder lowers the growth of tumors," says Erdman. "We know that broccoli does too. And we know they're better together. But it's going to take years to find out why."

1 cup, chopped (40 g)		
Calories: 9	Fiber: 1 g	
Protein: 1 g	Fat: 0 g	Carbs: 1 g
Vitamin K: 112%	Vitamin A: 21%	Vitamin C: 13%

1 oz (28 g)		
Calories: 10	Fiber: 0 g	
Protein: 1 g	Fat: 0 g	Carbs: 2 g
Vitamin C: 45%	Vitamin A: 10%	

Cruciferous Vegetables

A 5-STAR CHEF'S SECRET: KIMCHEE

"If you open my fridge at home, the first thing you'll smell is pickled cabbage," says chef Jean-Georges Vongerichten. "My wife is Korean, and she eats it with everything, from omelets to grilled meats to soup to pizza— and now so do I." Think of kimchee as sauerkraut's Eastern cousin. Traditionally a Korean dish, it's now a staple in most gourmet groceries. It has a spicy, pungent flavor, and can also be made with daikon radish, cucumber, or scallions.

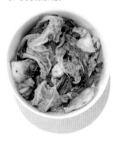

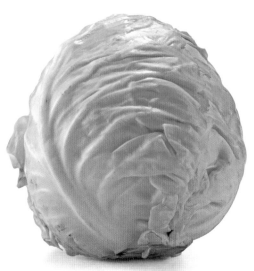

CABBAGE

One cup of chopped cabbage contains just 22 calories, and it's loaded with a type of isothiocyanates called sulforaphane that increases your body's production of enzymes that disarm cell-damaging free radicals. Sulforaphane actually boosts your levels of these cancer-fighting enzymes higher than any other plant chemical, according to Stanford University scientists.

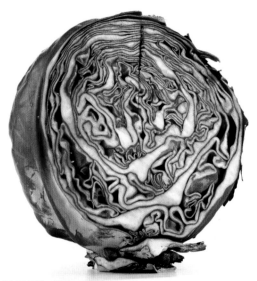

RED CABBAGE

You can't overlook red cabbage's bold color—its unique pigment delivers your body 15 times as much skin-protecting beta-carotene as its more common green relative. Eat red cabbage with a little fat to increase beta-carotene's absorption in the body.

SERVING SIZE	1 cup (89 g)			1 cup, chopped (89 g)		
Calories/Fiber	Calories: 22		Fiber: 2 g	Calories: 28		Fiber: 2 g
Macronutrients	Protein: 1 g	Fat: 0 g	Carbs: 5 g	Protein: 1 g	Fat: 0 g	Carbs: 7 g
Vitamins/Minerals	Vitamin K: 85%	Vitamin C: 54%	Folate: 10%	Vitamin C: 85%	Vitamin K: 42%	Vitamin A: 20%

Cruciferous vegetables belonging to the Brassica oleracea family—kale, cabbage, broccoli—are the equivalent of Rockefellers or Kennedys in America: they're rich and prestigious. Not financially or politically, of course, but nutritionally. They're divided into slightly different camps, but each contains proven anti-cancer compounds, including indole-3 and sulforaphanes. Here's the family tree's breakdown:

BRASSICA OLERACEA

Capitata group:
Cabbage

Italica group:
Broccoli

Acephala group:
Kale
Collard greens

Alboglabra group:
Chinese broccoli

Botrytis group:
Cauliflower
Broccoflower

Gemmifera group:
Brussels sprouts

Gongylodes group:
Kohlrabi

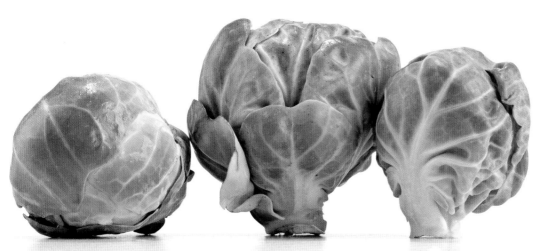

BRUSSELS SPROUT

Researchers at Tufts University in Massachusetts found that vitamin K—a nutrient found in abundance in brussels sprouts, as well as in other cruciferous vegetables such as broccoli—helps regulate insulin levels, an important ally in optimizing your blood sugar levels. Brussels sprouts also contain more glucosinolates than any other vegetable, sulfur-rich compounds that the body converts into isothiocyanates, which may reduce the risk of cancer.

1 cup (88 g)			
Calories: 38		Fiber: 3 g	
Protein: 3 g	Fat: 0 g	Carbs: 8 g	
Vitamin K: 195%	Vitamin C: 125%	Folate: 13%	

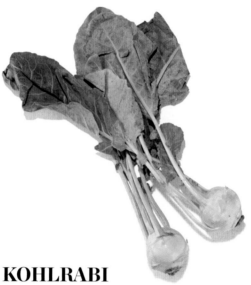

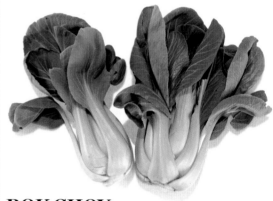

KOHLRABI

Kohlrabi tastes like the love child of a cabbage and a turnip. A 1-cup serving contains 14 percent of your daily requirement of potassium—which will help keep your blood pressure under control—along with glucosinolate, a phytochemical that may preven some cancers.

BOK CHOY

You might not recognize it without shrimp and brown sauce, but few vegetables pack more of a nutritional punch than this Chinese cabbage. For fewer calories than in a stick of gum, bok choy delivers a potent vitamin cocktail, including a big dose of rare cancer-fighting nitrogen compounds called indoles, as well as folic acid, iron, beta-carotene, and potassium. Potassium keeps your muscles and nerves healthy while lowering your blood pressure, and research suggests that beta-carotene can reduce the risk of both lung and bladder cancers, as well as macular degeneration.

SERVING SIZE	1 cup, raw (135 g)			1 cup, shredded		
Calories/Fiber	Calories: 36		Fiber: 5 g	Calories: 10		Fiber: 1 g
Macronutrients	Protein: 2 g	Fat: 0 g	Carbs: 8 g	Protein: 1 g	Fat: 0 g	Carbs: 2 g
Vitamins/Minerals	Vitamin C: 140%	Potassium: 14%	Vitamin B₆: 10%	Vitamin A: 60%	Vitamin C: 50%	

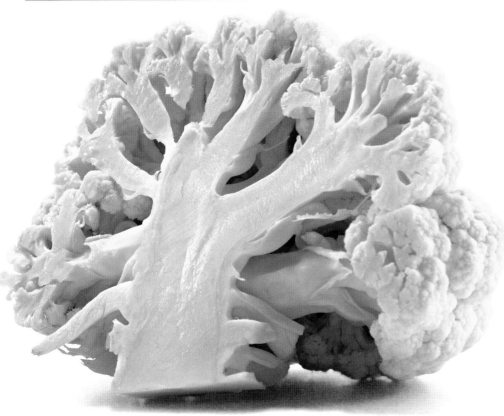

CAULIFLOWER

The florets in this ivory cluster contain detoxifying compounds called isothiocyanates, which offer protection against forms of prostate cancer. To boost your defenses even more, pair cauliflower with turmeric. The spice has prostate prestige on its own, but it becomes even more effective against cancer there when it's paired with cauliflower, according to a Rutgers University study. (The combination is particularly popular in Indian cuisine—order the cauliflower-and-potato dish aloo gobi.) Try orange-colored cauliflower, too. A hybrid variety, it's creamier, more tender, and bursting with cancer-fighting beta-carotene.

1 cup (100 g)			
Calories: 25		Fiber: 3 g	
Protein: 2 g	Fat: 0 g	Carbs: 5 g	
Vitamin C: 77%	Vitamin K: 20%	Folate: 14%	

Leafy Vegetables | THE HEALTHIEST FOODS IN THE WORLD

You can't go wrong with anything here. Some of these greens are surprisingly good sources of the bone-building, fat-burning mineral calcium. Others contain folic acid, a nutrient that helps maintain cardiovascular health and may battle depression. And almost all of them contain vitamin C to keep your immune system in shape, fiber to scour cholesterol, and potassium to repair muscles.

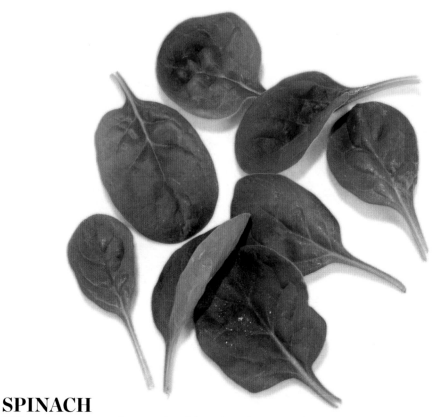

SPINACH

If there's one upgrade you should make when building a sandwich or salad, it's to swap iceberg lettuce for spinach, a renowned muscle builder. In a test-tube study, Rutgers researchers discovered that treating human muscle cells with a hormone found in spinach increased protein synthesis by 20 percent. The compound allows muscle tissue to repair itself faster, the researchers say. Spinach is also rich in vitamin K, calcium, phosphorus, potassium, zinc, and even selenium, which may help protect the liver and ward off Alzheimer's. One more reason to add it to your diet: A study in the *Journal of Nutrition* suggests that the carotenoid neoxanthin in spinach can kill prostate cancer cells.

SERVING SIZE	1 cup, raw (30 g)		
Calories/Fiber	Calories: 7		Fiber: 1 g
Macronutrients	Protein: 1 g	Fat: 0 g	Carbs: 1 g
Vitamins/Minerals	Vitamin K: 181%	Vitamin A: 56%	Folate: 15%

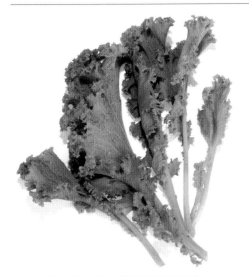

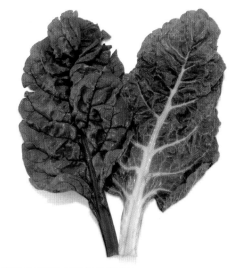

MUSTARD GREENS

Mustard greens, a staple in Southern cooking, contain antioxidants that help the body produce nitric oxide, which helps deliver oxygen to your blood. Other green leafy vegetables also share this characteristic, but turnip and mustard greens also contain the highest amounts of the B vitamin folate—a cup of either delivers almost twice as much as spinach. Researchers have linked folate deficiency to depression, fatigue, heart disease, dementia, Alzheimer's disease, and more. Mustard greens have a strong flavor, so try blanching them to reduce their bitterness.

SWISS CHARD

Native to the Mediterranean (not the Alps) and closely related to beets, Swiss chard is, like kale, one of nature's multivitamins, delivering substantial amounts of 16 vitamins and vital nutrients. For a mere 7 calories' worth of raw chard, you get more than triple the recommended daily intake of bone-strengthening vitamin K; half your vision-boosting vitamin A; and 16 percent of the hard-to-get vitamin E, which studies have shown may help sharpen mental acuity. It also contains 10 mg each of the vision-benefiting carotenoids lutein and zeaxanthin. Chard is tender enough to eat raw, and it makes a good substitution for spinach in most recipes.

1 cup (56 g)		
Calories: 15		Fiber: 2 g
Protein: 2 g	Fat: 0 g	Carbs: 3 g
Vitamin K: 348%	Vitamin A: 118%	Folate: 26%

1 cup, raw (36 g)		
Calories: 7		Fiber: 1 g
Protein: 1 g	Fat: 0 g	Carbs: 1 g
Vitamin K: 374%	Vitamin A: 44%	Vitamin C: 18%

SMOOTH YOUR SKIN

Researchers in Australia, Indonesia, and Sweden studied the diets of 400 elderly men and women, and found that those who ate the most leafy green vegetables and beans had the fewest wrinkles. The reason? Leafy greens and beans are full of compounds that help prevent and repair wear and tear on your skin cells as you get older.

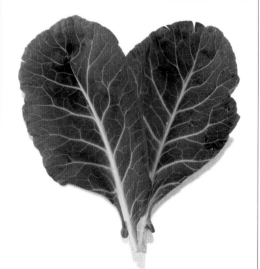

COLLARD GREENS

Collards are of the same plant family as broccoli and brussels sprouts, which puts them among the healthiest sides you can order with your barbecue. This side carries half a day's worth of vitamin A, 2 days' worth of vitamin K, and a heavy load of the cancer-fighting antioxidant sulforaphane.

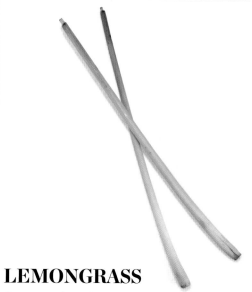

LEMONGRASS

Grown primarily in warm climates (tropical Asia, for example), this exotic grass exudes a lemon flavor after the stalks are chopped. It's loaded with antioxidants, which help protect against oxidative stress, one of the causes of heart disease and cancer. Try a stir-fry: Start with ½ tablespoon each of minced garlic, grated ginger, and minced lemongrass. Add vegetables, chicken, and soy sauce.

SERVING SIZE	1 cup, raw, chopped (36 g)			1 cup (67 g)		
Calories/Fiber	Calories: 11		Fiber: 1 g	Calories: 66		Fiber: 0 g
Macronutrients	Protein: 1 g	Fat: 0 g	Carbs: 2 g	Protein: 1 g	Fat: 0 g	Carbs: 17 g
Vitamins/Minerals	Vitamin K: 230%	Vitamin A: 48%	Vitamin C: 21%	Manganese: 175%	Iron: 30%	Potassium: 14%

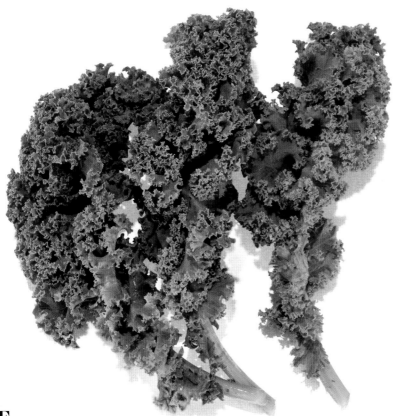

HOT AIR HELPS YOUR HEART

USDA researchers have discovered that steaming certain vegetables may make them even more potent at fighting high cholesterol than they are in their raw state. "The steaming process seems to improve the ability of vegetables to bind with bile acids in the intestine, a key factor in reducing cholesterol formation," says study author Talwinder Kahlon, PhD. Try it with the vegetables tested in the study: collard and mustard greens, kale, broccoli, green bell peppers, and cabbage.

KALE

Its green leaves are rich in vitamins A and C, potassium, calcium, iron, and folate, as well as the eye-healthy carotenoids lutein and zeaxanthin, pigments that accumulate in the retina and absorb damaging shortwave light rays. Kale also contains the flavonol kaempferol, which a study by Baylor College of Medicine researchers found helps stop pancreatic cancer cells from growing. Even cooked, 1 cup of kale is unsurpassed, containing more than 10 times your daily allotment of bone-strengthening vitamin K. If you don't like the curly variety, opt for the Russian or Lacinato kinds, which are more tender and have a milder flavor.

1 cup, cooked (130 g)			
Calories: 36		Fiber: 3 g	
Protein: 2 g	Fat: 1 g	Carbs: 7 g	
Vitamin K: 1,328%	Vitamin A: 354%	Vitamin C: 89%	

95

Lettuce comes in all kinds of sizes and colors, and many of them appear in flavorful packages of Mesclun, an assortment of young greens. But the best part of salad greens is the vitamin punch—A, C, and K, especially.

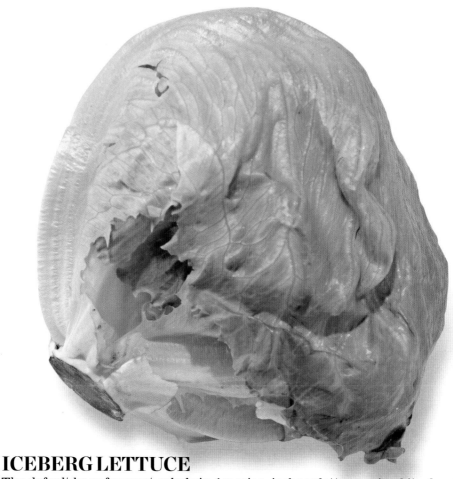

ICEBERG LETTUCE

The default base for most salads in America, iceberg lettuce gained its dominant foothold because it contains so much water and has such strong cell walls that it can last up to 3 weeks without wilting. But iceberg lettuce helps your diet as much as a real iceberg helped the Titanic, with just trace amounts of vitamins K and A, and folate. Upgrade to spinach, or Romaine if you like iceberg's crunchiness.

SERVING SIZE	1 cup, raw, shredded (72 g)		
Calories/Fiber	Calories: 10		Fiber: 1 g
Macronutrients	Protein: 1 g	Fat: 0 g	Carbs: 2 g
Vitamins/Minerals	Vitamin K: 22%	Vitamin A: 7%	Folate: 5%

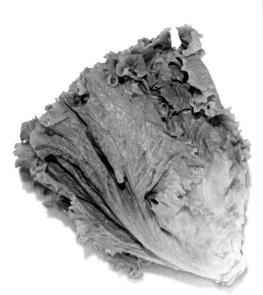

GREEN-LEAF LETTUCE

If nutrition facts accompanied bare heads of lettuce, you'd probably buy a lot more of the green-leaf variety. Compared to the most common types, green-leaf lettuce has the most vitamin C and K, and folate, as well as the minerals calcium and manganese.

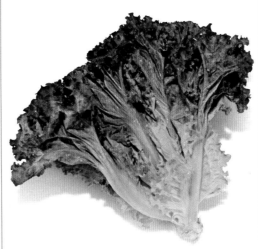

RED-LEAF LETTUCE

While dark colors usually coincide with the highest levels of nutrition, red-leaf lettuce is an exception to the rule. It doesn't lag too far behind green-leaf lettuce in most categories, however.

DO YOU NEED TO WASH BAGGED SALADS?

Don't bother. "Ready-to-eat salad is sanitized in a way far superior to any cleaning you can do at home," says Sam Beattie, PhD, a food safety specialist at Iowa State University. "It's washed in water and sanitizers such as chlorine compounds. Then it's rinsed thoroughly and spun dry—all at cold temperatures." But wouldn't washing it just be safer? No. "The first rule of produce microbiology is that once contaminated it is almost impossible to decontaminate," says Beattie. In reality, if there's a weak link in keeping prewashed greens clean, it's probably you. Wash your mitts with warm water and soap for at least 20 seconds before handling food, and don't ignore your nails. A British study found that 25 percent of men had harmful bacteria there.

1 cup, raw, shredded (36 g)		
Calories: 5		Fiber: 0 g
Protein: 0 g	Fat: 0 g	Carbs: 1 g
Vitamin K: 78%	Vitamin A: 53%	Vitamin C: 11%

1 cup, raw, shredded (28 g)		
Calories: 4		Fiber: 0 g
Protein: 0 g	Fat: 0 g	Carbs: 1 g
Vitamin K: 49%	Vitamin A: 42%	

Salad Greens

Salad Greens | THE HEALTHIEST FOODS IN THE WORLD

HEY GOOD-LOOKIN'

The National Institutes of Health found that people who consume the most lutein—found in leafy greens—are 43 percent less likely to develop macular degeneration. Enjoy your spinach and romaine lettuce!

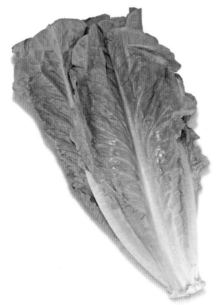

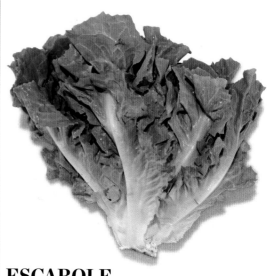

ROMAINE LETTUCE

Although similar in look and flavor to iceberg lettuce, Romaine is a nutritional powerhouse by comparison. Its robust, crunchy leaves—the foundation of Caesar salads—are low in calories and high in vitamin C and beta-carotene, which together prevent plaque from clogging arteries.

ESCAROLE

A head of broad-leafed, ragged-edged lettuce leaves with a yellow heart, escarole has a slightly bitter and nutty flavor. It's a good source of vitamin A, which helps maintain healthy eyes and skin, and may help support a strong immune system. It can be a good base for a salad, but, unlike most other salad greens, its also delicious cooked over moderate heat in a skillet.

SERVING SIZE	1 cup, raw, shredded (47 g)			1 cup, raw, chopped		
Calories/Fiber	Calories: 8	Fiber: 1 g		Calories: 10	Fiber: 2 g	
Macronutrients	Protein: 1 g	Fat: 0 g	Carbs: 2 g	Protein: 1 g	Fat: 0 g	Carbs: 2 g
Vitamins/Minerals	Vitamin A: 82%	Vitamin K: 60%	Vitamin C: 19%	Vitamin A: 20%		

9

TOP GREENS FOR FOLATE

1. Turnip greens
2. Spinach
3. Collard greens
4. Parsley
5. Mustard greens
6. Romaine lettuce
7. Asparagus
8. Brussels sprouts
9. Kale

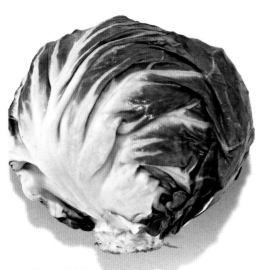

RADICCHIO

While radicchio looks like a miniature deep-red cabbage with white veins, it's actually more closely related to frisée and endive. Its tender, delicate leaves have a bittersweet flavor and are high in folate, which may help reduce dementia risk.

1 cup, raw, shredded (40 g)		
Calories: 9		Fiber: 0 g
Protein: 1 g	Fat: 0 g	Carbs: 2 g
Vitamin K: 128%	Copper: 7%	Folate: 6%

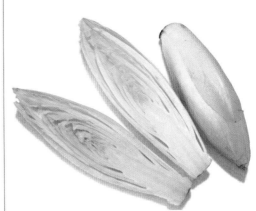

BELGIAN ENDIVE

These smooth, conical-shaped heads command a high price, but with the exception of vitamin K, they're even more nutritionally vacant than iceberg lettuce. Fault the plant's two-step growing process for both realities. Farmers plant the seed during spring, harvest the roots in the fall, and then force the pale yellow heads indoors in total darkness during winter—and without exposure to light, they never develop into nutrient-rich plants.

½ cup, raw, chopped (25 g)		
Calories: 4		Fiber: 1 g
Protein: 0 g	Fat: 0 g	Carbs: 1 g
Vitamin K: 72%	Vitamin A: 11%	

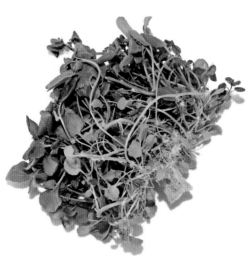

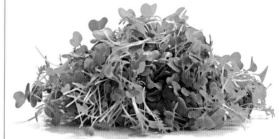

WATERCRESS

A member of the cabbage family, this leafy green will add a peppery kick to your salads and sandwiches. One cup of watercress has just 4 calories, but it's loaded with vitamins A, C, and K. A study in the *American Journal of Clinical Nutrition* also found that eating 3 ounces daily increases levels of the cancer-fighting antioxidants lutein and beta-carotene by 100 and 33 percent, respectively.

MIZUNA

A difficult-to-find Japanese mustard green with dark leaves, mizuna has a similar look and flavor to arugula, with less pungency. Plus it's got 10 times as much vitamin C, 8 times as much vitamin A, and twice as much protein as its rival.

SERVING SIZE	1 cup, raw, chopped (34 g)			1 cup, raw (56 g)		
Calories/Fiber	Calories: 4	Fiber: 0 g		Calories: 15	Fiber: 2 g	
Macronutrients	Protein: 1 g	Fat: 0 g	Carbs: 0 g	Protein: 2 g	Fat: 8 g	Carbs: 3 g
Vitamins/Minerals	Vitamin K: 106%	Vitamin C: 24%	Vitamin A: 22%	Vitamin A: 120%	Vitamin C: 70%	

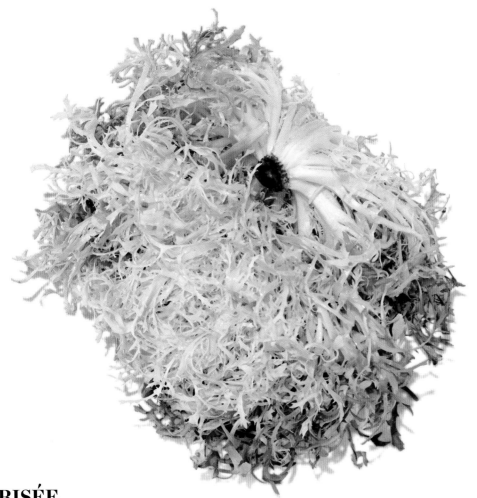

IMPROVE YOUR MOOD

Kale, spinach, Swiss chard, and other leafy greens are rich sources of B vitamins, which are part of the assembly line that manufactures feel-good hormones such as serotonin, dopamine, and norepi-nephrine. A lack of vitamin B_6 can even cause nervousness, irritability, and even depression, according to a study published in the *Journal of Neuroscience Nursing.*

FRISÉE

Also known as curly endive, this bitter green provides modest amounts of vitamins A and K, and folate. It can make a nice addition to salads because it packs such a bold flavor in such a small bite, and it pairs especially well with bacon and eggs.

1 cup, raw, chopped			
Calories: 17		Fiber: 3 g	
Protein: 1 g	Fat: 0 g	Carbs: 2 g	
Vitamin A: 20%	Potassium: 9%	Calcium: 5%	

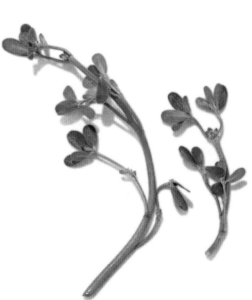

PURSLANE

Although the FDA classifies purslane as a broad-leaved weed, it's a popular vegetable and herb in many other countries, including China, Mexico, and Greece. It has the highest amount of heart-healthy omega-3 fats of any edible plant, according to researchers at the University of Texas at San Antonio. The scientists also report that this herb has 10 to 20 times more melatonin—an antioxidant that may inhibit cancer growth—than any other fruit or vegetable tested. Think of purslane as a great alternative or addition to lettuce.

DANDELION

Although you've probably long identified it as a lawn-wrecking weed, dandelion is as edible as any green in the grocery store (so long as it hasn't been doused with herbicides). Your eyes and bones will benefit from its high levels of vitamins A and K. Harvest the greens in the spring (before the plant flowers), or temper their bitterness by boiling them for a few minutes. You can also wilt the greens beneath hot-bacon dressing.

SERVING SIZE	1 cup (43 g)			1 cup, raw, chopped (55 g)		
Calories/Fiber	Calories: 7		Fiber: 0 g	Calories: 25		Fiber: 2 g
Macronutrients	Protein: 1 g	Fat: 0 g	Carbs: 1 g	Protein: 1 g	Fat: 0 g	Carbs: 5 g
Vitamins/Minerals	Vitamin C: 15%	Vitamin A: 11%		Vitamin K: 535%	Vitamin A: 112%	Vitamin C: 32%

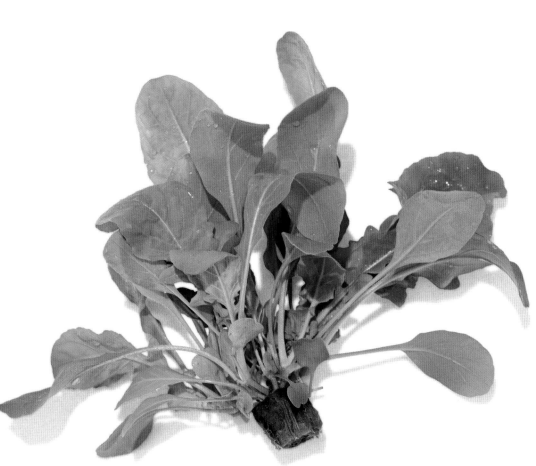

ARUGULA

These small and narrow leaves pack a spicy, pungent flavor that hits you with a mustard-like zing. They also contain glucosinolates—nutrient compounds that may help eliminate harmful toxins in the body. Arugula's peppery flavor complements sweet or acidic flavors, ranging from shrimp to citrus.

1 oz, raw (about 2⅓ cups, 28 g)		
Calories: 7		Fiber: 0 g
Protein: 1 g	Fat: 0 g	Carbs: 1 g
Vitamin K: 38%	Vitamin A: 13%	

BOOST YOUR IMMUNITY AND YOUR MUSCLES

Whether you're sautéing dark greens or making a salad, include a squeeze of citrus. "Vitamin C helps make plant-based iron more absorbable," says nutritionist Stacy Kennedy of the Dana Farber Cancer Institute. While too much isn't good for men, it's still an important nutrient because it carries oxygen to your red blood cells (staving off muscle fatigue). The inclusion of vitamin C is what allows the body to convert much of the plant-based iron into a form that's similar to what's found in fish and red meats.

Pair any of these vitamin C–rich choices . . .
Citrus fruits
Strawberries
Tomatoes
Bell peppers
Broccoli

. . . with any of these iron-heavy vegetables:
Leeks
Beet greens
Kale
Spinach
Mustard greens
Swiss chard

It's hard to tell what's more powerful about herbs: Their flavor or their antioxidant properties. For an example, check out how pizza-booster oregano (page 107) stacks up to blueberries. Herbal bonus: Calorie counts for most herbs are nonexistent. The same can't be said for other pizza toppings, like, say, sausage.

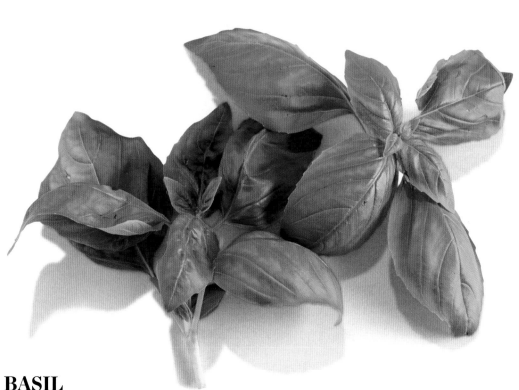

BASIL

Eating basil at dinner will help you remember a woman's name at the bar later that evening. The herb stimulates the brain's prefrontal cortex, which controls short-term memory, according to a study in *Critical Reviews in Food Science and Nutrition*. It also contains oils that prevent bacteria growth and inflammation, and it's rich in antioxidants that mop up cell-damaging free radicals inside the body. This can help prevent a host of unwanted conditions, such as osteoporosis, arthritis, and high cholesterol.

SERVING SIZE	¼ cup whole leaves (6 g)		
Calories/Fiber	Calories: 1		Fiber: 0 g
Macronutrients	Protein: 0 g	Fat: 0 g	Carbs: 0 g
Vitamins/Minerals	Vitamin K: 31%	Vitamin A: 6%	

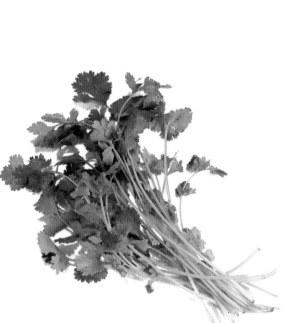

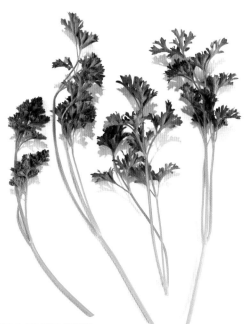

TRY TULSI

Holy basil, a popular Indian herb, is the ideal ingredient for infusing freshness and flavor into almost any meal. Animal studies have shown that natural chemicals in the plant, which is also known as tulsi, may help fight diabetes, heart disease, and cancer.

CILANTRO

A popular ingredient in Latin and Asian cuisines, cilantro has a fresh-and-zesty flavor—at least for most folks. But the plant does contain aldehydes, compounds that yield a soapy flavor to some people. (The plant's detractors even have a blog titled "I hate cilantro"!) The plant's seeds—known as coriander—contain kaempferol, an oil that researchers at Baylor College of Medicine claim may inhibit the growth of pancreatic cancer cells.

PARSLEY

These dainty leaves are highly concentrated with luteolin, a powerful flavonoid with anti-inflammatory properties. Researchers at the University of Illinois found that luteolin decreased inflammation in the brain, which helps prevent decline in cognitive function.

¼ cup, fresh (4 g)		
Calories: 1		Fiber: 0 g
Protein: 0 g	Fat: 0 g	Carbs: 0 g
Vitamin K: 16%	Vitamin A: 5%	Vitamin C: 2%

10 sprigs (10 g)		
Calories: 4		Fiber: 0 g
Protein: 0 g	Fat: 0 g	Carbs: 1 g
Vitamin K: 205%	Vitamin C: 22%	Vitamin A: 17%

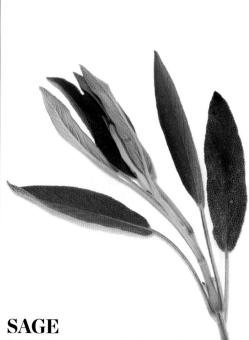

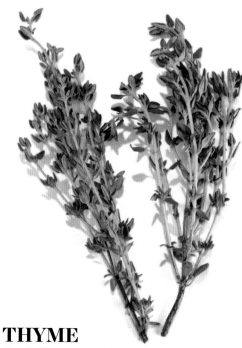

SAGE

Sage, like rosemary, is known to strengthen memory. The rosemerinic acid in these plants also works to preserve your body by protecting your cells from oxidative damage and alleviating the effects of asthma and arthritis.

THYME

Fresh thyme contains luteolin, a flavonoid linked to reduced brain inflammation, a risk factor for Alzheimer's. When dried it's also an incredibly rich source of iron, which is crucial to your body's ability to transport oxygen through your blood. And, as with oregano, seasoning with thyme helps protect food from bacterial contamination.

SERVING SIZE	1 Tbsp, dried, ground (2 g)			1 tsp, dried (1 g)		
Calories/Fiber	Calories: 6		Fiber: 1 g	Calories: 3		Fiber: 0 g
Macronutrients	Protein: 0 g	Fat: 0 g	Carbs: 1 g	Protein: 0 g	Fat: 0 g	Carbs:1 g
Vitamins/Minerals	Vitamin K: 43%			Vitamin K: 21%	Iron: 7%	

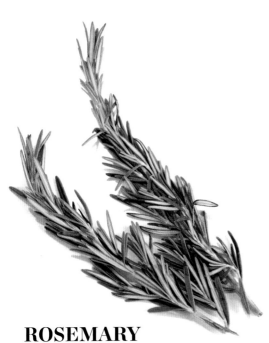

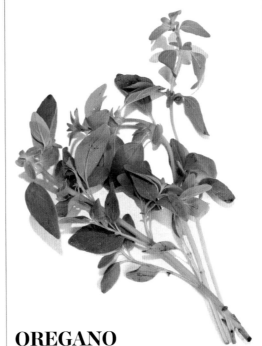

ROSEMARY

Call it the smart spice. Many people swear by rosemary's ability to increase cognitive functioning, and researchers in California have identified carnosic acid as an active ingredient in rosemary that can offset cognitive degeneration, protect against Alzheimer's, and prevent stroke.

OREGANO

Add a tablespoon of fresh oregano to your burgers and meat loaf. When researchers at Kansas State University mixed a variety of common household spices into ground beef to test their antibacterial properties, dried oregano was one of the best at wiping out E. coli. Your next pizza or pasta sauce could have big cancer-fighting potential, too: A USDA study also found that when adjusted for weight, oregano had four times the antioxidant activity of blueberries.

1 Tbsp, dried (3 g)		
Calories: 11	Fiber: 1 g	
Protein: 0 g	Fat: 0 g	Carbs: 2 g
Iron: 5%	Calcium: 4%	

1 tsp, dried, ground (2 g)		
Calories: 5	Fiber: 1 g	
Protein: 0 g	Fat: 0 g	Carbs: 1 g
Vitamin K: 14%		

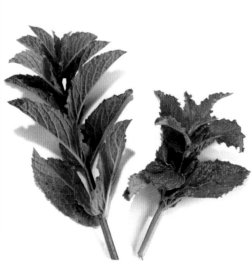

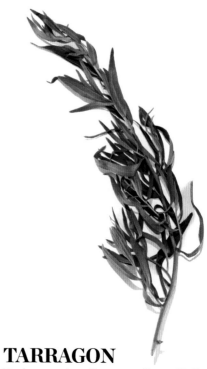

PEPPERMINT

Thank the menthol in peppermint for the plant's ability to battle cold symptoms, helping to clear mucus from the bronchial tract to facilitate easy breathing. Peppermint is also known to combat indigestion, gas, menstrual cramps, and irritable bowel syndrome. Use fresh mint to brew tea, or brighten up a batch of fruit salad with chopped leaves and a squeeze of lime.

TARRAGON

By increasing the secretion of bile and acids into the stomach, tarragon improves gastric efficiency and whets the appetite. Because of this, it's best used early in the meal to season an appetizer. It's also a modest source of kaempferol and quercetin, antioxidants that may defend against prostate cancer.

SERVING SIZE	2 Tbsp, fresh (3 g)			1 tsp, ground (2 g)		
Calories/Fiber	Calories: 2	Fiber: 0 g		Calories: 4	Fiber: 0 g	
Macronutrients	Protein: 0 g	Fat: 0 g	Carbs: 0 g	Protein: 0 g	Fat: 0 g	Carbs: 1 g
Vitamins/Minerals	Vitamin A: 3%	Manganese: 2%		Manganese: 2%	Iron: 1%	

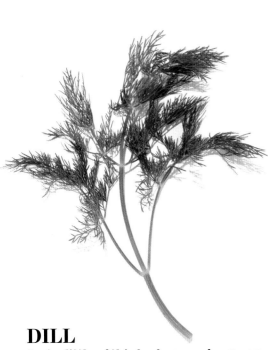

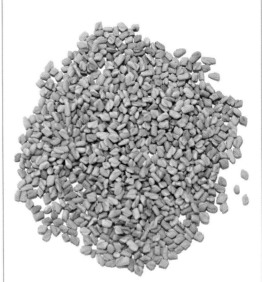

DILL

Just a little of this herb goes a long way, but it's an especially good source of the potent antioxidant quercetin, which may help reduce blood pressure, lower the risk of certain cancers, and stave off Alzheimer's disease.

FENUGREEK

This tangy, curry-scented spice is used in many tasty Indian dishes. Scientists think it may lower your blood-sugar response after a meal by delaying stomach emptying, which slows carbohydrate absorption and enhances insulin sensitivity. Fenugreek is a component of most curry powders. You can also mix a teaspoon of pure fenugreek powder into beef stew to kick up the flavor, or add whole seeds to a rice dish to create a Southeast Asian–style pilaf.

1 Tbsp, dried (3 g)		
Calories: 8	Fiber: 0 g	
Protein: 1 g	Fat: 0 g	Carbs: 2 g
Iron: 8%	Calcium: 5%	Vitamin A: 4%

1 Tbsp (11 g)		
Calories: 36	Fiber: 3 g	
Protein: 3 g	Fat: 1 g	Carbs: 6 g
Iron: 20%	Manganese: 7%	Copper: 6%

Squash come in so many varieties you'll never be short of ideas on how to add them to your diet year round: Cukes in your spring salad, zuchs on the summer grill, pumpkin in the fall, and in the winter? What else: Winter squash.

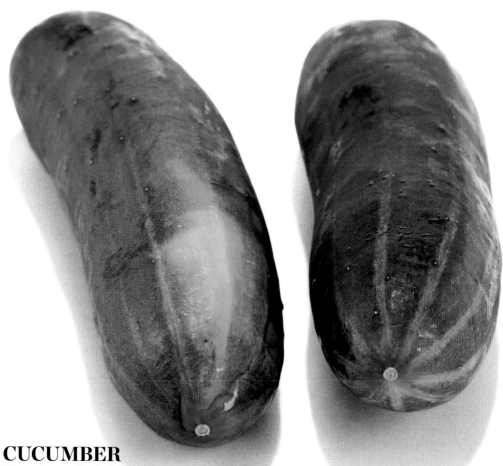

CUCUMBER

These low-calorie torpedoes will cleanse your palate and cool your mouth, but they're about 95 percent water—a number that comes in a few ticks higher than watermelon and nearly tops iceberg lettuce! Such high water content makes for a low nutrient density, although cukes do contain modest amounts of vitamin C and folate.

SERVING SIZE	1 cucumber, 8¼" (301 g)		
Calories/Fiber	Calories: 45		Fiber: 2 g
Macronutrients	Protein: 2 g	Fat: 0 g	Carbs: 11 g
Vitamins/Minerals	Vitamin K: 62%	Vitamin C: 14%	Potassium: 13%

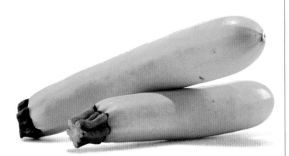

ZUCCHINI

Like the cucumber, zucchini is a low-calorie favorite. Although winter squash edge summer squash in most of the important nutritional categories, zucchini has a trump card in riboflavin, a B vitamin needed for red blood cell production and for converting carbohydrates to energy. A large one provides 27 percent of your daily requirement.

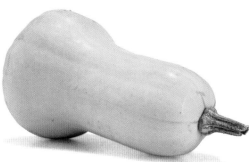

BUTTERNUT

Butternut squash is a gold mine of beta-carotene, although a cup still contains barely half the amount found in carrots. Still, researchers from Harvard found that men who consumed more beta-carotene over 15 years had significantly delayed cognitive aging. This winter squash is also a good source of potassium and fiber.

PICKING PICKLES

What happens when you take a nutritionally vacant cucumber and give it a long soak in a briny vinegar bath? You get a nutritionally vacant pickle with a sobering sodium problem. But pickles are fine in moderation, especially when you crave something crunchy and salty—and they're certainly a better choice than reaching for potato chips. And, other than their seasonings, there's not really that much of a difference between dill, kosher, and Polish, either. (In this instance, kosher means that garlic is one of the primary seasonings, not that a Rabbi oversaw the pickling process.) The one exception is that certain pickles, such as the bread-and-butter variety, are sometimes flavored with the wonder spice turmeric (or turmeric oleoresin, an organic extract), which is famed for its mental benefits. Chomping on that should chirp you up.

1 large (323 g)		
Calories: 52	Fiber: 4 g	
Protein: 4 g	Fat: 1 g	Carbs: 11 g
Vitamin A: 13%	Vitamin C: 92%	Riboflavin: 27%

1 cup, cubed (140 g)		
Calories: 63	Fiber: 3 g	
Protein: 1 g	Fat: 0 g	Carbs: 16 g
Vitamin A: 298%	Vitamin C: 49%	Potassium: 14%

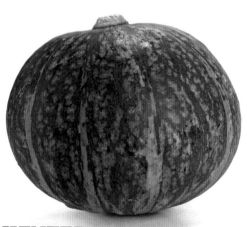

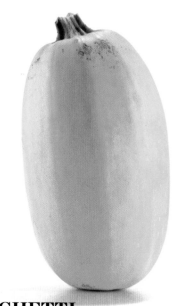

WINTER

Winter squash comes in a wide range of varieties, but always features a protective and inedible outer skin and yellow-orange flesh, and is a rich source of beta-carotene and vitamin C. Its flavor is enhanced best by roasting. Winter squash are also a good source of potassium, which can help alleviate high blood pressure.

SPAGHETTI

This squash is known for its spaghetti-like innards, which you can scoop out and use as a low-starch pasta alternative. If you're not making that faux Italian dish, however, pick a different type of winter squash. Other than its limited supply of fiber and vitamin C, spaghetti squash lacks standout qualities.

SERVING SIZE	1 cup, cubed (116 g)			1 cup, cubed (101 g)		
Calories/Fiber	Calories: 39		Fiber: 2 g	Calories: 31		Fiber: 0 g
Macronutrients	Protein: 1 g	Fat: 0 g	Carbs: 10 g	Protein: 1 g	Fat: 0 g	Carbs: 7 g
Vitamins/Minerals	Vitamin A: 32%	Vitamin C: 24%	Potassium: 12%	Manganese: 6%	Vitamin B6: 5%	Vitamin C: 4%

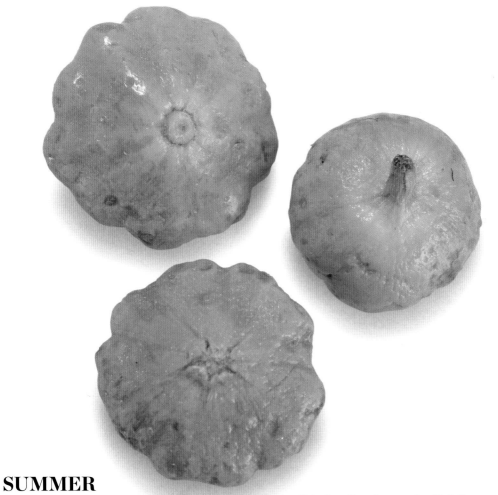

SUMMER

Their edible exteriors and softer interiors make this family of squash slightly easier to eat than their winter brethren, but summer squash's higher water content puts a few holes in their nutritional numbers. Vitamin C is the only noteworthy contribution to your diet.

1 cup, sliced (113 g)			
Calories: 18		Fiber: 1 g	
Protein: 1 g	Fat: 0 g	Carbs: 4 g	
Vitamin C: 32%	Vitamin B$_6$: 12%		

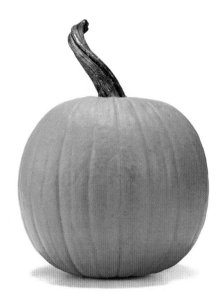

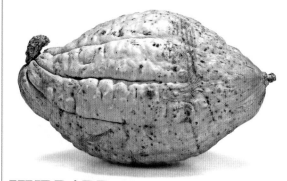

PUMPKIN

Think of these iconic orange squash as Halloween's only nutritious treat. But this is one instance where the canned kind (which has already been cooked) is even better than the real deal. One cup is loaded with iron and 7 grams of fiber, the crucial nutrient that most muscle-building, high-protein diets lack. It doesn't lack for oxidative stress-fighting antioxidants, either—it's even got more vitamin A than an equivalent amount of cooked carrots. But instead of pigging out on pumpkin pie, which is high in sugar and calories, try pouring canned pumpkin into your next protein shake.

HUBBARD

It's kind of ugly and warty-looking and has a hard skin that can't be eaten (like most winter squash), but its grainy, moist, orange-yellow flesh packs great flavor. Besides containing vitamins A and C, this squash is loaded with potassium, which can control blood pressure.

SERVING SIZE	1 cup, canned, no-salt (245 g)			1 cup, cubed (116 g)		
Calories/Fiber	Calories: 83		Fiber: 7 g	Calories: 46		Fiber: 0 g
Macronutrients	Protein: 3 g	Fat: 1 g	Carbs: 20 g	Protein: 2 g	Fat: 0 g	Carbs: 10 g
Vitamins/Minerals	Vitamin A: 763%	Vitamin K: 49%	Manganese: 18%	Vitamin A: 32%	Vitamin C: 21%	Potassium: 11%

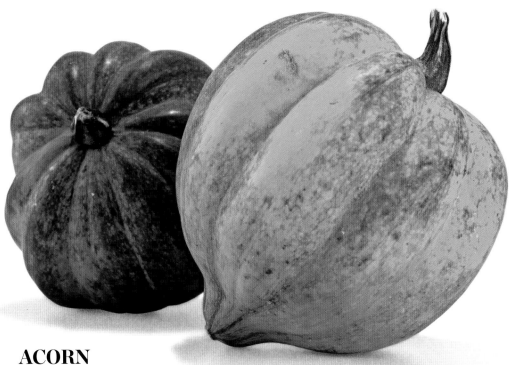

ACORN

Sweeter than pumpkins, these winter squash can be halved, seeded, and roasted in the oven for a quick-and-nutritious comfort meal. One 4" squash is a particularly good source of vitamin C and potassium, and it also supplies your body with a healthy dose of the B vitamin thiamin, which plays a central role in energy production and cognitive function.

1 cup, cubed (140 g)		
Calories: 56		Fiber: 2 g
Protein: 1 g	Fat: 0 g	Carbs: 15 g
Vitamin C: 26%	Potassium: 14%	Thiamin: 13%

Modern cooking would not exist without this category of vegetables. Consider onions and garlic: Never have two foods made so many people happy to have foul breath. The best part is that each of these entries brings terrific individual health benefits along with it.

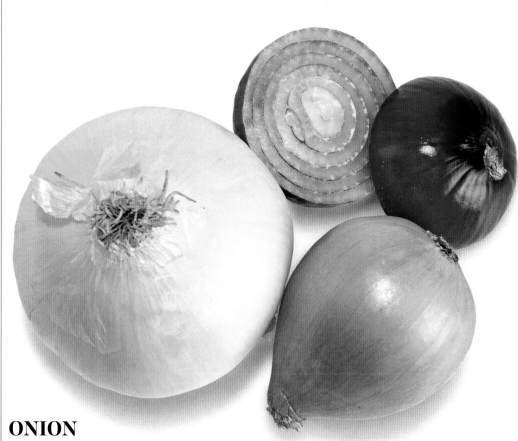

ONION

The ultimate wingman, the selfless onion serves to complement other foods—from bell peppers to liver. They're good sources of vitamin C, B₆, fiber, potassium, and manganese, but when raw, their pungent flavor can be overwhelming. (Which is why restaurants usually batter and fry them into submission.) While all onions are a good source of the flavanol quercetin, red onions contain more cyanidin, which may protect cells from harmful free radicals.

SERVING SIZE	1 cup, chopped (160 g)		
Calories/Fiber	Calories: 64		Fiber: 3 g
Macronutrients	Protein: 2 g	Fat: 0 g	Carbs: 15 g
Vitamins/Minerals	Vitamin C: 20%	Vitamin B₆: 10%	

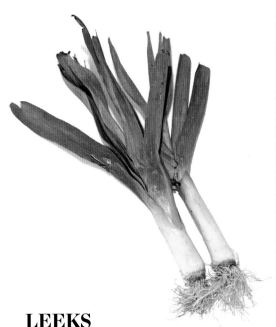

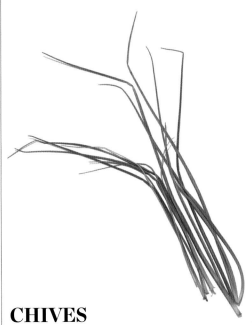

LEEKS

These large scallion-like cousins of garlic and onions pack healthy amounts of eye-protecting lutein, manganese, and vitamins A, C, and K. They also lend men some assistance down below. "Leeks can support sexual functioning and reduce the risk of prostate cancer," says Michael Dansinger, MD, an assistant professor of medicine and an obesity researcher at Tufts–New England Medical Center. "Slice the tender white part of a medium leek into thin ribbons and add it to soups, sautés, and salads."

CHIVES

Chives have a delicate, onion-like flavor, which you can enhance by finely slicing their green stalks before eating them. More herb than vegetable, chives contain modest amounts of the antioxidants kaempferol and isorhamnetin, the latter of which may reduce cancer risk, improve heart health, and ease diabetes complications.

1 leek (89 g)		
Calories: 54		Fiber: 2 g
Protein: 1 g	Fat: 0 g	Carbs: 13 g
Vitamin K: 52%	Vitamin A: 30%	Manganese: 21%

1 Tbsp, fresh, chopped (3 g)		
Calories: 1		Fiber: 0 g
Protein: 0 g	Fat: 0 g	Carbs: 0 g
Vitamin K: 8%	Vitamin A: 3%	Vitamin C: 3%

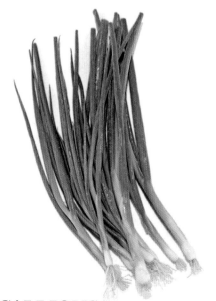

SCALLIONS

Also called green onions, scallions are long stalks attached to small onion-like bulbs. They contain less quercetin than regular onions but more vitamin K—just 2 tablespoons provide a third of your daily need. Unfortunately, scallions have earned a bad rap because of their dirty reputation. In the past decade they've triggered hepatitis A outbreaks in several states; researchers have also found them harboring cryptosporidium, shigella, and salmonella. Always wash the plant thoroughly before eating, but understand that heat is ultimately your best source of protection.

SHALLOTS

Shallots are similar in flavor to a mild white onion, yet grow in cloves like garlic. They're common in most world cuisines, especially Indian and Southeast Asian (in Iran, they add shallots to yogurt). Vitamins A, B_6, and manganese are plentiful in shallots, but you'd have to eat a ton of them (okay, several cups) to fulfill your daily amounts.

SERVING SIZE	1 cup, chopped (100 g)			1 Tbsp (10 g)		
Calories/Fiber	Calories: 32		Fiber: 3 g	Calories: 7		Fiber: 0 g
Macronutrients	Protein: 2 g	Fat: 0 g	Carbs: 7 g	Protein: 0 g	Fat: 0 g	Carbs: 2 g
Vitamins/Minerals	Vitamin K: 259%	Vitamin C: 31%	Vitamin A: 20%	Vitamin A: 2%	Vitamin B₆: 2%	Manganese: 1%

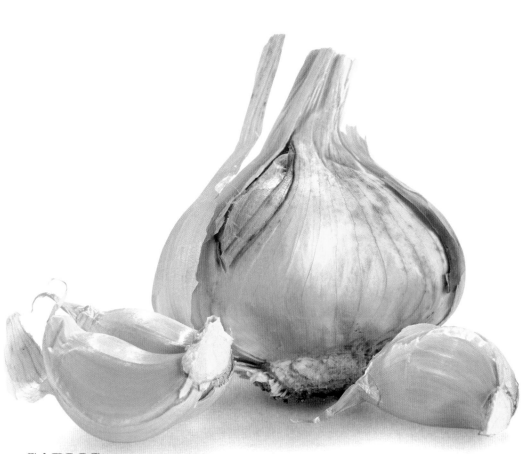

GARLIC

A culinary sidekick with serious health benefits, garlic deserves frequent inclusion in your meals. Enzymes in garlic increase the release of serotonin, a neurochemical that boosts your memory and aids relaxation, and the compound allicin is linked to lower cancer rates.

3 cloves (9 g)		
Calories: 13		Fiber: 0 g
Protein: 1 g	Fat: 0 g	Carbs: 3 g
Manganese: 8%	Vitamin B₆: 6%	Vitamin C: 5%

A handful of nuts every day can lower your heart-disease risk by a third, chop your Alzheimer's risk by two-thirds, and help you slim down. The best contain monounsaturated fat, the heart-healthy fats that help lower LDL (bad) cholesterol levels, while raising levels of HDL (good) cholesterol; protein, which will help you get lean; and plenty of vitamins, such as Vitamin E, calcium, and magnesium—nutrients that lower your risk of heart attack and improve your bone strength.

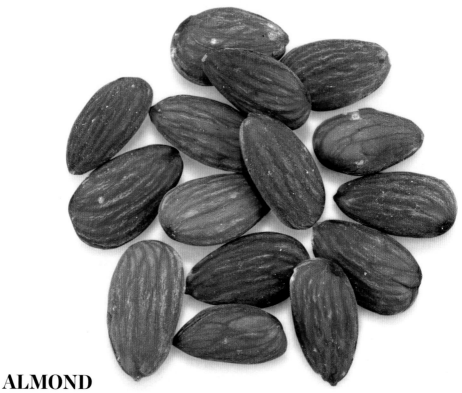

ALMOND

A true superfood, almonds are good for your brain, brawn, and belly. Much of the credit goes to a handful supplying half your daily value of the antioxidant vitamin E, which can increase memory and cognitive performance, according to researchers at New York–Presbyterian Hospital. A study published in the *Journal of the American Medical Association* also found that men who consumed the most vitamin E through their food had a 67 percent lower risk of Alzheimer's disease than those at the other end of the spectrum. Vitamin E's ability to fight free radicals also makes almonds a great post-workout snack because they help in muscle recovery, according to Jeff Volek, PhD. Plus, eating almonds seems to stimulate production of cholecystkinin, a hunger-suppressing hormone.

SERVING SIZE	1 oz, unsalted, dry-roasted (28 g)		
Calories/Fiber	Calories: 167		Fiber: 3 g
Macronutrients	Protein: 6 g	Fat: 15 g	Carbs: 5 g
Vitamins/Minerals	Manganese: 37%	Vitamin E: 36%	Magnesium: 20%

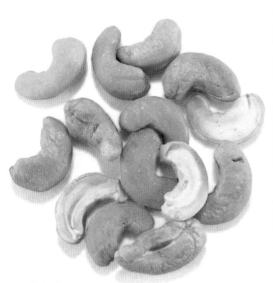

CASHEW

These rich, delicious nuggets contain slightly less monounsaturated fat and protein than almonds, but they get the edge in iron, which helps transport oxygen throughout the body and plays a critical role in energy production.

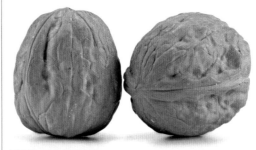

WALNUT

Think of the walnut as a true utility player: It's rich in heart-healthy omega-3s (a 1-ounce serving of walnuts packs 2,542 milligrams of omega-3!), features more anti-inflammatory polyphenols than red wine, and packs half as much muscle-building protein as chicken. Walnuts even make up for some of your bad habits. In one study, people who ate walnuts with large salami sandwiches reduced arterial inflammation caused by the lunchmeat and also improved their blood-vessel elasticity.

AN ALTERNATIVE TO ALMONDS

Almonds are great, but even greatest hits get old. Containing at least 3 grams of fiber and 7 grams of monounsaturated fat, hazelnuts, pistachios, and pecans are all good for your heart because they have the same artery-clearing combo found in almonds. Walnuts are lower in fiber and monounsaturated fat but high in omega-3 fatty acids. "Those four are interchange-able in their ability to keep your heart healthy, so mix them up," says Dawn Jackson Blatner, RD. To reap the rewards without gaining weight, eat a handful of one type daily, plus two Brazil nuts for cancer protection.

1 oz, unsalted, dry-roasted (28 g)		
Calories: 161	Fiber: 1 g	
Protein: 4 g	Fat: 13 g	Carbs: 9 g
Copper: 31%	Magnesium: 18%	Phosphorus: 14%

Calories: 183		Fiber: 2 g
Protein: 4 g	Fat: 18 g	Carbs: 4 g
Manganese: 48%	Copper: 22%	

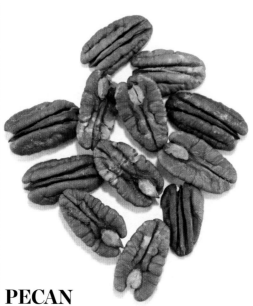

PECAN

The sweet old ladies who make delicious pies with these nuts probably don't know it, but pecans pack more anti-oxidants than any other nut. They're also rich in a form of vitamin E called gamma-tocopherol, which isn't in supplements or other varieties of nuts, according to Ella Haddad, PH, RD, a nutrition professor at Loma Linda University whose research shows that pecans help prevent arterial damage. Add them to your diet to reduce your risk of cancer, Alzheimer's disease, and heart disease.

BRAZIL NUT

Toxins in the air—whether from cigarettes or exhaust—have the potential to damage your sperm. But Brazil nuts pack more selenium (a mineral that helps keep sperm cells healthy) than any other food. When researchers in the United Kingdom had men with fertility problems increase their selenium intake, the men produced hardier, more viable sperm cells. Scientists at University of Arizona also found that selenium may prevent colon cancer in men.

SERVING SIZE	1 oz, unsalted, dry-roasted (28 g)			1 oz, dried, unblanched (28 g)		
Calories/Fiber	Calories: 199	Fiber: 3 g		Calories: 185	Fiber: 2 g	
Macronutrients	Protein: 3 g	Fat: 21 g	Carbs: 4 g	Protein: 4 g	Fat: 19 g	Carbs: 3 g
Vitamins/Minerals	Manganese: 55%	Copper: 16%		Selenium: 774%	Magnesium: 27%	Copper: 25%

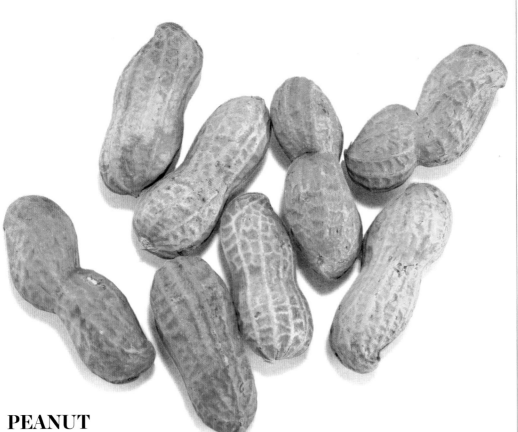

HEART THERAPY YOU CAN SPOON

Sure, peanut butter is high in calories, but that's because it's 43 percent fat. Surprisingly, half of that fat is the same heart-healthy, mono-unsaturated variety that gives olive oil its illustrious reputation. Olive oil does contain about twice as much monounsaturated fat, but it also turns your bread into a sponge and tastes pretty rotten with grape jelly. Do your body a favor by making peanut butter and celery sandwiches, and remember to limit your intake of white breads and other refined carbohydrates, which are far worse than the sticky stuff.

PEANUT

They're legumes, not nuts, but peanuts reduce the glycemic impact of a meal, increasing satiety and reducing food consumption later in the day, according to a study in the *Journal of the American College of Nutrition*. They also make a great go-to snack because of their high protein content. Just try to hold the salt, which transforms a reasonably healthy snack into a sodium disaster.

1 oz, unsalted, dry-roasted (28 g)		
Calories: 164		Fiber: 2 g
Protein: 7 g	Fat: 14 g	Carbs: 6 g
Manganese: 29%	Niacin: 19%	Magnesium: 12%

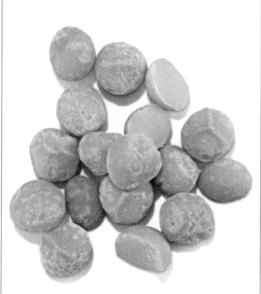

MACADAMIA

Australian scientists found that men with high cholesterol who ate 12 to 16 macadamia nuts a day raised their HDL (good) cholesterol levels by 8 percent. "Because macadamia nuts contain the highest amount of monounsaturated fat of all nuts, this degree of HDL-raising effect may be unique to them," says Manohar Garg, PhD, the study's author.

PISTACHIO

Snack on pistachios and you might be able to keep statins shelved. A daily serving or two can lower LDL (bad) cholesterol by up to 12 percent, according to Penn State University scientists. The lipid-lowering effect is likely due to the nuts' content of heart-healthy monounsaturated fats, fiber, and the plant cholesterol phytosterols, says study author Sarah Gebauer, PhD. Researchers have also reported greater weight-loss and blood fat reductions when dieters ate pistachios instead of unsalted pretzels.

SERVING SIZE	1 oz, unsalted, dry-roasted (28 g)			1 oz, unsalted, dry-roasted (28 g)		
Calories/Fiber	Calories: 203	Fiber: 2 g		Calories: 161	Fiber: 3 g	
Macronutrients	Protein: 2 g	Fat: 21 g	Carbs: 4 g	Protein: 6 g	Fat: 13 g	Carbs: 8 g
Vitamins/Minerals	Manganese: 43%	Thiamin: 13%		Copper: 19%	Manganese: 18%	Vitamin B6: 18%

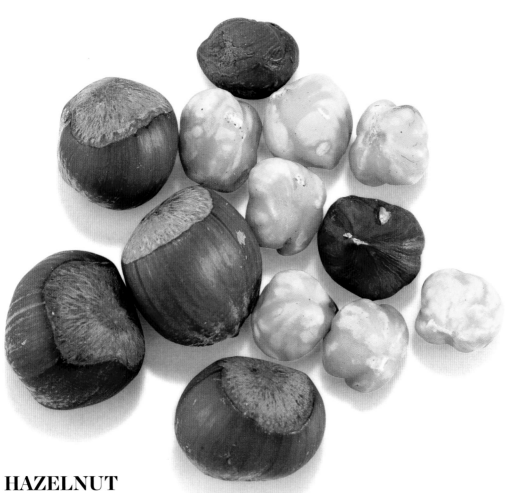

THE PERFECT SNACK FOOD

The high protein content in nuts makes them supremely satiating—the filling feeling that will keep you from overeating. And, according to a study in the *Journal of Nutrition*, your body simply can't absorb all the fat in nuts, so eating them won't cause extra pounds to weigh you down. Plus, researchers from Georgia Southern University found that eating a high-protein, high-fat snack can increase your calorie burn for more than 3 hours!

HAZELNUT

Men who ate a handful of hazelnuts daily boosted their HDL (good) cholesterol levels by 12 percent, according to a study in the *European Journal of Clinical Nutrition*. They're also rich in arginine, an amino acid that the body uses to build muscle as well as relax blood vessels, which in turn lowers blood pressure.

1 oz, unsalted, dry-roasted (28 g)		
Calories: 181		Fiber: 3 g
Protein: 4 g	Fat: 17 g	Carbs: 5 g
Manganese: 78%	Copper: 25%	Vitamin E: 21%

Seeds | THE HEALTHIEST FOODS IN THE WORLD

When you say seeds, you think birds. Don't. The foods in this section are serious nutritional powerhouses, and they are easy to add to so many other foods because, well, they're seeds. They're also easy to snack on all by themselves (just ask a finch).

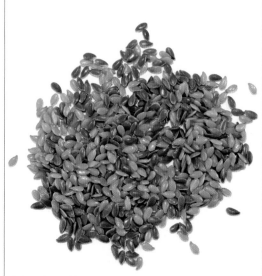

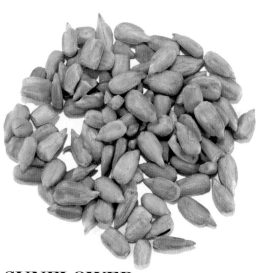

FLAXSEED

In addition to its protein and fiber, flaxseed—with 2,338 milligrams of omega-3 per serving—is a top source of alpha-linolenic acid (ALA), a type of omega-3 fatty acid that improves the workings of the brain's cerebral cortex, an area that processes sensory information. Your body doesn't process ALA as efficiently as the omega-3 fatty acids in fish oil, but ground flaxseed meal—a great addition to yogurt, cereals, salads, and smoothies—is more easily digested and also contains compounds called lignans that may help boost immune function by fostering healthier gut bacteria.

SUNFLOWER

Eating this snack at baseball games can help you turn back the clock. An ounce of sunflower seeds and almonds contain almost the same amount of vitamin E, which is one of the most important nutrients for looking younger, according to Barry Swanson, PhD, a professor of food science at Washington State University. "No antioxidant is more effective at fighting the aging effects of free radicals," he says. Just remember to wear sunscreen to prevent wrinkles—and opt for low-sodium seeds or those with no salt at all.

SERVING SIZE	1 Tbsp, whole (10 g)			1 oz (28 g)		
Calories/Fiber	Calories: 55		Fiber: 3 g	Calories: 168		Fiber: 3 g
Macronutrients	Protein: 2 g	Fat: 4 g	Carbs: 3 g	Protein: 5 g	Fat: 14 g	Carbs: 7 g
Vitamins/Minerals				Vitamin E: 37%	Selenium: 32%	Phosphorus: 32%

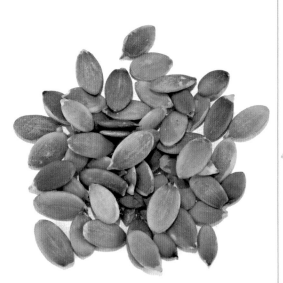

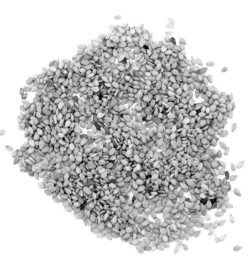

HEMP SEED

Look beyond the cannabis classification of these seeds and you'll appreciate them as an unheralded source of muscle-building protein. Unlike other plant sources that have incomplete proteins, hemp seeds provide all the essential amino acids, meaning their protein is comparable to meat, eggs, and dairy in both quality and amount per serving. Add them to your oatmeal or yogurt for an extra dose of muscle.

Per 4 Tbsp (30 g) serving:
*170 calories,
10 g protein, 5 g carbs,
0 g fiber, 12 g fat,
and RDI of 12% iron*

PUMPKIN SEED

You toss jack-o'-lantern innards into the trash each Halloween, but a few toasted spoonfuls of the seeds is probably the healthiest snack you'll never overlook again. Credit their magnesium, the lightweight mineral that plays a role in more than 300 bodily processes. Men with the highest levels of magnesium have a 40 percent lower risk of early death than those with the lowest levels, according to French researchers. And low levels may also increase your blood levels of C-reactive protein, a key marker of heart disease.

SESAME SEED

Most of us get our sesame seeds on hamburger buns, but sesame seeds are nutty additions (flavor-wise, not sanity-wise) to Indian, Middle Eastern, and Japanese foods. The seeds are rich in iron, copper, manganese, and calcium.

1 oz (28 g)		
Calories: 146	Fiber: 1 g	
Protein: 9 g	Fat: 12 g	Carbs: 4 g
Manganese: 42%	Magnesium: 37%	Iron: 23%

1 oz, whole, roasted and toasted (28 g)		
Calories: 158	Fiber: 4 g	
Protein: 5 g	Fat: 13 g	Carbs: 7 g
Copper: 35%	Calcium: 27%	Iron: 23%

Jelly beans are about the only beans that you shouldn't eat regularly. Try all these varieties for the fiber, protein, and nutritional power packed into such small packages. Plus, study after study reveals that bean eaters live longer and weigh less. In the National Health and Nutrition Examination Survey, scientists found that people who consumed beans were 23 percent less likely to have large waists than those who said they never ate them.

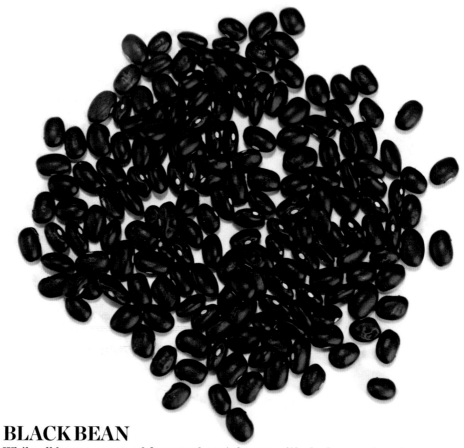

BLACK BEAN

While all beans are good for your heart, beans with darker seed coats possess the most antioxidants—a fact that earns the black variety top marks. Black beans are also the only beans that boost your brainpower, thanks to their being full of antioxidant compounds called anthocyanins, which dilate blood vessels and improve brain function. A cup of black beans also contains about 60 percent of your daily fiber and folate recommendations, as well as 30 percent of your protein. Order them instead of refried beans whenever you eat Mexican food.

SERVING SIZE	1 cup, boiled (172 g)			
Calories/Fiber	Calories: 227		Fiber: 15 g	
Macronutrients	Protein: 15 g	Fat: 1 g	Carbs: 41 g	
Vitamins/Minerals	Folate: 64%	Thiamin: 28%	Iron: 20%	

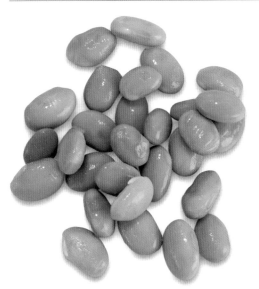

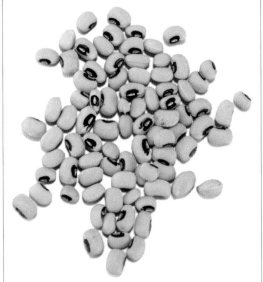

EDAMAME

This is the quintessential Japanese appetizer: soybeans so fresh that they're still in their shells. And unlike the hundreds of food products that contain soy—everything from milk products to veggie burgers—edamame makes a great start to your meal. Working them free from their pods keeps you from eating too quickly, and each bean provides a nourishing mix of protein, fiber, folate, and omega-3 fats.

BLACK-EYED PEA

Traditional Southern cooking takes a lot of potshots for unhealthy ingredients, but the black-eyed pea isn't one of them. They're high in protein and fiber, but if you buy them canned, be sure to drain and rinse them to lower the salt content.

1 cup, frozen, prepared (155 g)		
Calories: 189	Fiber: 8 g	
Protein: 17 g	Fat: 8 g	Carbs: 16 g
Folate: 121%	Vitamin K: 52%	Potassium: 19%

1 cup (260 g)		
Calories: 180	Fiber: 8 g	
Protein: 12 g	Fat: 2 g	Carbs: 32 g
Iron: 20%		

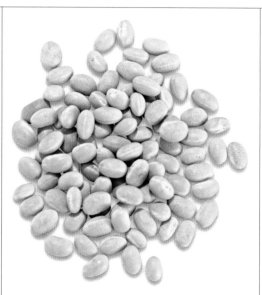

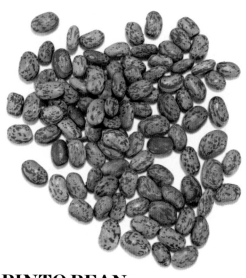

NAVY (WHITE) BEAN

Perfect little fiber bombs, white beans are one of the more versatile beans (baked beans are made out of them). They're also great in chili and stews.

PINTO BEAN

You take a small fiber hit with pinto beans compared with other beans, but they're still loaded with good stuff—the USDA ranks beans as one of the highest antioxidant foods out there.

SERVING SIZE	1 oz (28 g)			1 oz (28 g)		
Calories/Fiber	Calories: 94		Fiber: 6 g	Calories: 97		Fiber: 4 g
Macronutrients	Protein: 7 g	Fat: 0 g	Carbs: 17 g	Protein: 6 g	Fat: 0 g	Carbs: 18 g
Vitamins/Minerals	Folate: 25%			Folate: 37%		

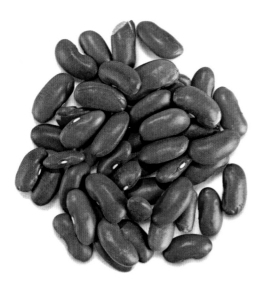

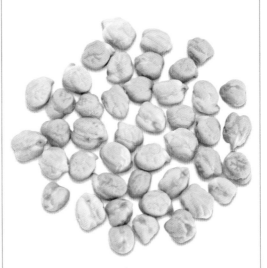

KIDNEY BEAN

These legumes are an excellent source of thiamin and riboflavin. Both vitamins help your body use energy efficiently, so you won't be nodding off mid-PowerPoint.

CHICKPEA/GARBANZO

Like all legumes, chickpeas bring to the table both protein and fiber, the sultans of satiety. Add to that a healthy dose of antioxidants and you have the makings of a salad-topping superstar. Also called garbanzo beans. Garbanzo beans: Also called chickpeas. Don't ask us why.

1 oz (28 g)		
Calories: 93	Fiber: 7 g	
Protein: 7 g	Fat: 0 g	Carbs: 17 g
Folate: 28%	Manganese: 14%	Thiamin: 10%

1 oz (28 g)		
Calories: 102	Fiber: 5 g	
Protein: 5 g	Fat: 2 g	Carbs: 17 g
Folate: 39%	Manganese: 31%	

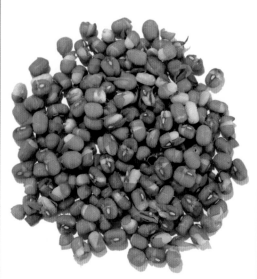

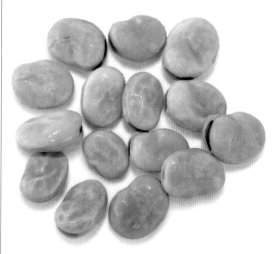

MUNG BEAN

Commonly eaten in China and India, these beans have a tender texture and a sweet flavor. Sure, they're high in potassium, iron, and fiber, but they're also 24 percent protein. What's more, unlike many other legumes, mung beans retain most of their vitamin C even after they're boiled. Toss boiled mung beans into your next salad. Their natural sweetness will add flavor without piling on excess calories or sodium.

FAVA

Also known as broadbeans, they may look like the lima beans you were fed as a kid, but with their big, meaty flavor and tons of protein, folate, and fiber, few legumes are more worthy of your adult palate. To prepare, remove the beans from their pods and boil them in water for 3 minutes. Drain and cool the beans, and peel off the white outer shells. Now you can scatter the beans on salads and pasta dishes. Or try this: Throw 2 cups of favas into a blender with a minced garlic clove, the juice of a lemon, and a drizzle of olive oil. Blend until smooth, season, and slather the puree on grilled salmon.

SERVING SIZE	1 oz (28 g)			1 cup, raw, in pod (126 g)		
Calories/Fiber	Calories: 97		Fiber: 5 g	Calories: 111		Fiber: 0 g
Macronutrients	Protein: 7 g	Fat: 0 g	Carbs: 18 g	Protein: 10 g	Fat: 1 g	Carbs: 22 g
Vitamins/Minerals	Folate: 44%	Manganese: 14%	Vitamin C: 2%	Folate: 47%	Manganese: 42%	

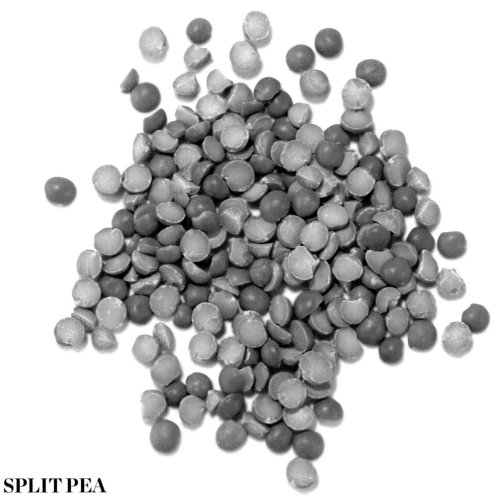

SPLIT PEA

Best known for making split-pea soup, split peas bring on the legume power with B vitamins (especially folate and thiamin), manganese, and a body-cleansing 16 grams of fiber per cup. When you're talking comfort food in the cold weather months, it's hard to find a healthier soup ingredient.

1 cup, cooked (196 g)		
Calories: 231		Fiber: 16 g
Protein: 16 g	Fat: 1 g	Carbs: 41 g
Manganese: 39%	Folate: 32%	

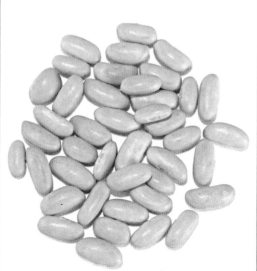

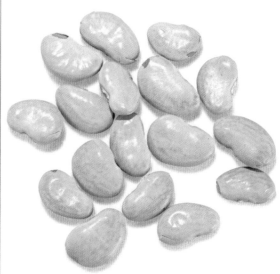

CANNELLINI BEAN

A classic Italian white bean that's great for soups and salads, bruschette and crostini. Be sure to drain and rinse the canned varieties to lower the salt content.

LIMA BEAN (BUTTER BEAN)

Originating in South America (named after Lima, Peru), their heartiness makes them a good soup bean. Try them in burritos, too.

SERVING SIZE	1 cup (262 g)			½ cup, boiled (188 g)		
Calories/Fiber	Calories: 200		Fiber: 10 g	Calories: 216		Fiber: 13 g
Macronutrients	Protein: 12 g	Fat: 2 g	Carbs: 34 g	Protein: 15 g	Fat: 1 g	Carbs: 39 g
Vitamins/Minerals	Iron: 20%			Manganese: 49%	Folate: 39%	

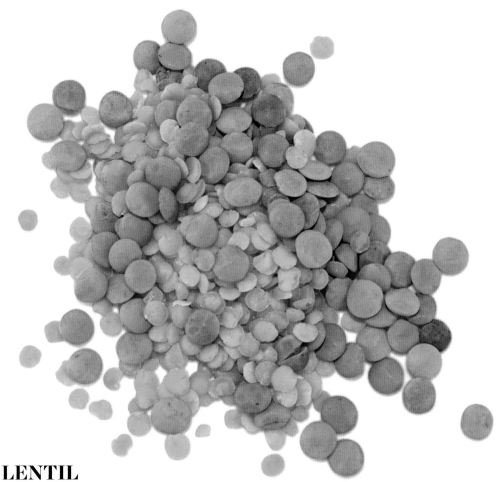

LENTIL

It's no surprise that these hearty legumes are good for you. But when was the last time you ate any? Boiled lentils have about 16 grams of belly-filling fiber in every cup. Cooked lentils also contain 27 percent more folate per cup than cooked spinach. They're also packed with protein, not to mention B vitamins and zinc, which are important for good sexual health.

1 cup, boiled, unsalted (198 g)		
Calories: 230		Fiber: 16 g
Protein: 18 g	Fat: 1 g	Carbs: 40 g
Folate: 90%	Iron: 37%	

Common Fruits | THE HEALTHIEST FOODS IN THE WORLD

You cannot escape the word "common" here. These fruits are available everywhere all year round, they're portable, and they're damn delicious, so you have no excuse for not sampling at least a couple a day (is there any better or easier 2 p.m. office snack than an apple?). Put a bowlful where you can see them.

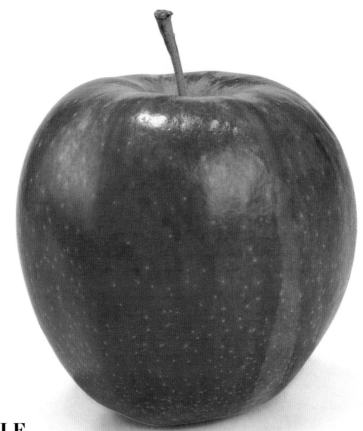

APPLE

The most popular source of antioxidants in our diet, one apple has an antioxidant effect equivalent to 1,500 milligrams of vitamin C. They lower bad cholesterol, thanks to plant sterols, and benefit diabetics by lowering blood sugar. They're also rich in amino acids, which bolster testosterone levels and muscle growth. An apple a day delivers quercetin, a flavonoid that reduces the risk of allergies, heart attack, Alzheimer's, Parkinson's, and prostate and lung cancers. Even the classic Red Delicious is a great choice. They contain the most inflammation-fighting antioxidants.

SERVING SIZE	1 medium (3" diameter)		
Calories/Fiber	Calories: 95		Fiber: 4 g
Macronutrients	Protein: 0 g	Fat: 0 g	Carbs: 25 g
Vitamins/Minerals	Vitamin C: 14%		

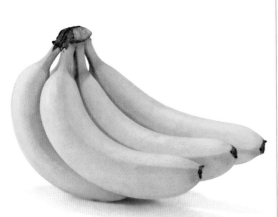

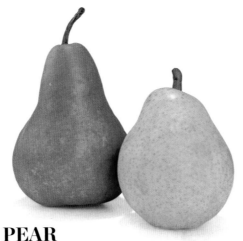

BANANA

One of the top food sources of vitamin B$_6$, bananas help reduce fatigue, depression, stress, and insomnia. Bananas are high in magnesium, which keeps bones strong, and potassium, which helps prevent heart disease and high blood pressure. Bananas also bolster the nervous system, boost immune function, and help the body metabolize protein.

PEAR

Pears aren't usually spoken about with the same nutritional "ooos" and "ahhhs" as apples, which are rightfully regarded as a superfood. Still, a single pear has more fiber than an apple, comparable vitamin C, and only a few more calories and carbs. When picking pears, you want a pleasant fragrance and some softness at the stem end. A bit of brown discoloration is fine. Ripen them at room temperature in a loosely closed paper bag.

1 medium (7"–8" long)		
Calories: 105	Fiber: 3 g	
Protein: 1 g	Fat: 0 g	Carbs: 27 g
Vitamin B$_6$: 22%	Vitamin C: 17%	Potassium: 12%

1 medium (178 g)		
Calories: 103	Fiber: 6 g	
Protein: 1 g	Fat: 0 g	Carbs: 28 g
Vitamin C: 12%	Vitamin K: 10%	

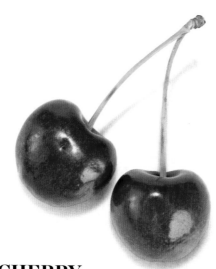

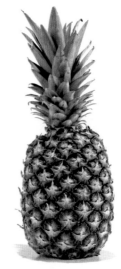

CHERRY

Research by the US Department of Agriculture shows that eating up to 45 bing cherries a day can lower the risk of tendinitis, bursitis, arthritis, and gout. (Forty-five is a lot, so focus on the "up to" part of that sentence.) Studies also suggest that they reduce the risk of chronic diseases and metabolic syndrome. They also taste great on yogurt or cereal.

PINEAPPLE

With its potent mix of vitamins, antioxidants, and enzymes (in particular, bromelain), pineapple is an all-body anti-inflammation cocktail. It also protects against colon cancer, arthritis, and macular degeneration. If only the "colada" part of the equation were as healthy.

SERVING SIZE	1 cup, with pits (138 g)			1 cup, chunks (165 g)		
Calories/Fiber	Calories: 87		Fiber: 3 g	Calories: 82		Fiber: 2 g
Macronutrients	Protein: 1 g	Fat: 0 g	Carbs: 22 g	Protein: 1 g	Fat: 0 g	Carbs: 22 g
Vitamins/Minerals	Vitamin C: 16%			Vitamin C: 131%	Manganese: 76%	

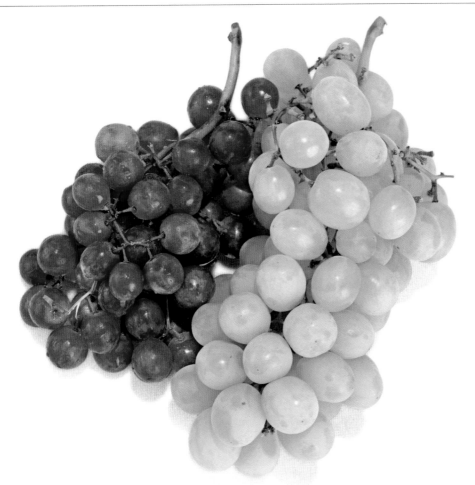

GRAPE LEAVES

You'll usually find these briny, refreshing staples of Greek and Middle Eastern cuisine sold in jars. Grape leaves are a good source of iron, vitamins A and C, and anthocyanins, the same flavonoids in wine that may protect you from disease. For an appetizer or snack, you can wrap them around a stuffing of rice, herbs, and spices. Find stuffed grape leaves (a.k.a. dolmas) at the olive bar in most supermarkets.

GRAPE (RED OR GREEN)

Red grapes and wine contain the potent antioxidant resveratrol, which is thought to fight cancer and heart disease. While this compound isn't as prevalent in the green grapes from which raisins are made, greenies are still a terrific source of vitamins C and K. Note: Most of the calories in grapes come from sugar.

1 cup, red or green (151 g)			
Calories: 104		Fiber: 1 g	
Protein: 1 g	Fat: 0 g	Carbs: 27 g	
Vitamin K: 28%	Vitamin C: 27%		

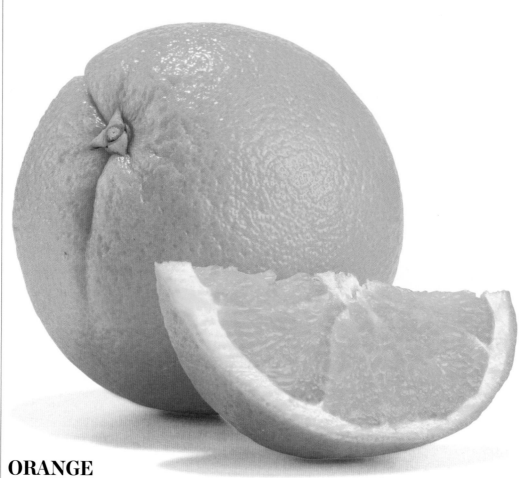

ORANGE

One of our finest natural sources of vitamin C. But the best way to get the full benefit of the fiber content is to avoid orange juice—which is usually stripped of fiber and packed with sugar—and eat the fruit itself.

SERVING SIZE	1 large (3" diameter)		
Calories/Fiber	Calories: 86		Fiber: 4 g
Macronutrients	Protein: 2 g	Fat: 0 g	Carbs: 22 g
Vitamins/Minerals	Vitamin C: 163%	Folate: 14%	

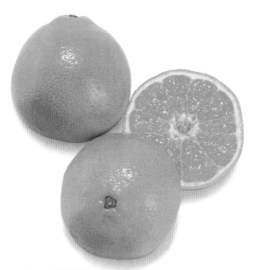

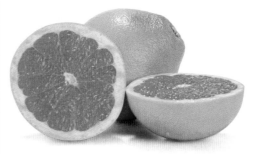

TANGERINE

When researchers recently analyzed the eating habits of 857 people who'd participated in a National Cancer Institute study, they discovered that those who took in three servings of lutein- and zeaxanthin-rich produce daily were 46 percent less likely to develop non-Hodgkin's lymphoma than the folks who ate less of those foods. Tangerines (along with spinach, kale, corn, broccoli, kiwi, and honeydew) made the list of recommended sources.

GRAPEFRUIT (PINK AND RUBY RED)

Just call it the better-body fruit. In a study of 100 obese people at the Scripps Clinic in California, those who ate half a grapefruit with each meal for 12 weeks lost nearly 4 pounds more than those who skipped grapefruit. (See "A Grapefruit Diet That Works?" at right.) Those who ate the grapefruit also exhibited a decrease in insulin levels, indicating that their bodies had improved upon the ability to metabolize sugar. Loaded with vitamin C, grapefruit also contains natural compounds called limonoids, which can lower cholesterol. The red varieties are a potent source of the cancer-fighting substance lycopene.

A GRAPEFRUIT DIET THAT WORKS?

Several studies have found that eating grapefruit three times a day leads to significant weight loss. In one study, subjects dropped pounds even though they hadn't deliberately altered any other part of their diets. They also lowered their blood pressure by 6 points, enough to reduce their risk of stroke by 40 percent. Although the mechanism isn't clear, researchers speculate that grapefruit's acidity may slow your rate of digestion, helping to keep you full longer. The scientists note that for weight loss, substituting 8 ounces of juice for each serving of the fruit is just as effective.

1 medium fruit (2½" diameter)		
Calories: 47	Fiber: 2 g	
Protein: 1 g	Fat: 0 g	Carbs: 12 g
Vitamin C: 39%	Vitamin A: 12%	

½ grapefruit (3¾" diameter)		
Calories: 52	Fiber: 2 g	
Protein: 1 g	Fat: 0 g	Carbs: 13 g
Vitamin C: 64%	Vitamin A: 28%	

ORANGE YA GLAD?

Citrus fruits are best known for vitamin C, of course, but they also deliver fiber and boost the blood's alkaline levels, which helps heal wounds faster, says Gay Riley, MS, RD, CCN, author of *The Pocket Personal Trainer*. They'll also make your blood less acidic, which cuts inflammation. If that's not enough? Collagen is abundant in connective tissues, tendons, bones, and muscles, and vitamin C is a key component of your body's collagen recipe.

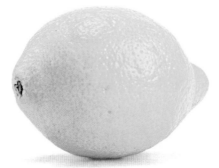

LEMON

Bursting with fiber and vitamin C, lemons are like a healthy version of salt: They enhance the flavor of everything. Italians love lemon juice so much that they use it instead of vinegar in salad dressings. For a quick pasta dish, mix the juice of three lemons with a tablespoon of olive oil and then toss it with spaghetti. Add Parmesan, pepper, a teaspoon of lemon zest, and chopped basil.

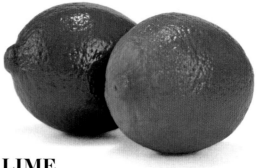

LIME

Limes are the classic ingredient. If you always keep a few on hand, your fish, homemade salsa, stir-fry, and even your domestic beers will taste better for it. The difference between a lemon and a lime? Lemons have about four times as much vitamin C.

SERVING SIZE	1 fruit, without seeds			1 fruit (2" diameter)		
Calories/Fiber	Calories: 22		Fiber: 5 g	Calories: 20		Fiber: 2 g
Macronutrients	Protein: 1 g	Fat: 0 g	Carbs: 12 g	Protein: 0 g	Fat: 0 g	Carbs: 7 g
Vitamins/Minerals	Vitamin C: 139%			Vitamin C: 32%		

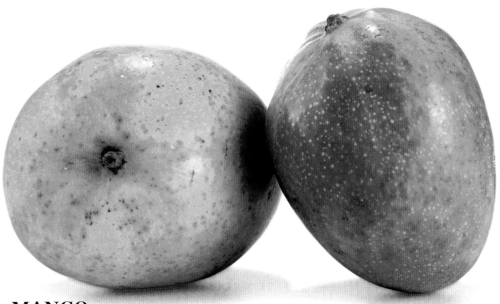

MANGO

Add some frozen mango to your next smoothie. Packed with vitamins A and C, mangoes add a healthy dose of beta-carotene, which may help prevent cancer and promotes healthy skin.

1 cup, sliced (165 g)			
Calories: 107		Fiber: 3 g	
Protein: 1 g	Fat: 0 g	Carbs: 28 g	
Vitamin C: 76%	Vitamin A: 25%	Vitamin B$_6$: 11%	

Stone Fruits | THE HEALTHIEST FOODS IN THE WORLD

Sweet, succulent, and loaded with vitamins, stone fruits (named that way because biting into their pits is like chomping on a rock) are generally available year-round, but when they're available locally in-season, there really is no substitute.

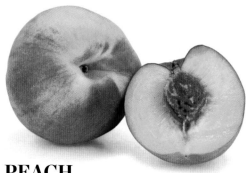

PEACH

Being pretty as a peach comes at a price. The fruit is often doused with pesticides in the weeks prior to harvest to ensure blemish-free skin. By the time it arrives in your supermarket's produce department, the typical peach can be coated with up to nine different pesticides, according to USDA sampling. At the supermarket: Fill your plastic produce bag with peaches that wear a "USDA Organic" sticker.

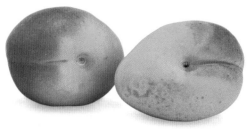

APRICOT

You won't find many low-calorie foods with the same nutritional payoff: 1 cup of apricot slices delivers 3 grams of fiber and more than half a day's worth of vitamin A. Plus, it's a good source of potassium—and all for 74 calories.

SERVING SIZE	1 medium fruit (2⅔" diameter)			1 cup, halved		
Calories/Fiber	Calories: 59		Fiber: 2 g	Calories: 74		Fiber: 3 g
Macronutrients	Protein: 1 g	Fat: 0 g	Carbs: 15 g	Protein: 2 g	Fat: 1 g	Carbs: 17 g
Vitamins/Minerals	Vitamin C: 17%			Vitamin A: 60%		

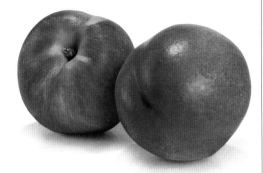

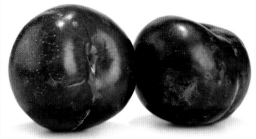

NECTARINE

There may be no more succulent treat than a ripe nectarine in summer. Not as nutritionally dense as peaches or apricots, they still supply small doses of vitamins A and C, and potassium.

PLUM

Nutritionally the weakest stone sister, with small amounts of vitamins A, C, and K, and potassium. But plums are still a low-calorie version of a Jolly Rancher. The next time you face a 2 p.m. office slump, scarf a plum and let the tart flavor wake you right up.

1 medium fruit		
Calories: 62	Fiber: 2 g	
Protein: 2 g	Fat: 0 g	Carbs: 15 g
Vitamin C: 13%	Vitamin A: 9%	Potassium: 8%

1 fruit		
Calories: 30	Fiber: 1 g	
Protein: 0 g	Fat: 0 g	Carbs: 8 g
Vitamin C: 10%	Vitamin K: 5%	Vitamin A: 5%

On first glance, you might think, what are these things? Answer: great additions to your diet. "Exotic fruits tend to be higher in vitamin C, higher in potassium, and lower in calories than typical American produce," says Leslie Bonci, MPH, RD, LDN, director of sports nutrition at the University of Pittsburgh Medical Center. Plus, they taste great. These are your best bets.

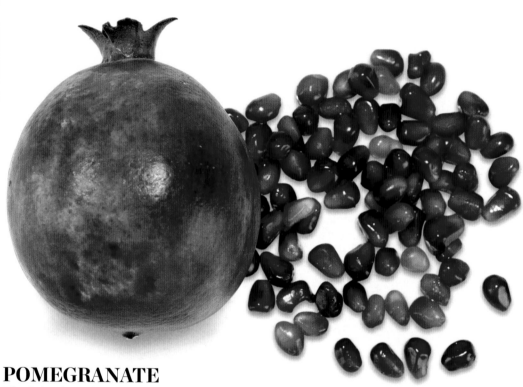

POMEGRANATE

The juice from the biblical fruit of many seeds can reduce your risk of most cancers, thanks to polyphenols called ellagitannins, which give the fruit its color. In fact, a recent study at UCLA found that pomegranate juice slows the growth of prostate cancer cells by a factor of six. It will liven up any protein you put under it: salmon, pork tenderloin, even that tired old turkey. Peak season: October to January.

SERVING SIZE	1 fruit (4" diameter)		
Calories/Fiber	Calories: 234		Fiber: 11 g
Macronutrients	Protein: 5 g	Fat: 3 g	Carbs: 53 g
Vitamins/Minerals	Vitamin K: 58%	Vitamin C: 48%	Folate: 27%

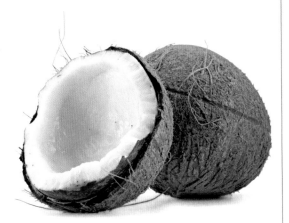

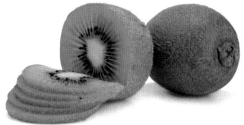

COCONUT

Ounce for ounce, coconut contains even more saturated fat than butter—119 percent of your recommended daily intake, per cup. Still, it appears to have a beneficial effect on heart-disease risk factors. One reason: More than 50 percent of its saturated-fat content is lauric acid. A recent analysis of 60 studies published in the *American Journal of Clinical Nutrition* reports that even though lauric acid raises LDL (bad) cholesterol, it boosts HDL (good) cholesterol even more. Overall, this means it decreases your risk of cardio-vascular disease.

KIWI

Ounce for ounce, kiwis pack more vitamin C than oranges do, says David Grotto, RD, the author of *101 Optimal Life Foods*. "Kiwis, which are actually giant berries, are also packed with fiber, potassium, and vitamin E," he says. "For maximum nutritional benefit, eat them like apples, skin and all."

1 cup, shredded (80 g)		
Calories: 283	Fiber: 7 g	
Protein: 3 g	Fat: 27 g	Carbs: 12 g
Manganese: 60%	Selenium: 12%	

1 medium fruit		
Calories: 46	Fiber: 2 g	
Protein: 1 g	Fat: 0 g	Carbs: 11 g
Vitamin C: 117%	Vitamin K: 38%	Potassium: 7%

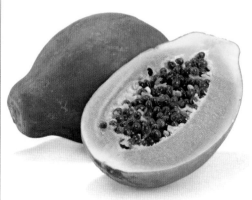

PAPAYA

With about a full day's worth of vitamin C, a medium-size papaya can help kick a cold right out of your system. The beta-carotene and vitamins C and E in papayas also reduce inflammation throughout the body, lessening the effects of asthma. Native to Central and South America, papaya is the best known source of papain—an enzyme so efficient at breaking down protein that it's used commercially to tenderize meat. Cut the fruit in half and scoop out the juicy flesh, or grind up the seeds and use them as a black-pepper substitute.

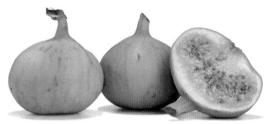

FIG

Excluding the eponymous cookie, most Americans have a strained relationship with the fig. Too bad, because they're explosively sweet and flavorful, and loaded with belly-filling fiber. Slice some raw and eat with a hunk of blue cheese and almonds. Peak season: June to August.

SERVING SIZE	1 cup, cubed (140 g)		
Calories/Fiber	Calories: 55	Fiber: 3 g	
Macronutrients	Protein: 1 g	Fat: 0 g	Carbs: 14 g
Vitamins/Minerals	Vitamin C: 144%	Vitamin A: 31%	Folate: 13%

SERVING SIZE	1 large fruit (2½" diameter)		
Calories/Fiber	Calories: 47	Fiber: 2 g	
Macronutrients	Protein: 0 g	Fat: 0 g	Carbs: 12 g
Vitamins/Minerals	Folate: 4%	Vitamin K: 4%	Potassium: 4%

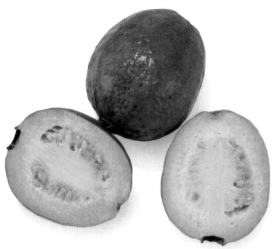

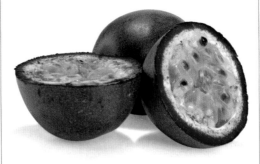

GUAVA

Guava is an obscure tropical fruit that's subtly acidic, with sweetness that intensifies as you eat your way to the center. Guava has a higher concentration of lycopene—an antioxidant that fights prostate cancer—than any other fruit or vegetable, including tomatoes and watermelon. In addition, 1 cup of the stuff provides 688 milligrams of potassium, which is 63 percent more than you'll find in a medium banana. And guava may be the ultimate high-fiber food: There's almost 9 grams of fiber in every cup. Down the entire fruit, from the rind to the seeds. It's all edible—and nutritious.

PASSION FRUIT

This South American fruit is packed with vision-protecting vitamin A and more cholesterol-lowering fiber than your average textile mill—a single serving has 25 grams, a full day's worth, plus potassium twice that of a banana. Cut the fruit in half and eat the pulp with a spoon, or use it as a topping for ice cream. Make sure you eat the seeds—that's where the fiber is stored.

1 cup (165 g)		
Calories: 112	Fiber: 9 g	
Protein: 4 g	Fat: 2 g	Carbs: 24 g
Vitamin C: 628%	Folate: 20%	Potassium: 20%

1 cup (236 g)		
Calories: 229	Fiber: 25 g	
Protein: 5 g	Fat: 2 g	Carbs: 55 g
Vitamin C: 118%	Vitamin A: 60%	Potassium: 23%

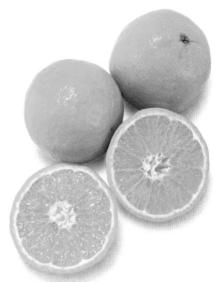

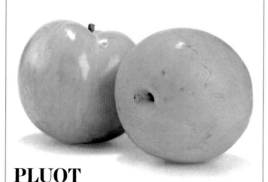

PLUOT

This luscious love child of an apricot and a plum (pronounced *plew-ott*) is one of our favorite signs of summer—a low-cal fiber delivery system. One bite and you'll understand why one of the most popular pluot varieties is called Flavor Grenade. Peak season: May to September.

LIMEQUAT

Snacking on three of these bite-size nuggets provides about 20 percent of your daily fiber, which may help tamp down your blood pressure and cholesterol levels and lower your risk of type-2 diabetes. Eat them as you would kumquats, skin and all. Season: July to November.

SERVING SIZE	1 fruit			3 fruits		
Calories/Fiber	Calories: 80		Fiber: 3 g	Calories: 60		Fiber: 6 g
Macronutrients	Protein: 1 g	Fat: 0 g	Carbs: 19 g	Protein: 0 g	Fat: 0 g	Carbs: 21 g
Vitamins/Minerals				Vitamin C: 106%		

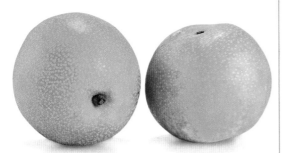

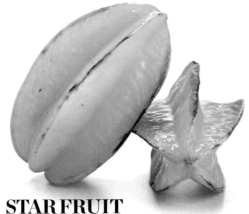

ASIAN PEAR

Subtly sweet, mildly tart, and perfectly crisp, the Asian pear just may be a flawless fruit. It packs a heavy punch of flavonoids, known to reduce the risk of cardiovascular disease. Quick recipe: Toss 4 cups mixed greens with a thinly sliced pear, half a sliced red onion, ¼ cup toasted pecans, ¼ cup crumbled goat cheese, and enough olive oil and balsamic vinegar to cover lightly.

STAR FRUIT

Native to Asia, star fruit—also known as carambola—is low in calories and high in vitamin C. It's also a great source of polyphenols, antioxidants that fight cardiovascular inflammation. Plus, it's unusually delicious—the flavor is best described as that of an ultrasweet tropical plum. It's in season from July through September. You can eat star fruit whole—skin included—or slice it into little stars and feel like a kid again.

1 fruit			
Calories: 51		Fiber: 4 g	
Protein: 1 g	Fat: 0 g		Carbs: 13 g
Vitamin C: 8%			

1 medium fruit (3⅝" long)			
Calories: 28		Fiber: 3 g	
Protein: 1 g	Fat: 0 g		Carbs: 6 g
Vitamin C: 52%	Potassium: 3%		Vitamin A: 1%

Berries are a must-eat food, dense with antioxidants and other powerful nutrients that defend against everything from cancer to memory loss. Eat by the handful, in a smoothie, or toss a pint of your favorite berries with a bag of mixed greens, toasted walnuts, and crumbled goat cheese.

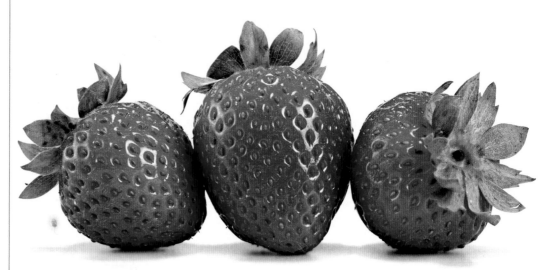

STRAWBERRY

During winter months, strawberries probably travel a long way to get to you. Seek out unblemished berries with a bright-red color extending to the stem, and a strong fruity smell. They're neither hard nor mushy. Ideal storage: Place unwashed berries in a single layer on a paper towel in a covered container in your refrigerator.

SERVING SIZE	1 cup, halves (152 g)		
Calories/Fiber	Calories: 49		Fiber: 3 g
Macronutrients	Protein: 1 g	Fat: 0 g	Carbs: 12 g
Vitamins/Minerals	Vitamin C: 149%	Manganese: 29%	

ARONIA BERRY (CHOKE-BERRY)

Once revered by Native Americans as a miracle fruit, this tiny, tart berry has resurfaced as a superfood. No fruit packs more anthocyanins, potent cancer-fighting antioxidants that lend the berry its deep purple color. Because of this, aronia has been shown to fight cardiovascular disease, chronic inflammation, and even liver damage in rats.

Per 1-cup serving:
*47 calories,
1.4 g protein,
9.6 g carbs, 5 g fiber,
0.5 g fat, and RDI
of 35 % vitamin C*

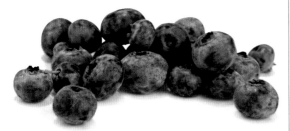

BLUEBERRY

"This potent little fruit can help prevent a range of diseases, from cancer to heart disease," says Ryan Andrews, the director of research at Precision Nutrition in Toronto, Canada. A mere 3.5 ounces contains more antioxidants than any other fruit. Drizzle with lemon juice and mix with strawberries for a disease-fighting supersnack.

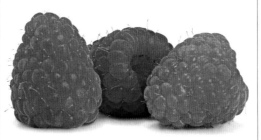

RASPBERRY

Don't let the tart sweetness fool you. Raspberries contain anthocyanins, which boost insulin production and lower blood sugar levels, providing a strong defense against diabetes.

1 cup (148 g)		
Calories: 84		Fiber: 4 g
Protein: 1 g	Fat: 0 g	Carbs: 21 g
Vitamin K: 36%	Vitamin C: 24%	Manganese: 25%

1 cup (123 g)		
Calories: 64		Fiber: 8 g
Protein: 1 g	Fat: 1 g	Carbs: 15 g
Vitamin C: 54%	Manganese: 41%	Vitamin K: 12%

153

BLACK CURRANTS

Fresh berries are always great, but black currant jelly is also a good source of quercetin—an antioxidant that Finnish researchers believe may improve heart health by preventing the buildup of the free radicals that can damage arterial walls and allow plaque to penetrate.

Per 1-cup (112 g) serving:
71 calories, 2 g protein, 17 g carbs, 0 g fiber, 0 g fat, and RDI of 338% vitamin C

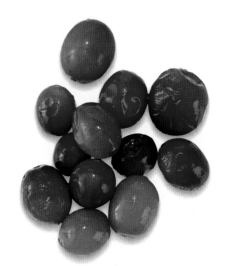

CRANBERRY

Cranberries have more antioxidants than most other common fruits and vegetables. One serving has five times the amount found in broccoli. Cranberries are a natural probiotic, enhancing good bacteria levels in the gut and protecting it from foodborne illnesses. But beware: They're so tart that most any cranberry products are loaded with sugar—so find ones with the least sugar content you can.

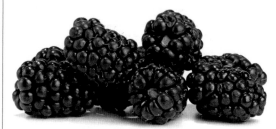

BLACK RASPBERRY (BLACKBERRY)

Shop around for black raspberries, which have 40 percent more antioxidants than the red kind, according to lab tests. They're so sweet and juicy you can substitute them for jelly in a PB&J.

SERVING SIZE	1 cup, whole (100 g)			1 cup (144 g)		
Calories/Fiber	Calories: 46		Fiber: 5 g	Calories: 62		Fiber: 8 g
Macronutrients	Protein: 0 g	Fat: 0 g	Carbs: 12 g	Protein: 2 g	Fat: 1 g	Carbs: 15 g
Vitamins/Minerals	Vitamin C: 22%	Manganese: 18%		Vitamin C: 50%	Manganese: 47%	Vitamin K: 36%

GOLDEN-BERRIES

These tangy, dark yellow berries are native to South America, where they're sold fresh or made into preserves. In the United States, you're more likely to find the fruit dried and bagged. Besides protein and fiber, they're also a great source of vitamin A and disease-fighting antioxidants. Snack on the dried berries alone like you would raisins, or toss a handful on a salad or your breakfast cereal.

Per 1-cup serving:
70 calories, 3 g protein, 16 g carbs, 4 g fiber, 1 g fat, and RDIs of 25% vitamin C and 20% vitamin A

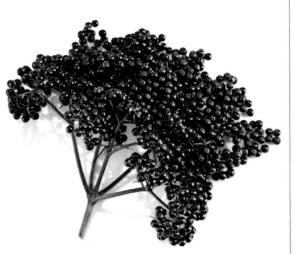

ELDERBERRY

The Monty Pythoners would have you believe that smelling of elderberries is an offensive thing. It's actually quite intelligent, assuming you've eaten them and not just smeared them on your tunic, as a cup will give you nearly a day's worth of vitamin C.

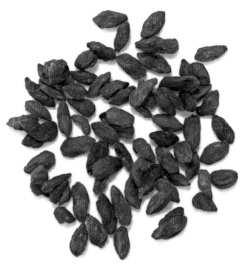

GOJI BERRY (WOLFBERRY)

No need to pay $35 for 1 liter of goji juice. Whole berries can be bought in many Asian markets for a fraction of the price. They taste like a cross between a cranberry and a cherry. The bitter-sweet berries are packed with the phytochemicals beta-carotene and zeaxanthin, which studies have shown reduce the risk of lung and bladder cancers. Goji berries are also unique among fruits for their ability to reduce LDL (bad) cholesterol and raise HDL (good) cholesterol. Serving tip: Use dried goji berries like cranberries. Add them to your favorite trail mix or sprinkle them on top of cereals and stews.

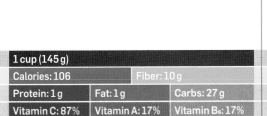

1 cup (145 g)			
Calories: 106		Fiber: 10 g	
Protein: 1 g	Fat: 1 g		Carbs: 27 g
Vitamin C: 87%	Vitamin A: 17%		Vitamin B₆: 17%

5 Tbsp (28 g)			
Calories: 112		Fiber: 3 g	
Protein: 1 g	Fat: 0 g		Carbs: 24 g
Vitamin A: 170%	Vitamin C: 20%		

155

Melons are a terrific sweet substitute for anyone who wants to follow the E-A-T-S plan (page 32) and cut down on added sugars. Cantaloupe and honeydew provide slow-digesting carbs that help assuage the craving for bread. Plus, the sweetness of a fresh scoop seems like dessert after you've cut down on candy and baked goods.

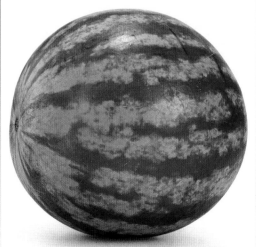

WATERMELON

Eating watermelon could help your heart. USDA scientists found that people who drank six 8-ounce cups of watermelon juice daily for 3 weeks experienced a 22 percent increase in their levels of arginine—an amino acid that boosts bloodflow to your ticker. Credit watermelon's high content of citrulline, a nutrient your body converts to arginine. Can't manage six cups? Smaller amounts help, too.

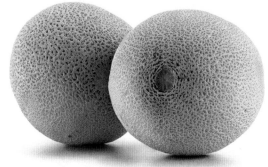

CANTALOUPE

When the FDA sampled domestically grown cantaloupe, it found that 3.5 percent of the melons carried salmonella and shigella, the latter being a bacteria normally passed person-to-person. When selecting melons, try to find perfect skin. Dents or bruising on the fruit can provide a path in for pathogens.

SERVING SIZE	1 cup, balled (154 g)			1 cup, balled (177 g)		
Calories/Fiber	Calories: 46		Fiber: 1 g	Calories: 60		Fiber: 2 g
Macronutrients	Protein: 1 g	Fat: 0 g	Carbs: 12 g	Protein: 1 g	Fat: 0 g	Carbs: 16 g
Vitamins/Minerals	Vitamin C: 21%	Vitamin A: 18%		Vitamin A: 120%	Vitamin C: 108%	Potassium: 14%

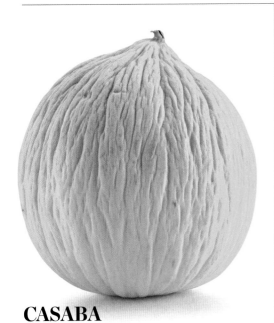

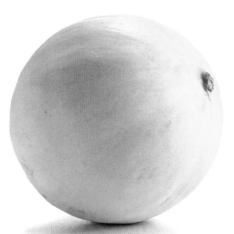

TUSCAN MELON

Boasting three parents, this fruit is a combination of the sweet cantaloupe, the aromatic Charentais melon, and the juicy muskmelon. Not only is the Tuscan melon rich in vision- and skin-fortifying vitamin A, but it's also high in vitamin C. Season: May to September

Per ¼ melon serving: *50 calories, 0 g protein, 12 g carbs, 1 g fiber, 0 g fat, with RDIs of 101% vitamin A and 80% vitamin C*

CASABA

The default picnic melons share these pages, but casaba—loaded up with B and C vitamins—are a sweet change from the old stalwarts. They're great raw. The flesh should be a rich yellow color with very little green. They should also be firm with a little give at the stem. Avoid soft flesh and blemishes.

HONEYDEW

In a study of 14,000 people, Cornell scientists found that those who ate the most candy also downed the most fruit. The connection, of course, is that both taste sweet. Honeydew and other melons are perfect substitutes for a guy with a sweet tooth, especially if you crave soft sweets like marshmallows.

1 cup, cubed (170 g)		
Calories: 48	Fiber: 2 g	
Protein: 2 g	Fat: 0 g	Carbs: 11 g
Vitamin C: 62%	Vitamin B₆: 14%	

1 cup, balled (177 g)		
Calories: 64 g	Fiber: 1 g	
Protein: 1 g	Fat: 0 g	Carbs: 16 g
Vitamin C: 53%	Potassium: 12%	

Snack smart. Hauling fresh produce around isn't always realistic. That's why dehydrated fruit is one of the best snacks—it's portable, it has the same nutrients as the hydrated version, and it's cool because astronauts eat it too.

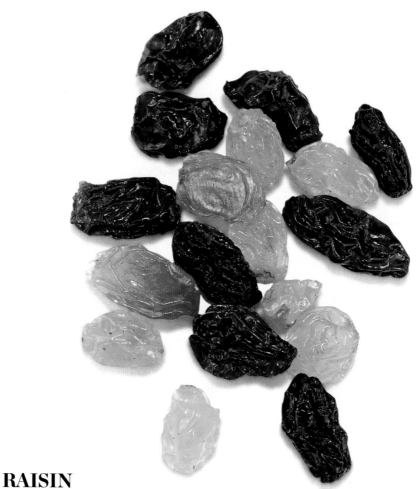

RAISIN

According to a University of Maine study, the drying process converts green grapes' fructose molecules to fructan, a type of fiber that can absorb cholesterol. Data suggests that eating a half cup of raisins daily can lower LDL (bad) cholesterol levels in patients with high cholesterol.

SERVING SIZE	1 oz (60 raisins)			
Calories/Fiber	Calories: 84		Fiber: 1 g	
Macronutrients	Protein: 1 g	Fat: 0 g	Carbs: 22 g	
Vitamins/Minerals	Potassium: 7%	Vitamin C: 3%		

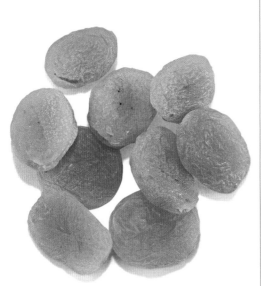

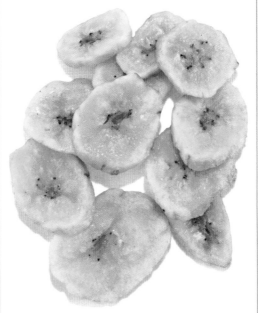

DRIED APRICOT

A portable food with a big nutritional payoff: 1 cup of dried apricot halves delivers 9 grams of fiber and almost your entire recommended daily intake of vitamin A, and is a good source of potassium and vitamin E.

BANANA CHIP

One of the top food sources of vitamin B_6, bananas help reduce fatigue, depression, stress, and insomnia. Bananas are high in magnesium, which keeps bones strong, and potassium, which helps prevent heart disease and high blood pressure. Bananas also bolster the nervous system, boost immune function, and help the body metabolize protein.

1 cup (130 g)		
Calories: 313	Fiber: 9 g	
Protein: 4 g	Fat: 1 g	Carbs: 81 g
Vitamin A: 94%	Potassium: 43%	Vitamin E: 28%

1 oz (¼ cup, 28 g)		
Calories: 145	Fiber: 2 g	
Protein: 1 g	Fat: 9 g	Carbs: 16 g
Manganese: 22%	Potassium: 4%	

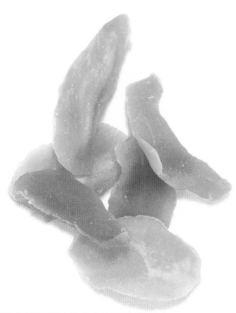

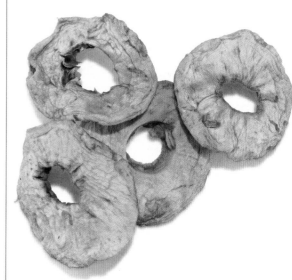

DRIED MANGO

A dried fruit salad is an underrated portable snack that's perfect for the office or a long trip—and antioxidant-packed dried mangos are an underrated dried fruit to add to that medley.

DRIED APPLE

People who eat apples are healthier, according to a study presented at the 2009 Experimental Biology Conference. Researchers found that people who had eaten apple products within the past 24 hours were 27 percent less likely to develop metabolic syndrome and had a 36 percent lower risk of high blood pressure. And one dried apple ring gives you 1 g of fiber for 15 calories. Chow down.

SERVING SIZE	4 pieces (40 g)			1 ring (6 g)		
Calories/Fiber	Calories: 130		Fiber: 0 g	Calories: 15		Fiber: 1 g
Macronutrients	Protein: 0 g	Fat: 1 g	Carbs: 32 g	Protein: 0 g	Fat: 0 g	Carbs: 4 g
Vitamins/Minerals	Vitamin A: 20%	Iron: 6%				

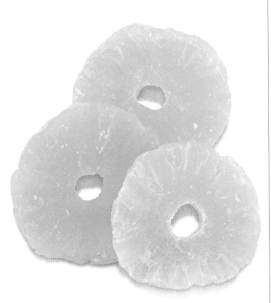

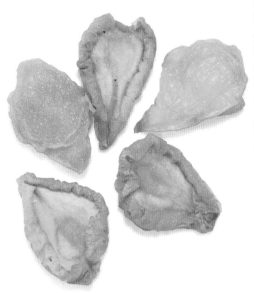

DRIED PINEAPPLE

These tropical rings boast a mix of vitamins, minerals, and enzymes, but read the label. Dried pineapple, like many dried fruits, can come coated in sugar.

DRIED PEAR

Sun-dried pears are a rare treat—sweet and dessert-like yet with all the nutritional fiber and potassium benefits.

1 oz (28 g)		
Calories: 130	Fiber: 1 g	
Protein: 0 g	Fat: 0 g	Carbs: 24 g
Potassium: 4%	Calcium: 2%	

50 g		
Calories: 64	Fiber: 3 g	
Protein: 0 g	Fat: 0 g	Carbs: 17 g
Potassium: 4%	Vitamin C: 3%	

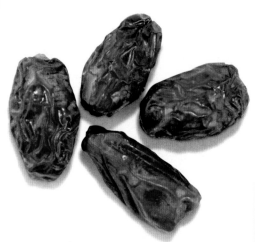

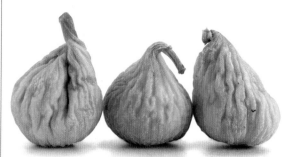

DATE (MEDJOOL)

Dates are little sugar bombs, but better than any processed sugary snack you'll find because of a potent load of fiber, potassium, vitamin B₆, and magnesium. Substitute them for cookies and candy and your kids won't complain.

DRIED FIG

Nutrients in figs help support proper pH levels in the body, making it more difficult for pathogens to invade. Plus, the fiber in figs can lower insulin and blood-sugar levels, reducing the risk of diabetes and metabolic syndrome. Select figs with dark skins (they contain more nutrients) and eat them alone or add them to trail mix.

SERVING SIZE	1 date, pitted (24 g)			1 fig (8 g)		
Calories/Fiber	Calories: 66	Fiber: 2 g		Calories: 21	Fiber: 1 g	
Macronutrients	Protein: 0 g	Fat: 0 g	Carbs: 18 g	Protein: 0 g	Fat: 0 g	Carbs: 5 g
Vitamins/Minerals	Potassium: 5%	Vitamin B₆: 3%	Magnesium: 3%	Potassium: 2%	Manganese: 2%	

FACTS OF LIFE:

100

Percentage more cell-repairing antioxidants in dried fruit than in fresh fruit.

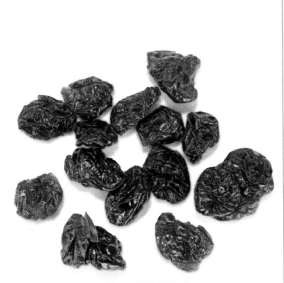

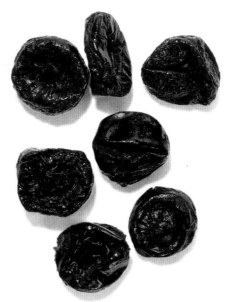

DRIED CHERRY

Research by the US Department of Agriculture shows that eating up to 45 bing cherries a day can lower the risk of tendinitis, bursitis, arthritis, and gout. Studies also suggest that they reduce the risk of chronic diseases and metabolic syndrome. Dried cherries also taste great in homemade trail mix.

DRIED PLUM/PRUNE

These dark shrivelers are rich in copper and boron, both of which can help prevent osteoporosis. Dried plums also contain high amounts of neochlorogenic and chlorogenic acids, antioxidants that are effective at combating the "superoxide anion radical." This nasty free radical causes structural damage to your cells that could bring on cancer.

¼ cup (40 g)		
Calories: 140	Fiber: 3 g	
Protein: 2 g	Fat: 0 g	Carbs: 16 g
Vitamin A: 10	Potassium: 10%	

1 oz (28 g)		
Calories: 95	Fiber: 1 g	
Protein: 1 g	Fat: 0 g	Carbs: 25 g
Vitamin A: 10%	Vitamin B₆: 10%	

Fish may be the healthiest food on the planet: omega-3 fatty acids are the key to their nutritional power. There is no protein that's quicker, more adaptable, and easier to cook. Plus, those who eat two servings of fish a week live longer and have lower rates of cardiovascular disease, greater mental capacity, and less abdominal fat than those who avoid seafood. So what kind of fish should you eat? Read on.

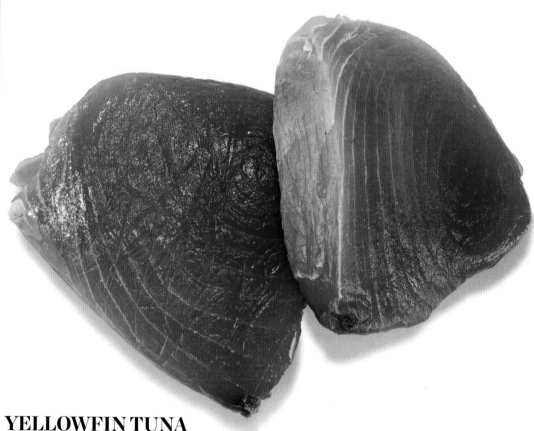

YELLOWFIN TUNA

When buying fresh tuna, avoid overfished bluefin tuna; opt for US Atlantic-caught yellowfin instead. At the fish counter, tuna is never brown. It should be bright red. An artificial-looking, pinkish color means they're putting a preserving gas on it.

SERVING SIZE	4 oz, boneless (112 g)		
Calories/Fiber/Omega-3	Calories: 120	Fiber: 0 g	Omega-3: 272 mg
Macronutrients	Protein: 28 g	Fat: 0 g	Carbs: 0 g
Vitamins/Minerals	Niacin: 56%	Vitamin: B$_6$ 52%	

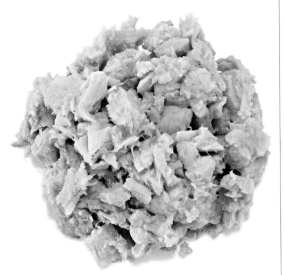

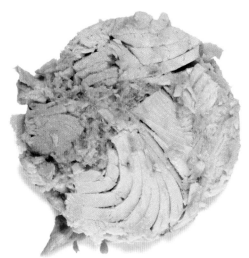

LIGHT TUNA CANNED IN WATER

Light tuna usually comes from a larger fish, the yellowfin, has a pinker color than albacore, and a stronger, fishier flavor. It also has a little secret: selenium. This nutrient helps preserve elastin, a protein that keeps your skin smooth and tight. The antioxidant is also believed to buffer against the sun (it stops the formation of free radicals created by UV exposure from damaging cells).

WHITE TUNA CANNED IN WATER

White tuna comes from albacore, a small tuna caught in both the Pacific and Atlantic oceans. It has a milder flavor and three times more omega-3 acids per ounce than light tuna. Fancy, or solid, is the top grade of canned tuna, cut in larger slabs.

1 can (165 g)		
Calories: 191	Fiber: 0 g	Omega-3: 460 mg
Protein: 42 g	Fat: 1 g	Carbs: 0 g
Selenium: 190%	Niacin: 110%	Vitamin B_{12}: 82%

1 can (172 g)		
Calories: 220	Fiber: 0 g	Omega-3: 1,636 mg
Protein: 41 g	Fat: 5 g	Carbs: 0 g
Selenium: 161%	Niacin: 50%	Vitamin B_{12}: 34%

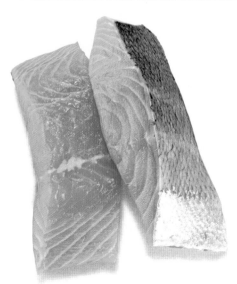

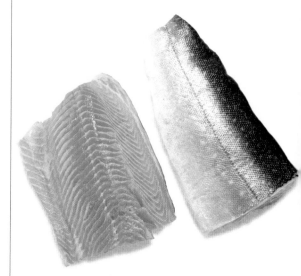

WILD ALASKAN SALMON (SOCKEYE)

Avoid farmed (or "Atlantic") salmon and opt for wild salmon whenever possible. Atlantic salmon's omega-3/omega-6 ratio is far less appealing than that of wild fish, a result of its grain-infused feed—feed that contains artificial pigments to make the fish's meat a more appealing shade of pink-orange. Meanwhile, a diet of heart-healthy fats, like those found in wild salmon, raises HDL (good) cholesterol levels. Wild salmon's huge dose of omega-3 fatty acids can ward off heart disease.

ARCTIC CHAR

Often considered a good substitute for salmon—its flesh is red or pink—char is both a fresh- and saltwater fish. If the water's cold—from Canada across Scandinavia and Siberia, even in the Alps—you'll find char.

SERVING SIZE	4 oz (112 g)			4 oz (112 g)		
Calories/Fiber/Omega-3	Calories: 172	Fiber: 0 g	Omega-3: 1,264 mg	Calories: 204	Fiber: 0 g	Omega-3: N/A
Macronutrients	Protein: 24 g	Fat: 8 g	Carbs: 0 g	Protein: 24 g	Fat: 8 g	Carbs: 0 g
Vitamins/Minerals	Vitamin B₁₂: 144%	Selenium: 48%	Niacin: 44%			

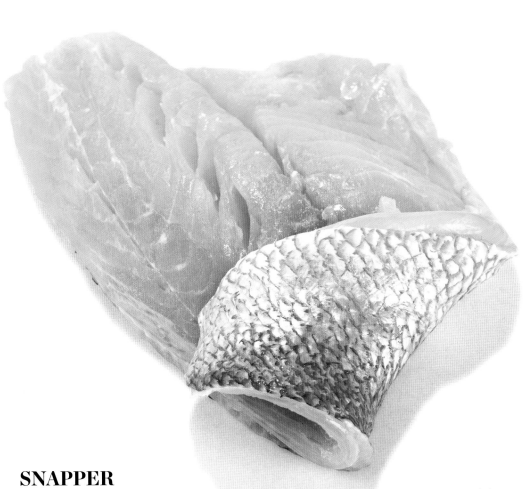

SNAPPER

Snapper is a delicious, lean fish that delivers a higher protein kick and lower fat payoff than the salmons and herrings of the world. It also delivers selenium and B vitamins by the finful.

1 fillet (7–8 oz, 218 g)		
Calories: 218	Fiber: 0 g	Omega-3: 829 mg
Protein: 45 g	Fat: 3 g	Carbs: 0 g
Selenium: 119%	Vitamin B_{12}: 109%	Vitamin B_6: 44%

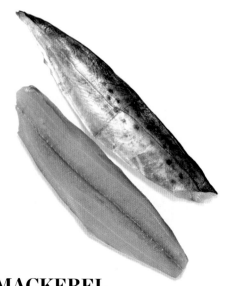

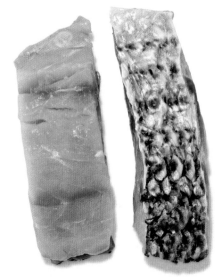

MACKEREL

You'd have to eat two salmon fillets to get the omega-3 power in one serving of mackerel. Grill it with olive oil, lemon, and sea salt.

STRIPED BASS, FARMED

Fish from cold waters are more fatty because of those lower temperatures, meaning more omega-3s. Stripers, because they travel the shoreline, are exposed to a lot of pesticide runoff. To help avoid exposure to pollutants, opt for farmed striped bass, which is designated as cleaner than wild.

SERVING SIZE	1 fillet, Atlantic (4 oz, 112 g)			1 fillet (5–6 oz, 159 g)		
Calories/Fiber/Omega-3	Calories: 230	Fiber: 0 g	Omega-3: 2,991 mg	Calories: 154	Fiber: 0 g	Omega-3: 1,223 mg
Macronutrients	Protein: 21 g	Fat: 16 g	Carbs: 0 g	Protein: 28 g	Fat: 4 g	Carbs: 0 g
Vitamins/Minerals	Vitamin B₁₂: 163%	Vitamin D: 101%	Phosphorus: 24%	Vitamin B₁₂: 101%	Selenium: 83%	

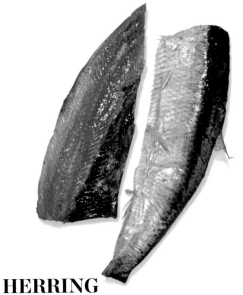

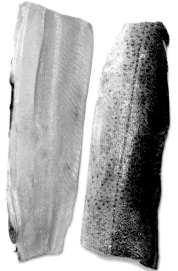

SKIN OR NO SKIN?

You're either a skin guy or you're not. We're skin guys. That's because fish skin helps insulate the flesh, keeping it moist during high-heat cooking like grilling and broiling. Plus, the skin can house some dense deposits of omega-3s. If it's crispy skin you seek, go with striped bass (farmed), red snapper, or wild salmon, and use a nonstick pan to help keep the fillet intact. Skin or not, be sure to pat your fish dry before cooking it; removing the moisture ensures even caramelization.

HERRING

Herring is another of the renowned "small, oily ocean fish" that pack massive doses of omega-3s, as well as vitamins D and B$_{12}$. Dig in and enjoy. Also, according to a certain group of British knights, the herring is an excellent tree-cutting tool.

RAINBOW TROUT

When shopping, remember that an extremely fresh fish stays flat, not floppy, when held out horizontally (before it's cut up, of course). Whole trout should be covered in a natural, clear, slick film. The fish's eyes should be bright and protruding.

4 oz, Atlantic (112 g)		
Calories: 180	Fiber: 0 g	Omega-3: 1,952 mg
Protein: 20 g	Fat: 12 g	Carbs: 0 g
Vitamin D: 460%	Vitamin B$_{12}$: 256%	

1 fillet, wild (4–5 oz, 159 g)		
Calories: 189	Fiber: 0 g	Omega-3: 1,291 mg
Protein: 33 g	Fat: 6 g	Carbs: 0 g
Vitamin B$_{12}$: 118%	Niacin: 43%	

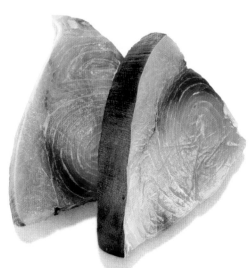

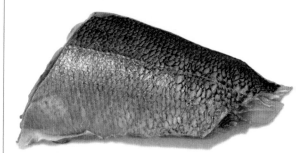

SWORDFISH

Swordfish flesh is typically white or tinged with pink, but not beige. The portions of dark meat in fillets should be red, not brown. Because of high mercury levels, limit consumption of swordfish to once a week or less. Avoid imported swordfish; its high level of bycatch (unwanted caught fish) wrecks havoc on our ocean's food chain.

BLUEFISH

Bluefish are a common sportfish on the East Coast of the US, but they swim in all climates. They're prepared in a variety of ways, and if you hook one that's more than 20 pounds—nice catch, Quint. You've caught an omega-3-rich fish that's packed with vitamins, too.

SERVING SIZE	1 piece (4½" x 2" x 1", 136 g)			1 fillet (5–6 oz, 150 g)		
Calories/Fiber/Omega-3	Calories: 165	Fiber: 0 g	Omega-3: 1,122 mg	Calories: 186	Fiber: 0 g	Omega-3: 1,250 mg
Macronutrients	Protein: 27 g	Fat: 5 g	Carbs: 0 g	Protein: 30 g	Fat: 6 g	Carbs: 0 g
Vitamins/Minerals	Selenium: 93%	Niacin: 66%	Vitamin B$_{12}$: 40%	Vitamin B$_{12}$: 135%	Selenium: 78%	

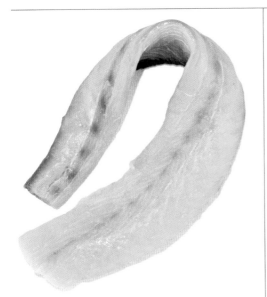

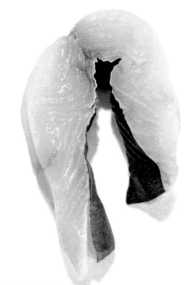

MAHIMAHI

These tropical sportfish are gorgeous, yellow or green tinged with a bold sailfin. The only place they look better is on your plate. Along with halibut, mahimahi carry one of the lowest contaminant loads of any common fish, thanks to their low-fat, high-protein flesh.

HALIBUT

A perfect halibut has the smell of aluminum. Alaskan halibut is snow-white; Eastern halibut is off-white to translucent white. Avoid fillets with patches of discoloration and cracks in the flesh, which signifies poor handling.

6 oz (168 g)		
Calories: 190	Fiber: 0 g	Omega-3: 250 mg
Protein: 40 g	Fat: 2 g	Carbs: 0 g
Iron: 15%		

½ fillet (204 g)		
Calories: 224	Fiber: 0 g	Omega-3: 1,065 mg
Protein: 42 g	Fat: 5 g	Carbs: 0 g
Selenium: 106%	Niacin: 60%	

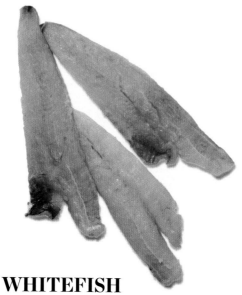

WHITEFISH

Most frozen fish dinners are made out of whitefish, a catchall phrase for a variety of fish such as cod, hake, and whiting that are used for fish fries. But fish sticks and other frozen fish must be baked, not battered, to be healthy. Still, the more fish, the better: when Canadian researchers compared a steady diet of the stuff with regular consumption of lean beef and chicken, the fish-eating folks experienced a 26 percent increase in HDL2, a more protective form of HDL. "Fish protein may increase insulin sensitivity, which in turn can elevate HDL2 cholesterol," says Helene Jacques, PhD, one of the study's authors.

CATFISH

An acquired taste for some—and a certified addiction to others—catfish is a staple in Southern cooking. If you avoid it deep-fried, you'll get a low-calorie dose of protein and vitamin D as well as omega-3s, B_{12}, selenium, and phosphorus.

SERVING SIZE	1 fillet, mixed species, raw (5–6 oz, 198 g)			1 fillet (5–6 oz, 159 g)		
Calories/Fiber/Omega-3	Calories: 265	Fiber: 0 g	Omega-3: 3,175 mg	Calories: 151	Fiber: 0 g	Omega-3: 851 mg
Macronutrients	Protein: 38 g	Fat: 12 g	Carbs: 0 g	Protein: 26 g	Fat: 4 g	Carbs: 0 g
Vitamins/Minerals	Phosphorus: 53%	Selenium: 36%	Vitamin B_{12}: 33%	Vitamin D: 199%	Vitamin B_{12}: 59%	Selenium: 29%

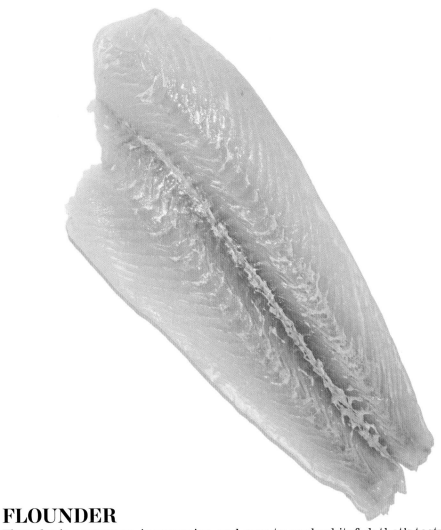

FLOUNDER

Flounder is a common, inexpensive, and easy-to-cook whitefish that's tasty as a fillet or can be creatively stuffed. It's particularly low in fat.

4 oz		
Calories: 104	Fiber: 0 g	Omega-3: 286 mg
Protein: 20 g	Fat: 0 g	Carbs: 0 g
Selenium: 52%	Vitamin B$_{12}$: 28%	

BARRAMUNDI (ASIAN SEABASS)

As a sportfish, Barramundi are known as fierce fighters. As food, they're common in Thai cuisine, are very popular in Australia, and have a white, flaky flesh.

Per 6-oz serving:
210 calories, 40 g protein, 0 g carbs, 0 g fiber, 5 g fat, and 1,300 mg omega-3

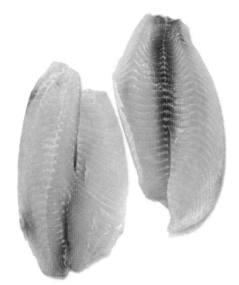

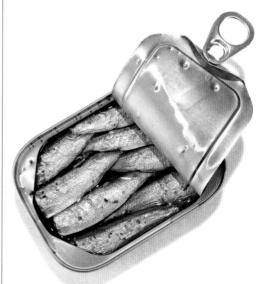

TILAPIA

A great light, low-calorie fish when caught from the wild, but avoid farmed tilapia. The critters are fattened with soy pellets, leaving them higher in common omega-6s than they are in heart-healthy, hard-to-find omega-3s. Tilapia is often served breaded and fried, adding more unhealthy fats. In fact, a study in the *Journal of the American Dietetic Association* recently warned people who are concerned about heart disease to avoid eating tilapia for just that reason.

SARDINES

This oily fish is a top source of omega-3 fats, rivaling even salmon. Plus, it's packed with bone-building calcium. Look for sardines packed in olive oil and eat 'em straight from the can. For a more sophisticated approach, wrap a sardine around an almond-stuffed olive.

SERVING SIZE	4 oz			1 can (3.75 oz, 92 g)		
Calories/Fiber/Omega-3	Calories: 108	Fiber: 0 g	Omega-3: 248 mg	Calories: 191	Fiber: 0 g	Omega-3: 1,362 mg
Macronutrients	Protein: 24 g	Fat: 0 g	Carbs: 0 g	Protein: 23 g	Fat: 11 g	Carbs: 0 g
Vitamins/Minerals	Selenium: 68%	Vitamin B12: 28%		Vitamin B12: 137%	Vitamin D: 63%	Calcium: 35%

Fish: A Purist's Guide

Omega-3 fatty acids, the superhealthy polyunsaturated fats, have been linked to lower rates of heart disease, depression, stroke, and possibly even Alzheimer's and some forms of skin cancer. But just because it lives below the waves doesn't mean it's the best choice to wave into home. Not all fish are created equal. The best are high in omega-3s, low in omega-6s, low in toxins like mercury and persistent organic pollutants (POPs—chemicals that have been linked to weight gain), and sustainable—meaning you're not putting the kebosh on your children's nutritional future by indulging. Below, we've rated some of the best and worst choices.

FISH (3 OZ SERVING)*	OMEGA-3S	OMEGA-6S	CONTAMINANTS*	SUSTAINABILITY*
THE BEST				
Wild Alaskan salmon	1,253 mg	114 mg	LOW (PCBs)	HIGH
Pacific halibut	444 mg	297 mg	LOW (mercury)	HIGH
Farmed rainbow trout	838 mg	506 mg	LOW (PCBs)	MEDIUM
US albacore/yellowfin tuna	207 mg	58 mg	MEDIUM (mercury)	HIGH
Dungeness crab	340 mg	0 mg	LOW (mercury)	HIGH
THE WORST				
Farmed (Atlantic) salmon	1,705 mg	1,900 mg	HIGH (POPs)	LOW
Farmed tilapia	185 mg	450 mg	LOW (PCBs)	MEDIUM
Chilean sea bass	570 mg	20 mg	MEDIUM (mercury)	LOW
Shrimp	284 mg	88 mg	HIGH (POPs)	LOW
Eel	712 mg	213 mg	HIGH (PCBs)	LOW

Information based on each fish's sustainability and chemical load, as monitored by the Monterey Bay Aquarium's Seafood Watch, The Environmental Defense Fund, the Marine Conservation Society Good Fish Guide, and the Blue Ocean Institute Seafood Guide

Once you get through their armor, the critters herein are highly nutritious (packed with selenium, for one), but they also bring an air of celebration and feasting with them as well. Lobsters, crabs, a couple dozen steamers—when else would you eat them except when surrounded by friends? For fun, throw a summer seafood party in the middle of winter.

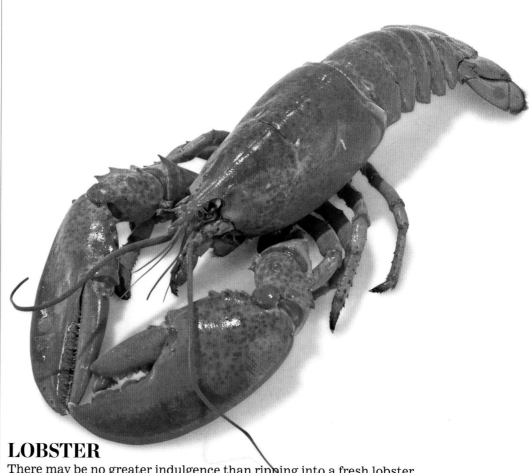

LOBSTER

There may be no greater indulgence than ripping into a fresh lobster. And rip with confidence, knowing it's good for you, too (look at that selenium). Just go easy on the butter.

SERVING SIZE	1 lobster (150 g)		
Calories/Fiber/Omega-3	Calories: 135	Fiber: 0 g	Omega-3: N/A
Macronutrients	Protein: 28 g	Fat: 1 g	Carbs: 1 g
Vitamins/Minerals	Copper: 125%	Selenium: 89%	Zinc: 30%

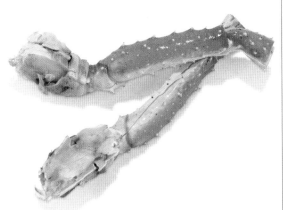

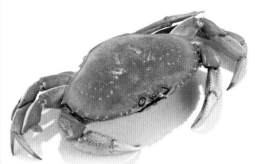

ALASKAN KING CRAB

High in protein and low in fat, the sweet flesh of the king crab is spiked with zinc—a whopping 7 milligrams per 3.5-ounce serving. "Zinc is an antioxidant, but more important, it helps support healthy bone mass and immune function," says Susan Bowerman, assistant director of the Center for Human Nutrition at the University of California at Los Angeles.

DUNGENESS CRAB

These crabs are the nutritional prince to the king crab, yet still share a royal dose of zinc, selenium, and a comparable amount of protein and B_{12}.

1 leg (172 g)		
Calories: 144	Fiber: 0 g	Omega-3: N/A
Protein 31 g	Fat: 1 g	Carbs: 0 g
Vitamin B_{12}: 258%	Zinc: 68%	

1 crab (163 g)		
Calories: 140	Fiber: 0 g	Omega-3: 517 mg
Protein: 28 g	Fat: 2 g	Carbs: 1 g
Vitamin B_{12}: 244%	Selenium: 86%	Zinc: 46%

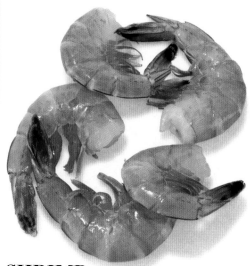

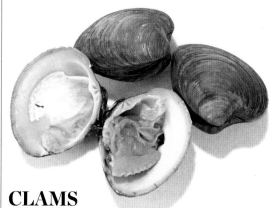

SHRIMP

Your basic shrimp cocktail is a great low-calorie appetizer, but shrimp are also one of our favorite and most versatile foods—sautéed, grilled, you name it, and you get a healthy portion of protein, selenium, and vitamin D. When possible, opt for wild-caught shrimp, which are lower in pesticides.

CLAMS

A nice batch of steamed clams is also a nutritional bonanza—with B_{12} and iron off the charts—as well as surprising amounts of vitamin C and potassium. Clams also stock your body with magnesium, which is important in metabolism, nerve function, and muscle function.

SERVING SIZE	4 large (28 g)			1 cup (227 g)		
Calories/Fiber/Omega-3	Calories: 30	Fiber: 0 g	Omega-3: 151 mg	Calories: 168	Fiber: 0 g	Omega-3: 449 mg
Macronutrients	Protein: 6 g	Fat: <1 g	Carbs: 0 g	Protein: 29 g	Fat: 2 g	Carbs: 6 g
Vitamins/Minerals	Selenium: 15%	Vitamin D: 11%		Vitamin B_{12}: 1,870%	Vitamin C: 49%	Potassium: 20%

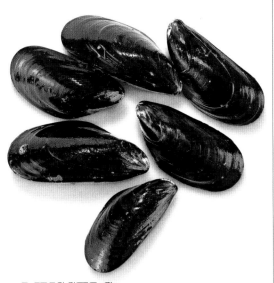

MUSSELS

Another superstar seafood combination of omega-3s, protein, B$_{12}$, and a host of other nutrients, yet mussels are often upstaged by clams. Sub them in for a nice change.

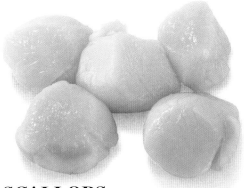

SCALLOPS

Though lobster and shrimp get all the love, scallops remain some of the most delicious shellfish to grace the seas. With 75 calories and 14 grams of protein per 3 ounces, sea scallops offer a great calorie value for the nutrition they provide, including plenty of cancer-fighting B$_{12}$.

1 cup (150 g)		
Calories: 129	Fiber: 0 g	Omega-3: 724 mg
Protein: 18 g	Fat: 3 g	Carbs: 6 g
Vitamin B$_{12}$: 300%	Manganese: 255%	Selenium: 96%

3 oz (about 6 large or 15 small)		
Calories: 75	Fiber: 0 g	Omega-3: 65 mg
Protein: 14 g	Fat: 1 g	Carbs: 2 g
Selenium: 27%	Vitamin B$_{12}$: 22%	

HOW TO BUY OYSTERS

At the fish market: Buy from the same beds that a chef stakes his reputation on. Sandy Ingber, executive chef and seafood buyer for Grand Central Oyster Bar in New York City, buys Blue Point, Chincoteague, Glidden Point, Narragansett Bay, Pemaquid, and Wellfleet oysters in the winter months. During summer, he buys Coromandel oysters from New Zealand. The reason for the seasonal shift: More than three-quarters of food illness outbreaks involving raw oysters occur in the Northern Hemisphere's warm-water months. At home: Eat only thoroughly cooked oysters. If you must slurp, do so only after following the buying advice above.

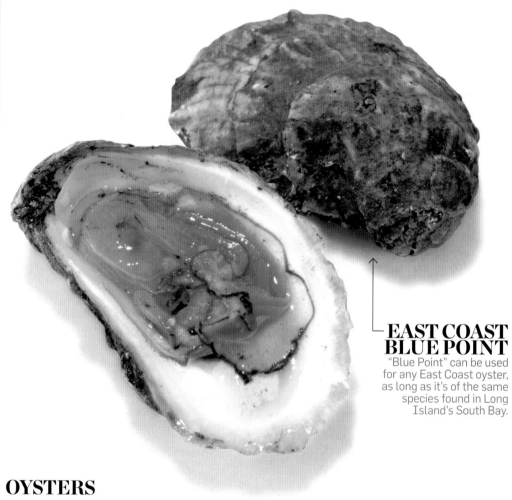

EAST COAST BLUE POINT

"Blue Point" can be used for any East Coast oyster, as long as it's of the same species found in Long Island's South Bay.

OYSTERS

Shellfish, in general, are an excellent source of zinc, calcium, copper, iodine, iron, potassium, and selenium. But the creamy flesh of oysters stands apart for its ability to elevate testosterone levels and protect against prostate cancer.

SERVING SIZE	6 medium, Eastern, wild, raw (84 g)		
Calories/Fiber/Omega-3	Calories: 57	Fiber: 0 g	Omega-3: 565 mg
Macronutrients	Protein: 6 g	Fat: 2 g	Carbs: 3 g
Vitamins/Minerals	Zinc: 509%	Vitamin B$_{12}$: 272%	Copper: 187%

ISLAND CREEK
Small, mild, and easy to eat, the Island Creek is a perfect choice raw or poached.

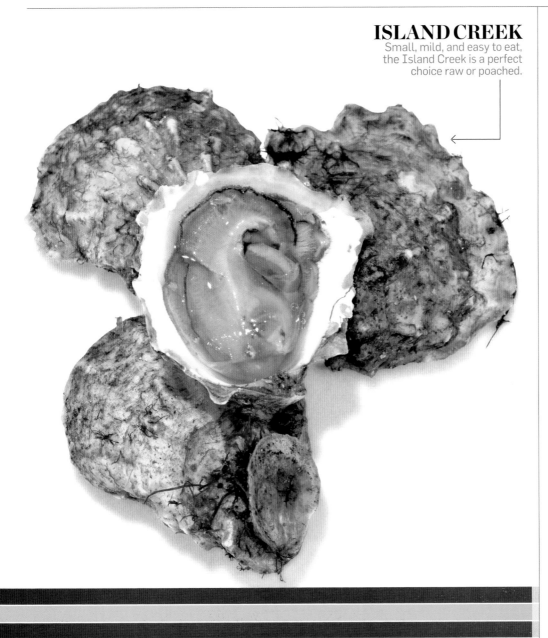

THE OYSTER CONNOIS-SEUR

While there are some 200 unique appellations in North America, there are only five species of oysters. Pacific varieties such as kumamotos and shigokus contain more omega-3s and protein than the Eastern species Crassostrea virginica.

Kumamoto:
Sweet, with a clean and fruity finish, these are the perfect date oysters.

Island Creek:
Small, firm, salty, and clean-flavored, they're the best choice for beginners.

Beausoleil:
These New Brunswick beauties have a crisp, fresh taste with a light finish.

Shigoku:
Small but mighty, Shigokus have a strong sea flavor with a cucumber finish.

Totten Virginica:
This plump, meaty variety is crammed with flavor.

Oils & Butter Guide

When deciding which oils to choose in cooking or dressings, look at the omega ratio. Corn, soybean, and other vegetable oils have high levels of omega-6s. These polyunsaturated fats aren't bad when they're balanced with similar amounts of omega-3 fatty acids, like the ones found in fish. "We now consume 20 to 1 omega-6s to omega-3s," says Jonny Bowden, PhD, author of *The 150 Healthiest Foods on Earth*. A high intake of omega-6 fats relative to omega-3 fats increases inflammation, which may increase your risk of heart

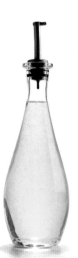
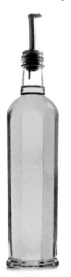
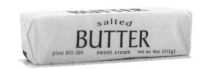

	CANOLA OIL	OLIVE OIL	BUTTER
OMEGA-6 TO OMEGA-3 RATIO:	2:1	13:1	7:1
Key fact:	A near-perfect omega ratio	Loaded with disease-fighting antioxidants	May fight cancer; won't adversely affect cholesterol
What you need to know:	This should be your go-to option for everyday frying, sautéing, and baking. Canola oil can withstand relatively high heat, and its neutral flavor won't dominate a recipe.	Extra-virgin has a robust flavor and should be saved to dress salads, vegetables, and cooked dishes. For cooking, regular or light olive oil is fine. (Note: "Light" in this case refers to color, not fat or calorie content.)	It's a logical choice for baked goods and adds a rich note to sautes and sauces. What's more, fat, like that in butter, is necessary in order to help your body absorb fat-soluble vitamins, such as vitamins A, D, E, and K.

disease, diabetes, and cancer, according to a 2008 review of studies by the Center for Genetics, Nutrition and Health.

Use this chart as a reference. These fats have roughly the same number of calories (120 per tablespoon), but they aren't all equal in other aspects. Favor the first few in this section; use the later ones sparingly, if at all.

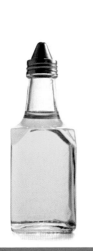
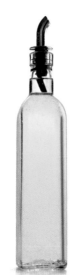
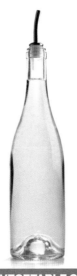
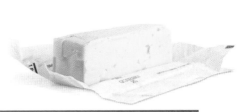

PEANUT OIL	SESAME OIL	VEGETABLE OIL	MARGARINE
Not enough omega-3 to count	138:1	Varies	11:1
May boost your HDL (good) cholesterol	Contains antioxidants, but high in omega-6s	Avoid! Beware of it in processed foods	Avoid, unless it's a spread with healthy fats
Because of its high smoke point, peanut oil should be your choice for wok cooking, stir-frying, and pan-searing meat or fish.	Use the dark variety, made from toasted sesame seeds, as a condiment over Asian noodle dishes. Save the light variety for high-heat cooking.	This label can mean many things. It usually refers to soybean or corn oil, or a blend that may also include sunflower or canola oil.	Never use margarine that contains trans fat. Butter is better, or find a healthier version, like Smart Balance Buttery Spread with Flax Oil.

When Harvard University researchers analyzed the diets of more than 27,000 people over 8 years, they discovered that those who ate whole grains daily weighed 2.5 pounds less than those who ate only refined-grain foods. But remember: Just because the label says "whole grain" doesn't mean it's healthy; a product only needs to be made of 51 percent whole-grain flour in order to carry this label. You want to see the word "whole" next to every type of flour in the ingredients.

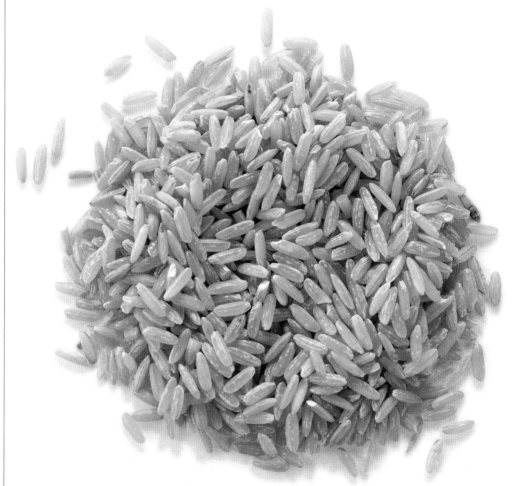

BROWN RICE, MEDIUM GRAIN

Plain brown rice has virtually no salt and a strong dose of minerals and fiber. And just about any food expert will tell you that you should sub it in for white rice every time.

SERVING SIZE	1 cup, cooked (195 g)		
Calories/Fiber	Calories: 218		Fiber: 4 g
Macronutrients	Protein: 5 g	Fat: 2 g	Carbs: 46 g
Vitamins/Minerals	Manganese: 107%	Magnesium: 21%	Vitamin B₆: 15%

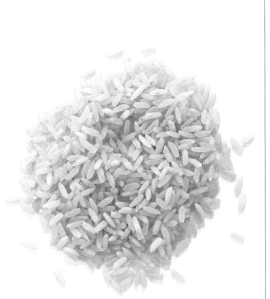

WHITE RICE, MEDIUM GRAIN, UNENRICHED

Other than a dose of manganese, white rice is virtually devoid of nutritional value. What's more, it's a high-glycemic food—53 g of carbs with no fiber content to offset it. With so many easy, nutritious substitutes available, you never have to touch the stuff.

QUINOA

The South American grain quinoa (*KEEN-wah*) has about twice as much protein as brown rice, and its protein consists of a complete set of branch chain and essential amino acids, making it a tissue- and muscle-building powerhouse. All that protein and fiber—in conjunction with a handful of healthy fats and a comparatively small dose of carbohydrates—help insure a low impact on your blood sugar. Quinoa's soft and nutty taste is easy to handle for even picky eaters and it cooks just like rice, ready in about 15 minutes.

1 cup, cooked (186 g)		
Calories: 242		Fiber: 0 g
Protein: 4 g	Fat: 0 g	Carbs: 53 g
Manganese: 35%		

1 cup, cooked (185 g)		
Calories: 222		Fiber: 5 g
Protein: 8 g	Fat: 4 g	Carbs: 39 g
Manganese: 58%	Magnesium: 30%	Folate: 19%

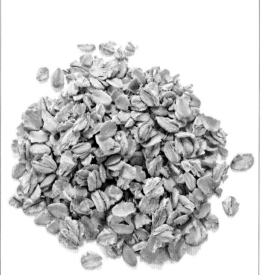

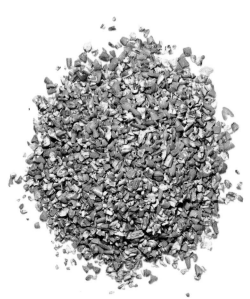

ROLLED OATS (INSTANT AND OLD-FASHIONED)

Instant oatmeal is really rolled oats cut up to cook faster. Old-fashioned oatmeal is groats (the hulled grain) rolled into flakes; it takes about 5 minutes to cook. Oats are one of the easiest ways to get more fiber into your diet. They reduce your risk of heart disease, high blood pressure, and type 2 diabetes and deliver a muscle-building protein punch. Just beware of the sugar in "flavored" instant oatmeal. Go for plain and sweeten with fruit.

STEEL-CUT OATS

Steel-cut oats are groats that are cut up but not rolled. It's nutty and toothsome, but takes a half hour to cook unless you soak it overnight. Still, they are worth the extra time and effort. "The enzymes in your gastrointestinal tract take a longer time to penetrate the unrolled groats in steel-cut oatmeal," says David Jenkins, MD, PhD, a nutrition and metabolism researcher at the University of Toronto. "This results in a slower uptake of glucose, and that makes steel-cut oatmeal better, especially for people who are at risk of diabetes."

SERVING SIZE	1 cup, cooked with water (234 g)			1 cup, uncooked (80 g)		
Calories/Fiber	Calories: 166		Fiber: 4 g	Calories: 300		Fiber: 8 g
Macronutrients	Protein: 6 g	Fat: 4 g	Carbs: 32 g	Protein: 10 g	Fat: 5 g	Carbs: 54 g
Vitamins/Minerals	Manganese: 68%	Selenium: 18%		Magnesium: 27%	Potassium: 4%	

CEREALS: THE GREAT SUGAR SWINDLE

Just because your favorite cereal doesn't have a cartoon character on the box doesn't mean it isn't a total sugar bomb. Not even heart-smart logos and bloated health claims can salvage the contents of boxes like Post Raisin Bran, General Mills Basic 4, or Multi-Bran Chex, all of which have more sugar than the same-size bowl of Froot Loops. Stick to cereals with high fiber-to-sugar ratios to ensure a low-sugar-impact start to your morning.

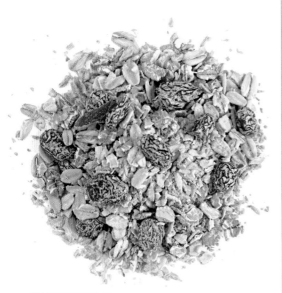

MUESLI

Originating in Switzerland, muesli is a fiber-and-protein power combination of rolled oats, dried fruits, and nuts. Though 1 cup pushes 300 calories, the payoff in vitamins and minerals across the board makes it a hearty meal.

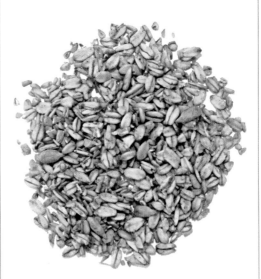

GRANOLA

Though granola's rich in many nutrients, it's now nearly impossible to find a box of the stuff with less sugar per serving than a plate of cookies. Deflect granola's unruly sugar load by scanning the cereal aisle for cereal-and-granola hybrids—or mix-and-match your bowls by yourself.

1 cup (85 g)		
Calories: 289		Fiber: 6 g
Protein: 8 g	Fat: 4 g	Carbs: 66 g
Vitamin B₆: 52%	Vitamin B₁₂: 52%	Vitamin E: 31%

1 cup (122 g)		
Calories: 597		Fiber: 11 g
Protein: 18 g	Fat: 29 g	Carbs: 65 g
Manganese: 247%	Vitamin E: 68%	Phosphorus: 56%

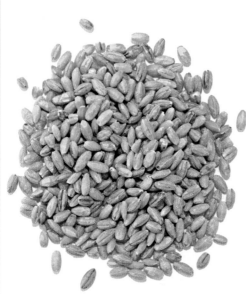

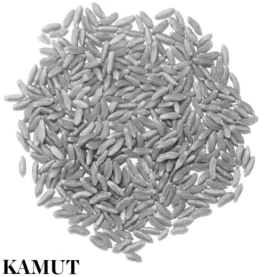

BARLEY (PEARLED)

It's not just for soups. Swedish researchers found that if you eat barley for breakfast, the fibrous grain cuts blood sugar response by 44 percent at lunch and 14 percent at dinner. And the less your sugar spikes, the more stable your energy (and hunger) levels will be.

KAMUT

This cousin of durum wheat was once considered the food of pharaohs. It's now embraced by mere mortals as an alternative to brown rice. Kamut has higher levels of heart-healthy fatty acids than most grains. It also has up to 40 percent more protein than wheat.

SERVING SIZE	1 cup, cooked (157 g)			1 cup, cooked (172 g)		
Calories/Fiber	Calories: 193		Fiber: 6 g	Calories: 251		Fiber: 7 g
Macronutrients	Protein: 4 g	Fat: 1 g	Carbs: 44 g	Protein: 11 g	Fat: 2 g	Carbs: 52 g
Vitamins/Minerals	Manganese: 20%	Selenium: 19%	Niacin: 16%	Niacin: 24%	Thiamin: 14%	

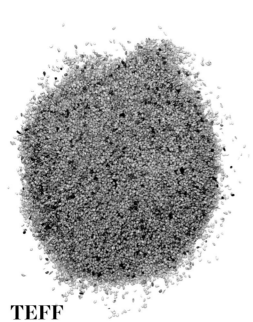

TEFF

In Amharic, the official language of Ethiopia, the word teff means "lost," which is exactly what will happen to a teff seed if you drop it. It's gluten-free, making it an excellent wheat alternative for people with celiac disease.

1 cup, cooked (252 g)		
Calories: 255		Fiber: N/A
Protein: 10 g	Fat: 2 g	Carbs: 50 g
Thiamin: 31%		

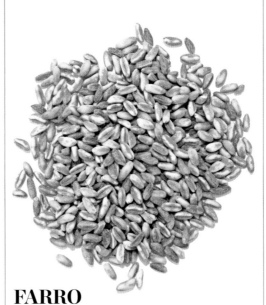

FARRO

Farro—a staple for ancient Egyptians and modern-day Italians alike—has everything you need: nearly twice the protein and fiber of brown rice, along with calcium and iron. "But it's really the soulful flavor and chewy texture that make it so special," says Scott Conant, chef at New York City's Scarpetta restaurant. Conant stirs cooked farro into soups and stews, tosses it with roasted vegetables to make salads, and replaces rice with farro in pilafs and risottos.

½ cup, cooked (60 g)		
Calories: 100		Fiber: 4 g
Protein: 4 g	Fat: 1 g	Carbs: 26 g

FIBER'S FINER POINTS

Fiber is the secret to losing weight without hunger. One US Department of Agriculture study found that those who increased their daily fiber intake from 12 grams to 24 grams absorbed 90 fewer calories per day than those who ate the same amount of food but less fiber. Do nothing other than add more of the rough stuff and you could lose 9 pounds in a year.

But beware: Sneaky food marketers often add isolated fibers such as inulin and maltodextrin to foods so that they can claim a food is "high in fiber."

But these fake-food additives are no substitute for whole grains such as oats. When you eat whole grains, the fiber is part of the carbohydrate. Your body has to work to break the whole thing down, which means you're digesting the whole food slowly. But when marketers just add isolated fiber on top of a refined carbohydrate, you don't get the same effect. You're still getting a pure sugar rush, not a whole-grain food.

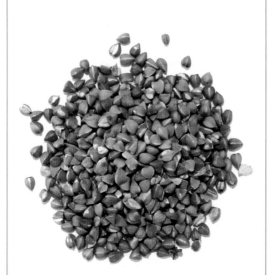

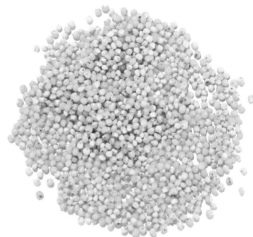

BUCKWHEAT

A concentrated nutritional punch:
A mere ounce of buckwheat delivers
3 grams of fiber and 4 grams of protein
and is rich in a host of minerals.

MILLET

This Asian grain has roughly the
same protein content as wheat and is
gluten-free. It also is rich in B vitamins,
calcium, and iron.

SERVING SIZE	1 oz, dry (28 g)			1 oz (28 g)		
Calories/Fiber	Calories: 96	Fiber: 3 g		Calories: 106	Fiber: 2 g	
Macronutrients	Protein: 4 g	Fat: 1 g	Carbs: 20 g	Protein: 3 g	Fat: 1 g	Carbs: 20 g
Vitamins/Minerals	Manganese: 18%	Copper: 15%	Magnesium: 16%	Manganese: 23%	Copper: 10%	Vitamin B6: 5%

AMARANTH

Gram for gram, few grains can compete with amaranth's nutritional portfolio. It's higher in fiber and protein than brown rice, it's loaded with vitamins, and it's been shown in studies to help lower blood pressure and cholesterol. Also, amaranth is one of the few grains that is a "complete protein," meaning it has all eight essential amino acids.

Per 1 cup, cooked (246 g) serving:
251 calories, 9 g protein, 46 g carbs, 5 g fiber, 4 g fat, and RDIs of 105% manganese, 40% magnesium, 36% phosphorus, and 29% iron

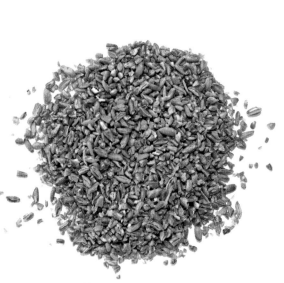

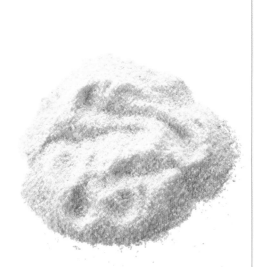

BULGUR

This whole grain, a type of cracked wheat, is common in Middle Eastern cuisine. It has a light, nutty flavor and is a terrific source of fiber and minerals. It's also a great substitute for rice or couscous.

CORNMEAL (WHOLE GRAIN, YELLOW)

Ground from dried corn, cornmeal isn't as nutritionally packed as wheat or other grains in this section. Still, it remains a staple especially in Southern cooking and is good source of magnesium, selenium, and thiamin.

1 oz (28 g)		
Calories: 96	Fiber: 5 g	
Protein: 3 g	Fat: 0 g	Carbs: 21 g
Manganese: 43%	Magnesium: 11%	

1 oz (28 g)		
Calories: 101	Fiber: 2 g	
Protein: 2 g	Fat: 1 g	Carbs: 22 g
Magnesium: 9%	Thiamin: 7%	Selenium: 6%

The largest single source of calories in the American diet isn't fast food, or desserts and sweets, or even meat and potatoes. In fact, it isn't even a food. Nearly 25 percent of our calories—about 450 calories a day—come from sodas, sweetened teas, and the like. Instead of sugar-sweetened beverages, try these metabolism-boosting, mind-sharpening, heart-protecting weight-loss beverages.

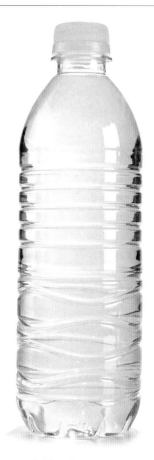

WATER

According to a study in the journal *Obesity Research,* those who drink water regularly consume almost 200 fewer calories a day than those who opt for sweeter beverages. Plus, a study in the *Journal of the American Dietetic Association* found that drinking a glass of water before breakfast may help reduce daily food intake by 13 percent. Flavored water isn't usually a smart choice, though, as most have added sweeteners. Get flavor without the sugar by adding citrus wedges, chopped mint, or crushed fresh or frozen berries to seltzer water.

SERVING SIZE	1 cup (8 oz)		
Calories/Fiber	Calories: 0 g		Fiber: 0 g
Macronutrients	Protein: 0 g	Fat: 0 g	Carbs: 0 g
Vitamins/Minerals			

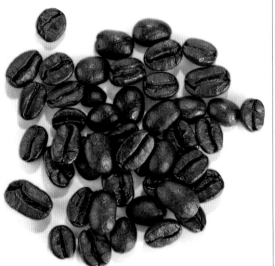

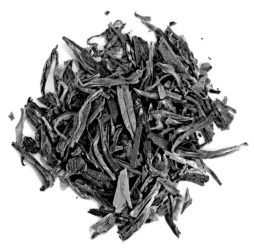

COFFEE (UNSWEETENED)

Coffee reduces your appetite, increases your metabolism, and gives you a shot of antioxidants—for almost zero calories. A study published in the journal *Physiology & Behavior* found that the average metabolic rate of people who drink caffeinated coffee is 16 percent higher than that of those who drink decaf. But those equations change when you order fancifully named coffee drinks from a chain like Starbucks. In fact, gourmet-coffee drinkers consume, on average, 206 more calories a day than people who sip regular joe. For best results, try it black.

GREEN TEA (UNSWEETENED)

Green tea is high in an antioxidant called ECGC, which may reduce the risk of most cancers, and also promotes fat burning. In one study, people who consumed the equivalent of 3 to 5 cups a day for 12 weeks decreased their body weight by 4.6 percent. According to other studies, consuming 2 to 4 cups of green tea a day may torch an extra 50 calories. That translates into about 5 pounds a year. Not bad for a few bags of leaves, eh? For maximum effect, let your tea steep for 3 minutes and drink it while it's still hot.

1 cup (8 oz)		
Calories: 2	Fiber: 0 g	
Protein: 0 g	Fat: 0 g	Carbs: 0 g
Riboflavin: 11%		

1 cup (8 oz)		
Calories: 0	Fiber: 0 g	
Protein: 0 g	Fat: 0 g	Carbs: 0 g

CAFFEINE: WHY EVERYONE LOVES COLA

Your preference for Pepsi over Sprite may have nothing to do with the flavor. Australian researchers determined that even though caffeine can't be tasted in soft drinks, it does make you like them more. "Caffeine is a mildly addictive compound that causes you to subconsciously favor beverages that contain it," says study author Russell Keast, PhD. "The added benefit to soft-drink manufacturers is that it may also lead you to consume more."

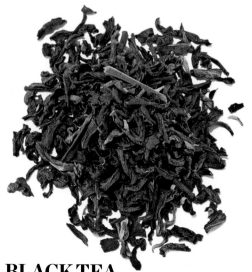

BLACK TEA (UNSWEETENED)

Drinking black tea makes high-carbohydrate meals a little healthier, according to a new study in the *Journal of the American College of Nutrition*. People who drank 1 cup of black tea after eating high-carb foods decreased their blood-sugar levels by 10 percent for 2.5 hours after the meal. Escaping the dreaded sugar spike and crash means you'll feel full longer and eat less. The researchers say the polyphenolic compounds in the tea increase circulating insulin, which lowers blood sugar.

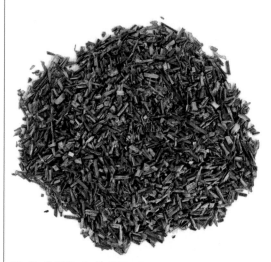

ROOIBOS TEA

Think of rooibos (*ROY-bus*) as the new green tea, although it's red, made from a root, and packed with even more digestion-enhancing phytochemicals and disease-fighting antioxidants. A Japanese study found that it might even help prevent allergies and fight cancer. Look for Celestial Seasonings rooibos teas (we recommend Madagascar Vanilla Red), or order organic varieties online at adagio.com.

SERVING SIZE	1 cup (8 fl oz)			1 cup (8 fl oz)		
Calories/Fiber	Calories: 2		Fiber: 0 g	Calories: 0		Fiber: 0 g
Macronutrients	Protein: 0 g	Fat: 0 g	Carbs: 0 g	Protein: 0 g	Fat: 0 g	Carbs: 0 g
Vitamins/Minerals	Maganese: 26%					

How to read tea leaves

CHOOSING TEA AT A COFFEE HOUSE CAN BE CONFUSING, ESPECIALLY FOR THOSE OF US STILL TRYING TO GRASP "VENTI." HERE'S A CHEAT SHEET.

Mighty Leaf Bombay Chai

Best for: Kickstarting your day. Contains caffeine and bold flavors.

Adagio Roobios

Best for: Chilling out. This South African herbal tea is caffeine-free, tastes naturally and subtly sweet, and comes in 13 flavors. For similar alternatives, try honeybush and chamomile teas.

Stash Peppermint

Best for: Post-meal. A cup or two of this refreshing herbal tea is a great finish.

Tazo Sweet Cinnamon Spice

Best for: Right before bed. It's spicy, but not overwhelmingly so, with a touch of sweetness.

Tazo Tea

Best for: A Starbucks alternative. Besides water, it's the only other drink on Starbucks' menu that has 0 calories. Just make sure you order the plain version—not the syrup-spiked, juice-infused, or latte kinds, all of which contain added sugar and calories.

Genmaicha

Best for: An afternoon pick-me-up. This Japanese green tea is mixed with roasted rice kernels. It has a savory smell, almost like popcorn.

Sur le Nil

Best for: After-dinner relaxing. Its flavor is more delicate than that of many green teas. Think of it as chamomile-plus, with hints of lemon and spice.

High Mountain Oolong

Best for: Relaxing after work. It's made with thick tea leaves, which gives it a full floral flavor with an earthy finish—a good balance for before dinner.

Wood Dragon Oolong

Best for: Guys who've quit coffee. Because it contains more stem than leaf, this strong, woodsy brew has significantly less caffeine than other oolong teas.

Honey Phoenix Oolong

Best for: Wintertime defrosting. It's a robust tea, with a flavor almost like a cherry pit. That makes it sweet, with a tinge of bitterness.

Vanilla Rooibos

Best for: Dessert—and not just because it's free of caffeine. You'll taste a light sweetness followed by a creamy finish.

Cassis

Best for: Snapping awake on a cold morning. This black tea is rich and powerful. You'll taste black currants, with a sweet, dry finish.

Pu-erh Tuocha

Best for: Coffee drinkers. It's strong and earthy, and has a kick of caffeine. The black tea comes pressed into nuggets, which break apart when you boil them.

Sencha

Best for: Green-tea beginners. It's sweet and mellow, without the bitter bite of some other green brews. Sip it with sushi or dessert.

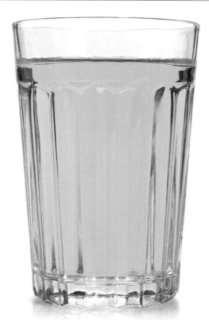

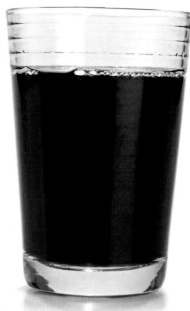

APPLE JUICE

Most of the apple juices you'll find in the supermarket have added vitamin C (ascorbic acid), but also added sugar. So read your labels before buying to avoid extra calories. That said, apple juice might be good brain food. A recent University of Massachusetts Lowell study showed that apple juice may improve memory by preventing the decline of acetylcholine, a neurotransmitter that can help slow Alzheimer's disease.

GRAPE JUICE

Besides providing protection from heart attack and stroke, grape juice can also help keep your middle-aged skin from sagging. Grapes are filled with antioxidant polyphenols that help to keep your skin flexible and elastic. But grape juice is another juice loaded up with sugar by manufacturers. Read your labels.

SERVING SIZE	1 cup (8 fl oz)			1 cup (8 fl oz)		
Calories/Fiber	Calories: 114		Fiber: 0 g	Calories: 152		Fiber: 1 g
Macronutrients	Protein: 0 g	Fat: 0 g	Carbs: 28 g	Protein: 1 g	Fat: 0 g	Carbs: 37 g
Vitamins/Minerals	Manganese: 9%	Vitamin C: 4%		Manganese: 30%	Potassium: 8%	

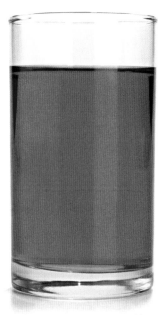

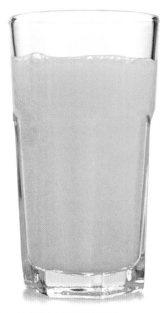

CRANBERRY JUICE

Cranberries have more antioxidants than other common fruits and vegetables. One serving has five times the amount in broccoli. But know that converting berries to juice, processing, and adding ascorbic acid (vitamin C) and pounds of sugar dilute much of the natural nutritional content. Go with low-sugar varieties.

ORANGE JUICE

Pour a glass of prevention: Orange juice may be the best drink to lower your risk of kidney stones, say researchers at University of Texas Southwestern medical center. While other fruit drinks, such as lemonade, can be helpful because they contain citrate—a compound that prevents calcium in urine from crystallizing into stones—the scientists found that people responded best to OJ. Why? It contains a type of citrate that better guards against the formation of the painful stones, says study author Clarita V. Odvina, MD.

1 cup (8 fl oz)		
Calories: 116	Fiber: 0 g	
Protein: 1 g	Fat: 0 g	Carbs: 31 g
Vitamin C: 39%	Vitamin E: 15%	

1 cup (8 fl oz)		
Calories: 112	Fiber: 0 g	
Protein: 2 g	Fat: 0 g	Carbs: 26 g
Vitamin C: 207%	Vitamin A: 10%	

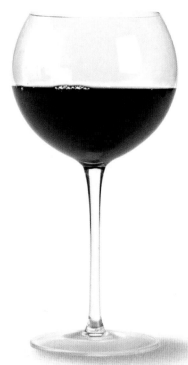

WINE

Oxidative stress plays a major role in aging, and an antioxidant in red wine called resveratrol may help extend life by neutralizing disease-causing free radicals. Pop a pinot noir: It packs the most resveratrol per glass. Additionally, the polyphenols found in grape skins—part of the red-wine-making process—are potent weapons against heart disease. But if you prefer white wine, you're still doing yourself a favor: A study published in the *Journal of Agricultural and Food Chemistry* found that giving white wine to rats both protected against heart attack and aided in recovery following an attack. However, that doesn't mean you have permission to go full-on Hasselhoff in your consumption: Canadian researchers found that, by dilating blood vessels, a single drink of wine allows your heart to work less. But the second drink was found to increase heart rate and blood flow without additional dilation, causing researchers to warn that repeated high consumption can lead to higher risk of heart attacks.

SERVING SIZE	1 glass (5 fl oz)		
Calories/Fiber	Calories: 125		Fiber: 0 g
Macronutrients	Protein: 0 g	Fat: 0 g	Carbs: 4 g
Vitamins/Minerals	Manganese: 10%	Potassium: 5%	Vitamin B₆: 4%

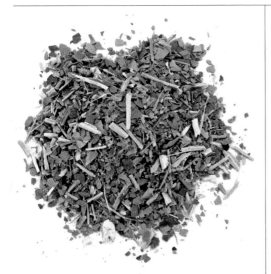

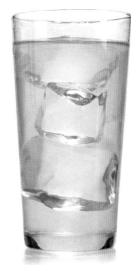

YERBA MATÉ

Yerba maté leaves steeped in hot (not boiling) water produce a traditional South American drink that is usually shared among friends from a hollow gourd. The taste is comparable to green tea, with half the caffeine of coffee. Nutritionally, it's green tea on steroids, with up to 90 percent more powerful cancer-fighting antioxidants, a cache of B vitamins, and plenty of chromium, which helps stabilize blood-sugar levels. Plus, its bolstering effect on metabolism is so valued that many diet pills list maté as an ingredient. For the strongest dose of maté's medicine, buy it in loose-leaf form.

*All values based on Eco Tea Organic Yerba Maté

1 cup (8 fl oz)		
Calories: 0		Fiber: 0 g
Protein: 0 g	Fat: 0 g	Carbs: 0 g
Chromium: 130%	Niacin: 15%	Iron: 15%

COCONUT WATER

Coconut water is the clear liquid inside young coconuts, and is a health food unto itself. At 46 calories a cup, it's a low-cal option that delivers 3 grams of fiber as well as good doses of potassium, magnesium, manganese, and vitamin C.

1 cup (24 oz)		
Calories: 46		Fiber: 3 g
Protein: 2 g	Fat: 0 g	Carbs: 9 g
Vitamin C: 10%	Potassium: 17%	

Not all peppers will burn your mouth (or fingers…or eyes…or worse if you don't wash your hands after handling the nasty ones). But they all bring the nutrition, whether from vitamin C or capsaicin—more about that on the next page. A meal with hot chilies increases your metabolic rate by 23 percent, which causes an increased burning of calories.

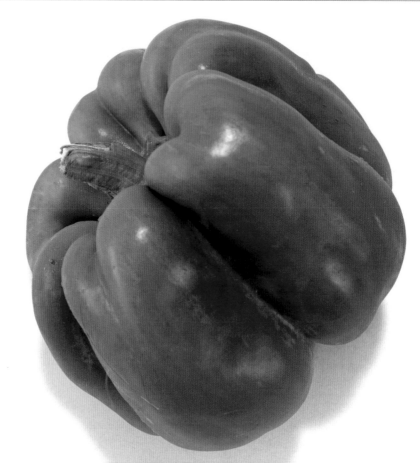

BELL PEPPER (GREEN)

Nutritionally, this pepper barely answers the bell. All bells are the same thing—the fruit of the pepper plant Capsicum annuum. The green ones just aren't ripe yet. Ripe, red bell peppers have nearly twice the vitamin C of green peppers (three times more than in an orange) and nine times the amount of vitamin A, because they've been soaking up the sun longer. They're also sweeter—and more expensive.

SERVING SIZE	1 cup, chopped (149 g)		
Calories/Fiber	Calories: 30		Fiber: 3 g
Macronutrients	Protein: 1 g	Fat: 0 g	Carbs: 7 g
Vitamins/Minerals	Vitamin C: 200%	Vitamin A: 11%	

How to pick a pepper

People don't eat jalapeño peppers because they like the sensation of mucous membranes being seared raw. Chile aficionados like the evil little vegetables because they cause the brain to produce endorphins, morphine-like substances that significantly alter your mental state.

Capsaicin, the chemical compound that gives chili peppers their heat, is actually odorless and tasteless; it simply stimulates the receptive points for pain on the tongue and in the mouth. Scoville heat units (SHU) gauge the level of capsaicin, and the higher the number is, the hotter the burn—and the greater the benefits. A recent Korean lab study found that capsaicin can help kill colon-cancer cells. Eating about 1 tablespoon of chopped red or green chiles boosts the activity of your sympathetic nervous system (responsible for our fight-or-flight response), resulting in a metabolism spike of 23 percent.

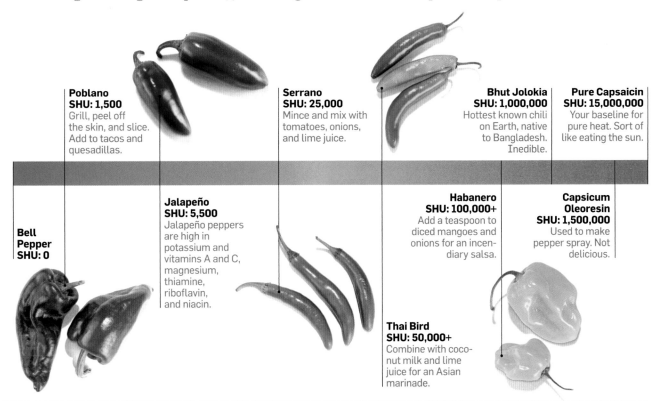

Poblano
SHU: 1,500
Grill, peel off the skin, and slice. Add to tacos and quesadillas.

Serrano
SHU: 25,000
Mince and mix with tomatoes, onions, and lime juice.

Bhut Jolokia
SHU: 1,000,000
Hottest known chili on Earth, native to Bangladesh. Inedible.

Pure Capsaicin
SHU: 15,000,000
Your baseline for pure heat. Sort of like eating the sun.

Bell Pepper
SHU: 0

Jalapeño
SHU: 5,500
Jalapeño peppers are high in potassium and vitamins A and C, magnesium, thiamine, riboflavin, and niacin.

Habanero
SHU: 100,000+
Add a teaspoon to diced mangoes and onions for an incendiary salsa.

Capsicum Oleoresin
SHU: 1,500,000
Used to make pepper spray. Not delicious.

Thai Bird
SHU: 50,000+
Combine with coconut milk and lime juice for an Asian marinade.

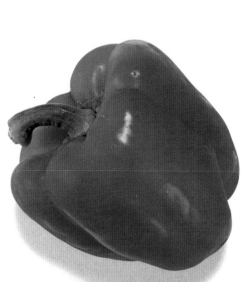

BELL PEPPER (RED, YELLOW, ORANGE)

All peppers are loaded with antioxidants, but none so much as the brightly colored reds, yellows, and oranges. These colors result from carotenoids concentrated in the flesh of the pepper, and it's these same carotenoids that give tomatoes, carrots, and grapefruits their healthy hues. The range of benefits provided by these colorful pigments include improved immune function, better communication between cells, protection against sun damage, and a diminished risk for several types of cancer.

PEPERONCINI

These are the tangy yellow pickled peppers you can get at the grocery store or thrown on your hoagie and antipasto at delis. They're an easy way to add some pepper benefits to just about any meat, fish, or vegetable sandwich. Keep a jar on the top shelf of the fridge.

SERVING SIZE	1 cup, chopped, red (149 g)			3 to 4 peppers (28 g)		
Calories/Fiber	Calories: 46		Fiber: 3 g	Calories: 10		Fiber: 0 g
Macronutrients	Protein: 1 g	Fat: 0 g	Carbs: 9 g	Protein: 0 g	Fat: 0 g	Carbs: 2 g
Vitamins/Minerals	Vitamin C: 317%	Vitamin A: 93%		Sodium: 14%		

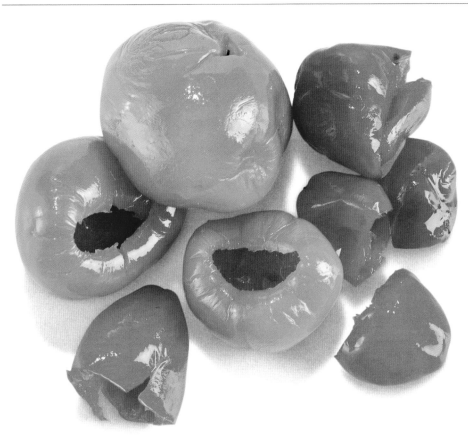

YOUR STOMACH LOVES CHILES

A review published in the *American Journal of Natural Medicine* found that people who ate the most chiles also had the fewest ulcers. "Capsaicin stimulates the production of saliva, which can help fight flatulence, dry mouth, and stomach cramps, and can even relieve indigestion," says Mark Blumenthal, executive director of the American Botanical Council. Capsaicin may also reduce inflammation and even kill headaches.

PEPPADEW PEPPER

This sweet-and-spicy fruit looks like a cross between a cherry tomato and a red pepper. Native to Africa, they're popular with chefs in the United States. Just $\frac{1}{3}$ cup of Peppadews packs heart-protecting vitamin B_6, cancer-fighting lycopene, and a day's worth of vitamin C. Toss Peppadews in a salad with avocado and blue cheese or in a simple pasta with olive oil and garlic. For a killer snack or appetizer, try filling them with a hunk of mozzarella or goat cheese. You'll find them in the salad section of upscale grocers.

⅓ cup (30 g)			
Calories: 40		Fiber: 1 g	
Protein: 0 g	Fat: 0 g	Carbs: 9 g	
Vitamin C: 100%			

No wonder rats always look so young. "Cheese is one of the best foods you can eat for your teeth," says Matthew Messina, DDS, an American Dental Association spokesman. "It's a good source of calcium, to keep your teeth strong. Plus, eating cheese can lower the levels of bacteria in your mouth and keep your teeth clean and cavity-free," he says. Cheese is also packed with protein and fat, which keep you full. And it's versatile and convenient—making it a great snack.

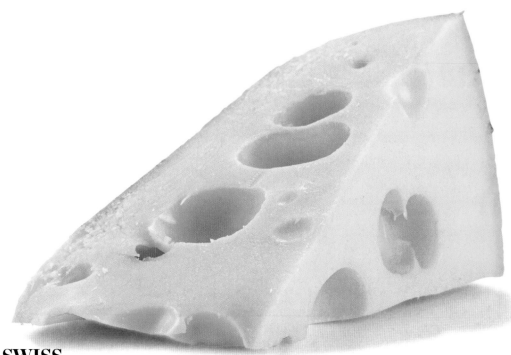

SWISS

Not only do you get calcium and protein, you also get a big dose of B_{12} with your slice. And is there any better taste in the world than a fresh slice of Swiss cheese? Have one melted over an open-faced tuna and tomato sandwich.

SERVING SIZE	1 slice (28 g)		
Calories/Fiber	Calories: 106		Fiber: 0 g
Macronutrients	Protein: 8 g	Fat: 8 g	Carbs: 2 g
Vitamins/Minerals	Calcium: 22%	Vitamin B₁₂: 16%	Phosphorus: 16%

AMERICAN

Not the ideal cheese. American has a third less calcium than most cheeses, and double the salt. It's a serviceable fallback position—and kid-friendly—but with so many other options, shop around.

Per 1, low-fat slice (21 g) serving: *38 calories, 5 g protein, 1 g carbs, 0 g fiber, 1 g fat, and RDIs of 17% phosphorus, 14% calcium, and 13% sodium*

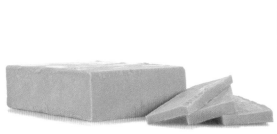

CHEDDAR

The classic cheese is a little higher in calories than the average cheese, but you lose none of the calcium and protein—and its versatility makes it a popular and tasty addition to dozens of meals.

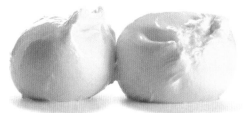

MOZZARELLA (PART SKIM)

Mozzerella is lower in calories than most common cheeses, which makes it the perfect app or snack. Try fresh mozzarella sliced with tomato and fresh basil with balsamic vinaigrette. Or eat as string cheese between meals at work.

1 slice (28 g)			
Calories: 113		Fiber: 0 g	
Protein: 7 g	Fat: 9 g		Carbs: 0 g
Calcium: 20%	Phosphorus: 14%		

1 oz (28 g)			
Calories: 71		Fiber: 0 g	
Protein 7 g	Fat: 4 g		Carbs: 1 g
Calcium: 22%	Phosphorus: 13%		

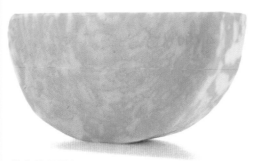

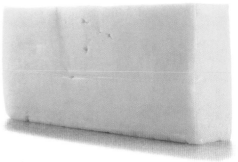

COLBY

Named after the town in Wisconsin where it was created, Colby is milder than cheddar and a great table cheese. It also goes well grated with salads.

MONTEREY JACK

Jack is a soft, milder cheese that melts well and is nice on sandwiches. It's probably best known in pepperjack form (hot pepper flakes inside the cheese), which has made it ubiquitous at tailgates and sporting-event parties, which means you probably eat a lot more of it than you should. Take small pieces and savor slowly—you'll enjoy more and eat less.

SERVING SIZE	1 oz (28 g)			1 oz (28 g)		
Calories/Fiber	Calories: 110	Fiber: 0 g		Calories: 104	Fiber: 0 g	
Macronutrients	Protein: 7 g	Fat: 9 g	Carbs: 1 g	Protein: 7 g	Fat: 8 g	Carbs: 0 g
Vitamins/Minerals	Calcium: 19%	Phosphorus: 13%		Calcuim: 20%		

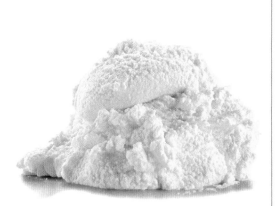

RICOTTA (PART SKIM)

Made from whey, this lower-calorie cheese is rich in amino acids, which speed muscle recovery after a workout. Put half a cup in a blender with skim milk and fruit for a postworkout cheese-cake-flavored smoothie.

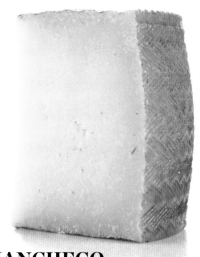

MANCHEGO

Manchego is a meticulously crafted Spanish cheese from sheep's milk that can only be produced in designated parts of the country on registered farms—though you can find it in most upscale grocery stores.

1 oz (28 g)		
Calories: 39	Fiber: 0 g	
Protein: 3 g	Fat: 2 g	Carbs: 1 g
Calcium: 8%		

1 oz (28 g)		
Calories: 120	Fiber: 0 g	
Protein: 7 g	Fat: 10 g	Carbs: 0 g
Calcium: 30%		

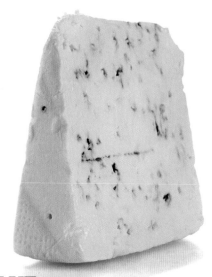

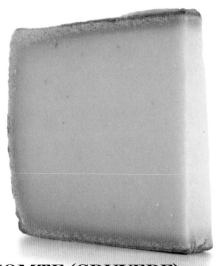

BLUE

One tasty cheese, but blue has more sodium than most cheese. It's best used paired with fruits such as figs, with nuts, or as crumbles over salad. Blue cheese dressing, however, contains more unhealthy fats than the cheese itself.

COMTE (GRUYERE)

The classic French cheese. A little-known health fact: Gruyere is low in sodium compared with other cheeses (1 ounce has 94 milligrams salt, 4 percent of your recommended daily intake) because strict production regulations say that salt can only be added to the surface of the cheese.

SERVING SIZE	1 oz (28 g)			1 oz (28 g)		
Calories/Fiber	Calories: 99	Fiber: 0 g		Calories: 116	Fiber: 0 g	
Macronutrients	Protein: 6 g	Fat: 8 g	Carbs: 1 g	Protein: 8 g	Fat: 9 g	Carbs: 0 g
Vitamins/Minerals	Calcium: 15%	Sodium: 16%		Calcium: 28%	Phosphorus: 17%	

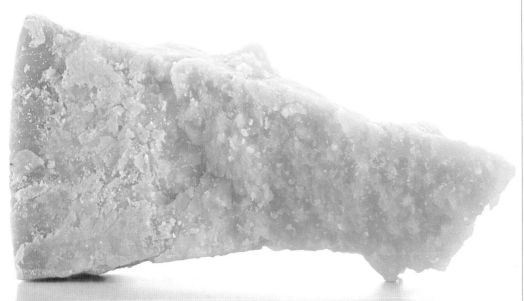

PARMESAN

"It's the MSG of Italian cooking," says Marco Canora, chef at Hearth and Insieme in New York City. "It makes everything from roasted asparagus and scrambled eggs to pasta and soup taste better." Look for Parmesan that has been aged at least 16 months, and be leery of cheese that is too pale.

1 oz, hard (28 g)		
Calories: 110		Fiber: 0 g
Protein: 10 g	Fat: 7 g	Carbs: 1 g
Calcium: 33%	Phosphorus: 19%	Sodium: 19%

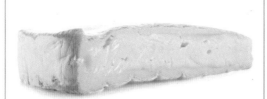

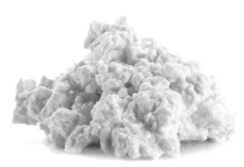

BRIE

Brie is delicious, but doesn't bring the
nutrition to the table like other cheeses,
with significantly less calcium.

COTTAGE

A half-cup of cottage cheese is
a good low-calorie, high-protein snack,
but a regular version would also pack
about 20 percent of your day's salt.
Stick with low-sodium versions.

SERVING SIZE	1 oz (28 g)			1 oz (28 g)		
Calories/Fiber	Calories: 94		Fiber: 0 g	Calories: 20		Fiber: 0 g
Macronutrients	Protein: 6 g	Fat: 8 g	Carbs: 0 g	Protein: 3 g	Fat: <0g	Carbs: 1 g
Vitamins/Minerals	Riboflavin: 9%	Vitamin B₁₂: 8%	Calcium: 5%	Sodium: 5%	Selenium: 4%	Phosphorus: 4%

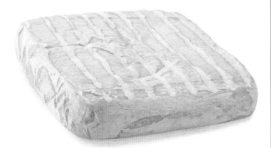

ROBIOLA

Step away from the Cheez Whiz: Robiola is a much healthier way to top a Triscuit. This Italian cheese is soft, like Brie, and it tastes as rich as butter. Spread it on a whole-grain cracker or baguette slice, and round out the snack with grapes or cantaloupe.

1 oz (28 g)		
Calories: 90	Fiber: 0 g	
Protein: 4.5 g	Fat: 8 g	Carbs: 0 g

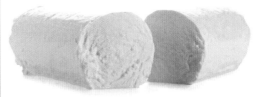

GOAT (CHEVRE)

Looking for something low in saturated fat? Skip Cheddar and Brie and try 2 ounces of soft cheese, such as fresh goat cheese or feta, in a salad of romaine and sliced pears tossed with olive oil and balsamic vinegar.

1 oz, semisoft (28 g)		
Calories: 102	Fiber: 0 g	
Protein: 6 g	Fat: 8 g	Carbs: 1 g
Riboflavin: 11%	Phosphorus: 10%	Calcium: 8%

Drinking two to three glasses of milk a day, whether it's fat-free, 2 percent, or whole, lowers the likelihood of both heart attack and stroke—a finding confirmed by British scientists. Also, because milk contains bone-strengthening calcium and muscle-building protein, it's a worthy beverage to work into your daily calorie allotment. The majority of scientific studies show that drinking whole milk will still improve cholesterol levels, just not as much as drinking skim does.

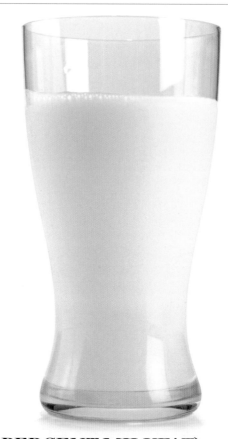

WHOLE (3.25 PERCENT MILKFAT)

While you've probably always been told to drink reduced-fat milk, the majority of scientific studies show that drinking whole milk actually improves cholesterol levels, just not as much as drinking fat-free does. One recent exception: Danish researchers found that men who consumed a diet rich in whole milk experienced a slight increase in LDL cholesterol (6 points). However, it's worth noting that these men drank six 8-ounce glasses a day, an unusually high amount. Even so, their triglycerides—another marker of heart disease risk—decreased by 22 percent.

SERVING SIZE	1 cup (244 g)		
Calories/Fiber	Calories: 146		Fiber: 0 g
Macronutrients	Protein: 8 g	Fat: 8 g	Carbs: 13 g
Vitamins/Minerals	Calcium: 28%	Riboflavin: 26%	Vitamin D: 24%

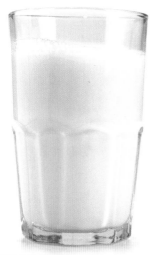

2 PERCENT

The best milk option, if you want to cut calories, is to go for lower-fat milk varieties—1 cup of 2 percent milk has 24 fewer calories than 1 cup of whole milk (and a cup of skim milk has 36 fewer calories than this 2 percent). But 2 percent isn't a poor nutritious choice—it still comes with belly-filling protein and is loaded with 286 milligrams of calcium, which meets nearly a third of your daily calcium needs. In a Purdue University study, women who took in at least 780 milligrams of calcium a day maintained their weight over a 2-year period, regardless of their exercise habits. But women who took in less than that gained weight—again, regardless of whether they exercised or not!

1 PERCENT

The USDA recommends that adults ages 19 to 50 get at least 1,000 milligrams of calcium a day, and teens and those over 50 should get at least 1,300. The truth is, the less fat in your milk, the more calcium you'll get—but it's a fairly negligible difference. One cup of whole milk has 276 milligrams of calcium, whereas 1 cup of 1 percent milk has 290 milligrams. Skim milk has the most—301 milligrams.

1 cup (244 g)		
Calories: 122	Fiber: 0 g	
Protein: 8 g	Fat: 5 g	Carbs: 12 g
Calcium: 29%	Riboflavin: 27%	Vitamin D: 26%

1 cup (244 g)		
Calories: 102	Fiber: 0 g	
Protein: 8 g	Fat: 2 g	Carbs: 13 g
Vitamin D: 32%	Calcium: 29%	Riboflavin: 27%

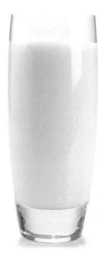

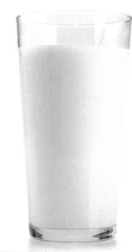

FAT-FREE

Fat-free milk has the most calcium, the least fat, and the fewest calories of all the milk varieties. Whichever you choose, here's one more pitch for drinking the stuff: Milk is one of the best muscle foods on the planet. The protein in milk is about 80 percent casein and 20 percent whey. Both are high-quality proteins, but whey is known as a "fast protein" because it's quickly broken down into amino acids and absorbed into the bloodstream. That makes it a very good protein to consume after your workout. Casein, on the other hand, is digested more slowly. So it's ideal for providing your body with a steady supply of smaller amounts of protein for a longer period of time, such as between meals or while you sleep.

BUTTERMILK (CULTURED OR FERMENTED)

Yogurt gets all the press for packing probiotics, but the healthy bacteria can be found in any fermented milk product, including buttermilk. Buttermilk also carries more calcium and protein than milk.

SERVING SIZE	1 cup (245 g)			1 cup (245 g)		
Calories/Fiber	Calories: 86	Fiber: 0 g		Calories: 137	Fiber: 0 g	
Macronutrients	Protein: 8 g	Fat: 0 g	Carbs: 12 g	Protein: 10 g	Fat: 5 g	Carbs: 13 g
Vitamins/Minerals	Calcium: 30%	Phosphorus: 25%	Riboflavin: 20%	Calcium: 35%	Riboflavin: 30%	Phosphorus: 20%

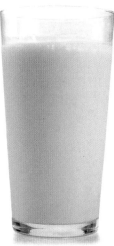

KEFIR

Similar to yogurt, this fermented dairy beverage is made by culturing fresh milk with kefir grains. Kefir's gut-friendly bacteria has been shown to help lower cholesterol, improve lactose digestion, and enhance the immune system. In addition, University of Washington scientists recently demonstrated that kefir was more effective than fruit juice or other dairy beverages at helping people control hunger. Look for kefir in the health-food section of your local supermarket.

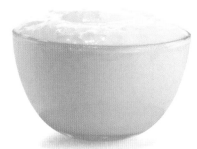

YOGURT

Probiotics and enzymes, those friendly bacteria found in yogurt, not only help the digestive system work properly, but also have a profound effect on the metabolism, according to a new study in *Molecular Systems Biology*. But not all yogurts are probiotic, so make sure the label says "live and active cultures." And beware of flavored and "fruit on the bottom" yogurts that make sugar a primary ingredient. Better to eat plain yogurt with fresh fruit.

THIS MILK'S NO DUD

A 2006 study in the *International Journal of Sport Nutrition and Exercise Metabolism* found that chocolate milk is as good as or better than Gatorade for replacing glucose in fatigued muscles. Why? Because it has more electrolytes and higher fat content. Research also shows that the balance of fat, protein, and carbs in chocolate milk makes it one-third more effective at replenishing muscles after a workout than other recovery beverages.

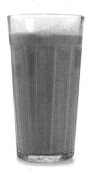

1 cup (244 g)		
Calories: 160		Fiber: 3 g
Protein: 10 g	Fat: 8 g	Carbs: 12 g
Calcium: 30%	Vitamin D: 25%	Vitamin A: 10%

1 cup (245 g)		
Calories: 154		Fiber: 0 g
Protein: 13 g	Fat: 4 g	Carbs: 17 g
Calcium: 45%	Phosphorus: 35%	Riboflavin: 31%

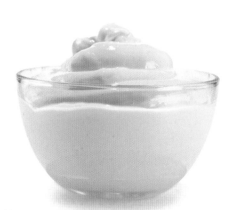

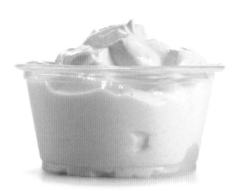

GREEK YOGURT

Greek yogurt has been separated from the watery whey that sits on top of regular yogurt, and the process has removed excessive sugars such as lactose and almost doubled the concentration of protein. That means it fills your belly more like a meal than a snack, with all the probiotic benefits of regular yogurt.

SOUR CREAM

For years, you've been told to avoid sour cream or to eat the light version because 90 percent of its calories are derived from fat, at least half of which is saturated. But 2 tablespoons of sour cream has only two-thirds the calories of a single tablespoon of mayonnaise—and less saturated fat than you'd get from drinking a 12-ounce glass of 2 percent reduced-fat milk. More important, sour cream is a close relative of butter, which means you're eating natural animal fat, not dangerous trans fat.

SERVING SIZE	1 cup (227 g)			2 Tbsp (24 g)		
Calories/Fiber	Calories: 130	Fiber: 0 g		Calories: 46	Fiber: 0 g	
Macronutrients	Protein: 23 g	Fat: 0 g	Carbs: 9 g	Protein: 0	Fat: 4 g	Carbs: 0 g
Vitamins/Minerals	Calcium: 30%	Riboflavin: 30%	Phosphorus: 30%			

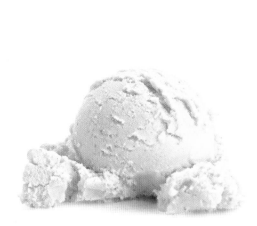

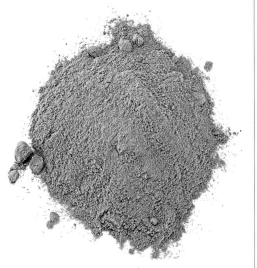

VANILLA EXTRACT

It's the secret ingredient that made nearly everything your mom baked taste better. A couple of drops will do the same for your protein shake.

ICE CREAM

A ½ cup of vanilla ice cream gives you about 17 milligrams of choline, which recent USDA research shows lowers blood levels of homocysteine—an amino acid that can hinder the flow of blood through blood vessels—by 8 percent, which translates to increased protection from cancer, heart attack, stroke, and dementia. A scoop (the size of a tennis ball) every few days isn't the diet saboteur it's made out to be. But ignore tricked-out designer ice creams packed with added sugar and preservatives. Pick a single-word ice cream—vanilla, chocolate, coffee, whatever—then add crumbled dark chocolate, berries, or crushed nuts.

WHEY AND CASEIN PROTEIN POWDER

Whey and casein are the primary proteins found in milk, at about 20 and 80 percent, respectively. Either will provide your muscles with the raw materials for growth, but combining quickly digested whey with slowly digested casein allows you to optimize your protein intake.

½ cup (66 g)		
Calories: 137		Fiber: 0 g
Protein: 2 g	Fat: 7 g	Carbs: 16 g
Riboflavin: 9%	Calcium: 8%	Phosphorus: 7%

1 oz, mixed (30 g)		
Calories: 109		Fiber: 0 g
Protein: 22 g	Fat: 1 g	Carbs: 3 g
Calcium: 15%	Phosphorus: 11%	Potassium: 6%

What kind of bread is healthiest? Flip around to the ingredient list. Is the first ingredient a whole grain? Does each slice have 2 or more grams of fiber? Do "inulin" or "polydextrose" show up? The correct answers are yes, yes, and no. "With whole grain, nothing is stripped away," says Jim White, RD, of the American Dietetic Association. That means you're noshing on natural fiber, not inulin or polydextrose, two additives used to artificially boost fiber.

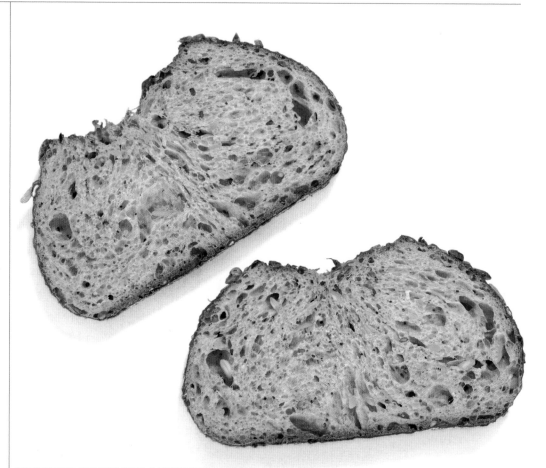

WHOLE WHEAT BREAD

When choosing a bread, always opt for whole wheat instead of white. That's because it comes with more fiber than the white-flour bread, which has essentially been stripped of all its good stuff. Fiber slows your digestion and helps you stay full for longer. That said, make sure not to fall for label hype. "Whole grains" or "multi-grain" don't necessarily indicate whole wheat. Make sure the label says "100%."

SERVING SIZE	1 slice (28 g)		
Calories/Fiber	Calories: 69		Fiber: 2 g
Macronutrients	Protein: 4 g	Fat: 2 g	Carbs: 12 g
Vitamins/Minerals	Manganese: 30%	Selenium: 16%	

GO WITH THE GRAIN

To understand what "whole grain" means, imagine a kernel of corn. That pale coating on the outside is the bran: it contains most of the fiber of the kernel. The little tiny bud in the middle is the germ: that's where the vitamins and minerals are hiding out. And the rest of the kernel is the endosperm, which is basically an energy storage facility full of carbohydrates. The same structure is found in other grains like wheat and oats. Combine the three parts of the grain and you get a perfect food. "Refine" the grain—eliminating the germ and the bran—and you get Wonder Bread.

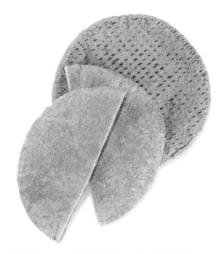

WHOLE WHEAT PITA

You should be careful with pitas just as you should be careful with tortilla wraps—they may be flat, but they're bloated with a surprising number of calories. Always check the packaging to make sure that the pita you choose comes with a load of fiber and protein. And, as with all starches, verify that you're buying 100 percent whole wheat, and not just "wheat."

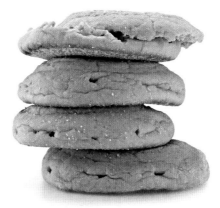

WHOLE WHEAT ENGLISH MUFFIN

One English muffin—two halves—has half as many calories as two slices of bread. So this is by far the best option for the outsides of your breakfast sandwich. One thing to watch out for, though: Most English muffins not only raise blood sugar significantly, but are nearly devoid of fiber, protein, and vitamins. Check the label before you buy, to make sure you're not purchasing what amounts to truly empty calories. One-hundred percent whole-wheat English muffins are a good start, but we'd recommend you take that a step further—we like the kind made from sprouted grains, which contain no flour and are packed with nutrients.

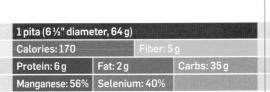

1 pita (6 ½" diameter, 64 g)		
Calories: 170	Fiber: 5 g	
Protein: 6 g	Fat: 2 g	Carbs: 35 g
Manganese: 56%	Selenium: 40%	

1 muffin (66 g)		
Calories: 134	Fiber: 4 g	
Protein: 6 g	Fat: 1 g	Carbs: 27 g
Manganese: 59%	Selenium: 38%	Calcium: 17%

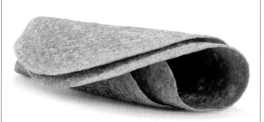

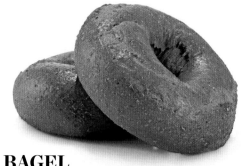

WHOLE WHEAT WRAP/TORTILLA

Be careful with wraps: They've grown to enormous proportions, and now come with as much as 300 calories—before you've added the innards! And when they're large, they also invite you to load more toppings and goodies into your sandwich than you would between two slices of bread. Keep the wraps or tortillas limited in diameter—6 inches, say, instead of 12—and you'll better be able to control your portion sizes.

BAGEL

Bagel shop bagels are massive, and even whole wheat and oat bran versions have somewhat fuzzy ingredients, so mind your serving size. MIT researchers analyzed blood samples from people who had eaten either a high-protein or a high-carbohydrate breakfast. Two hours after eating, the carb eaters had tryptophan levels 11 percent higher than before, and the people who had eaten protein dropped their tryptophan levels by 37 percent. The higher your tryptophan level, the more likely you are to feel tired and sluggish.

SERVING SIZE	1 wrap			1 medium bagel (4" diameter, 105 g)		
Calories/Fiber	Calories: 70		Fiber: 2 g	Calories: 289		Fiber: 2 g
Macronutrients	Protein: 3 g	Fat: 0 g	Carbs: 20 g	Protein 11 g	Fat: 2 g	Carbs: 56 g
Vitamins/Minerals	Potassium: 16%	Iron: 4%		Manganese: 28%	Sodium: 23%	

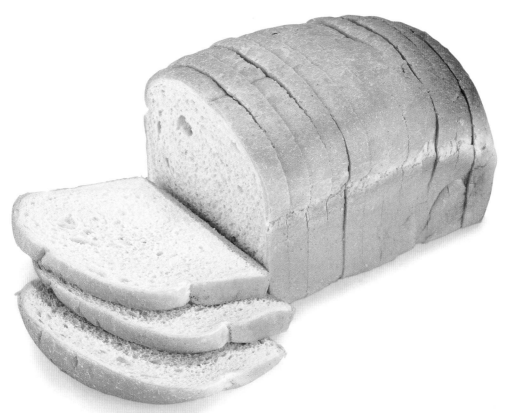

WHITE BREAD

If you must eat white bread, toast it. According to a UK study, when participants ate bread that had been frozen, thawed, and toasted, their blood sugar rose 39 percent less than it did when they consumed fresh slices. Freezing and toasting also worked on their own, reducing glycemic response by at least 26 percent each. It could be that these processes chemically alter starch and prevent it from breaking down into sugar, say the researchers. Store your loaves in the freezer and let slices defrost overnight at room temperature before toasting.

1 slice (25 g)		
Calories: 66		Fiber: 1 g
Protein: 2 g	Fat: 1 g	Carbs: 13 g
Thiamin: 8%	Folate: 7%	Selenium: 6%

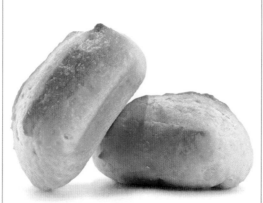

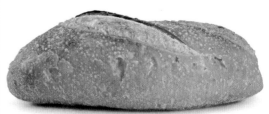

FRENCH (ROLL AND BAGUETTE)

Not as nutritious as whole grain breads, but French bread can be a terrific vehicle for other healthy foods, from olive oil dipping to soup soaking to bruschetta noshing. Be creative.

SOURDOUGH

Like white and French bread, sourdough is more about what it's eaten with. A great comfort food: clam chowder in a sourdough bowl.

SERVING SIZE	1 slice (32 g)			1 slice (32 g)		
Calories/Fiber	Calories: 92	Fiber: 1 g		Calories: 92	Fiber: 1 g	
Macronutrients	Protein: 4 g	Fat: 1 g	Carbs: 18 g	Protein: 4 g	Fat: 1 g	Carbs: 18 g
Vitamins/Minerals	Selenium: 12%	Folate: 12%		Selenium: 12%	Folate: 12%	

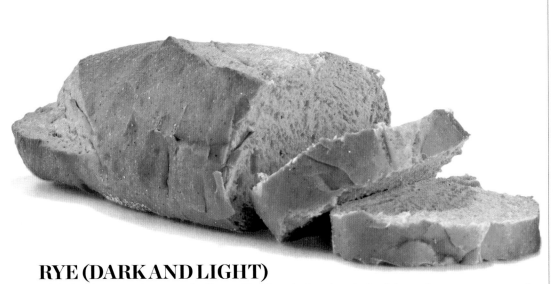

RYE (DARK AND LIGHT)

High in fiber, rye is a great alternative to whole wheat. Arabinoxylan—a compound found in abundance in rye—may enhance the growth of beneficial bacteria in your digestive tract, according to one study. Rye bread in lesser quantities may also promote digestive health, says Reetta Holma, PhD, the lead author of the study.

1 slice (32 g)			
Calories: 83		Fiber: 2 g	
Protein: 3 g	Fat: 1 g	Carbs: 15 g	
Selenium: 14%	Manganese: 13%		

Pasta has varying nutritional merits depending on the variety, but its real job is delivering an amazing and almost limitless variety of foods along with it—meat, vegetables, herbs, cheeses. Of all the foods in this book, pasta is the one that most rewards a daring imagination.

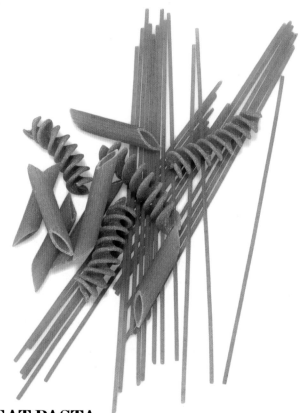

WHOLE WHEAT PASTA

Switching to whole grain pasta from white pasta can melt away your gut. Penn State researchers compared two groups of overweight dieters: One group swapped white bread and pasta for whole wheat products, while the other ate the same number of calories as the first group but didn't make the switch. Although all the dieters lost about 10 pounds in 3 months, the whole grain eaters dropped twice as much abdominal fat. The study's authors credit the extra fiber and antioxidants in whole grains, which help control inflammation and insulin (a hormone that tells your body to store belly fat).

SERVING SIZE	1 cup, cooked, spaghetti (140 g)		
Calories/Fiber	Calories: 174		Fiber: 6 g
Macronutrients	Protein: 7 g	Fat: 1 g	Carbs: 37 g
Vitamins/Minerals	Manganese: 97%	Selenium: 52%	

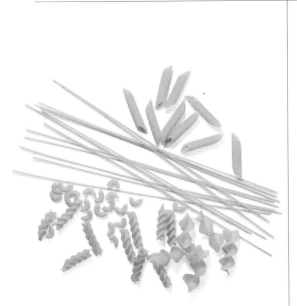

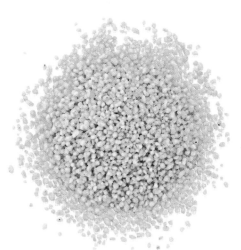

SHIRATAKI: THE NO-CARB NOODLE

Unfortunately, men tend to eat pasta in mounds, not moderation. But what if a noodle existed that was not only Atkins-approved but had virtually no calories? It's called shirataki. This translucent noodle, which is made from the powdered root of the Asian konjac yam, consists mostly of a no-calorie, highly soluble fiber called glucomannan. According to a study review by University of Connecticut researchers, glucomannan helps lower LDL (bad) cholesterol, triglycerides, fasting blood sugar, and even body weight. What's more, scientists in Thailand found that just 1 gram has the power to significantly slow the absorption of sugar into your bloodstream after you eat a carb-loaded meal. Translation: This noodle can make almost any meal healthier.

ENRICHED PASTA

The next best kind of pasta after whole wheat is the enriched kind. While white-flour pasta doesn't have the whole grain goodness that you'll get from whole wheat, the fact that it's enriched means that you're not consuming entirely empty calories. Before you go for the first package that boasts "enriched" right on the front, though, be sure to read the label to see exactly what it's been enriched with—and compare.

COUSCOUS

A diet too low in starches may restrict mood-boosting serotonin in your brain, a study in the *Archives of Internal Medicine* suggests. The right starches have fiber, vitamins, and heart-healthy phytochemicals. The wrong kinds mess with blood sugar. Think of couscous as tiny pasta. You want whole wheat couscous, rather than white, if possible. And when you mix it with vegetables, that makes the dish even better for you.

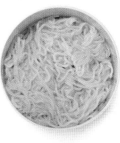

1 cup, cooked, spaghetti (140 g)		
Calories: 221	Fiber: 3 g	
Protein: 8 g	Fat: 1 g	Carbs: 43 g
Selenium: 53%	Folate: 26%	Thiamin: 26%

2 oz (57 g)		
Calories: 221	Fiber: 3 g	
Protein: 8 g	Fat: 1 g	Carbs: 43 g
Selenium: 62%		

The Sweet Stuff Guide

Yes, sugar takes most of the blame for the obesity epidemic. But sugar is important. The sugar in our bodies, glucose, is a fundamental fuel for body and brain, says David Levitsky, PhD, a professor of psychology and nutritional sciences at Cornell University. The problem: "Sweetened foods tend to make us overeat. And that threatens the energy balance in our bodies."

How off is the average American's energy balance? Doctors test for prediabetes and diabetes by having patients consume 75 grams of glucose to see how their system processes sugar. It's a kind of metabolic stress test—processing that kind of sugar load is not something your body should normally do.

And yet a 24-ounce regular soda often contains more than 75 grams of sugar. You'd have to eat four apples in order to ingest roughly the same amount of fructose in one large McDonald's Coke.

Corn Syrup

Corn syrup isn't as sweet as other sugars (not that you'd notice). It's primarily made up of glucose, which can be burned up as a source of immediate energy, stored in your liver and muscles for use later, or, as a last resort, turned into fat. It makes terrific fake blood with red food dye, but it's still just empty calories.

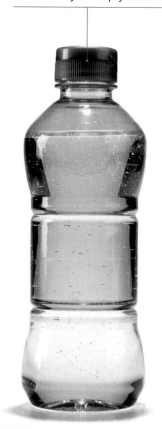

Refined Sugar

Even in quantities as large as one cup (200 g), granulated table sugar accumulates virtually no nutritional value whatsoever (okay, 2% of your recommended daily intake of riboflavin and selenium, but still). Avoid it as much as you can.

Brown Sugar

A teaspoon has 11 calories. One cup (packed, 220 g) has 18% of your recommended daily intake of calcium, 9% of iron, and 8% of potassium. But it'll cost you 836 calories to get there!

Honey

The bee's gift to cardiology. Researchers at the University of Illinois found that honey has powerful antioxidant qualities that help combat cardiovascular disease. Sugar, on the other hand, can lower your levels of HDL (good) cholesterol, potentially increasing your risk of heart-related disorders.

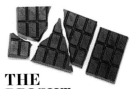

THE BRIGHT SIDE OF DARK CHOCOLATE

Research shows that dark chocolate can improve heart health, lower blood pressure, reduce LDL (bad) cholesterol, and increase the flow of blood to the brain. But there's a reason that chocolate has a reputation as an aphrodisiac. It also boosts serotonin and endorphin levels, which are associated with improved mood and greater concentration. Perhaps best of all, dark chocolate is full of anandamide and phenylethylamine, two compounds that cause the body to release the same feel-good endorphins triggered by sex and physical exertion. Look for chocolate that is 60 percent cocoa or higher.

Per 1 oz (28 g) serving: *162 calories, 11 g fat, 2 g protein, 15 g carbs, 2 g fiber, and RDIs of 19% selenium, 17% copper, and 10% iron*

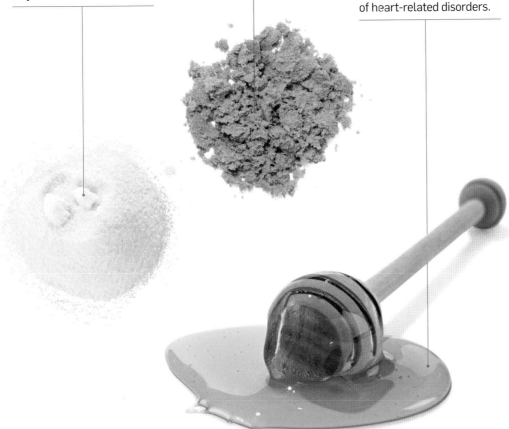

HIGH-FRUCTOSE CORN SYRUP

See page 363 to understand what HFCS is and how it differs (and doesn't) from regular table sugar.

Molasses

Sugarcane syrup is separated at a refining plant into sucrose (which is crystallized into white sugar) and molasses, which has most of the nutrients from the plant, including vitamin B6, iron, potassium, and calcium. But you'd have to drink a glass of the goo to accumulate meaningful levels.

Maple Syrup

Natural is always better. The artificial stuff is typically corn syrup with flavoring added. It has a less intense flavor, so most people wind up using more of it to achieve an ideal taste.

Agave Syrup

Most commonly served distilled with a side of lime, the nectar from the agave cactus is also a sweetener. The honeylike syrup has twice the sweetness and half the calories of sugar, but it is digested slowly, so it won't cause swings in energy. Agave is also one of the only nondairy foods to contain digestion-enhancing bifidobacteria.

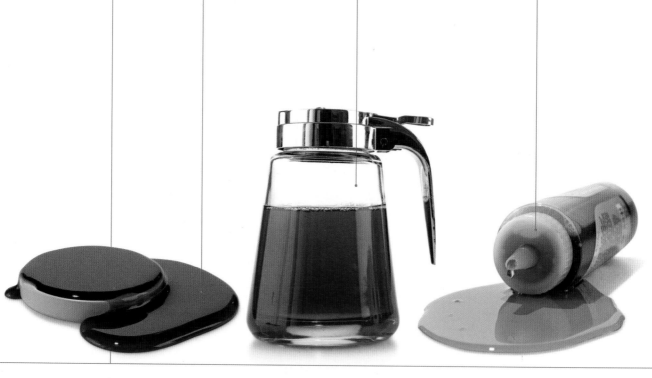

Your Guide to Artificial Sweetners

Some research seems to indicate that artificial sweeteners aren't the weight-loss wonders we once thought. A 2005 study at the University of Texas found that people who drank one can of diet soda per day had a 37 percent greater risk of obesity. Preliminary animal studies have even indicated that fake sugars can lower metabolism.

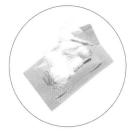
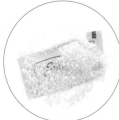
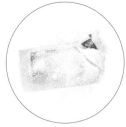

SACCHARIN (SWEET'N LOW)

What it is: Product of a reaction between sulfur dioxide, chlorine, ammonia, and two biochemical acids. Found in Crest and Colgate.

Calories: 0

Flavor profile: Metallic and bitter aftertaste; 300 to 500 times sweeter than sugar

Possible side effects: Linked to cancer in rats, but not in humans; FDA removed warning labels

SUCRALOSE (SPLENDA)

What it is: Sugar molecules blended with chlorine. Found in Arizona brand diet iced teas.

Calories: 0

Flavor profile: Slightly chemical; 600 times sweeter than sugar

Possible side effects: None

ASPARTAME (NUTRA-SWEET AND EQUAL)

What it is: A combination of two amino acids: aspartic acid and phenylalanine. Found in most diet sodas.

Calories: 0

Flavor profile: Chemical; 180 times sweeter than sugar

Possible side effects: None, unless you have a rare genetic sensitivity to it

STEVIA (PUREVIA AND TRUVIA)

What it is: Dried leaves of the naturally sweet but sugar-free stevia plant.

Calories: 0

Flavor profile: Licorice-like; 150 to 400 times sweeter than sugar

Whether you've sworn off meat or simply like as wide a variety of foods as you can find, meat alternatives are a staple and deliver a protein punch. Another bonus: They're ripe for more culinary experimentation than regular meat.

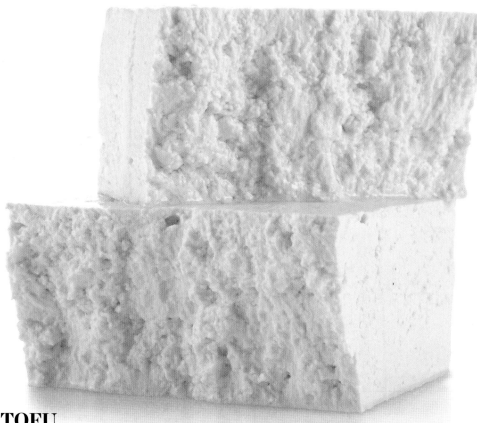

TOFU

Made from soybeans, tofu was once the bastion of vegetarians. But the plant protein in these pressed bean curds—available firm or soft, and delicious when marinated and tossed into salads—provides a full complement of amino acids, as well as isoflavone, which helps muscles recover from exercise.

SERVING SIZE	1 oz, raw (28 g)		
Calories/Fiber	Calories: 21		Fiber: 0 g
Macronutrients	Protein: 2 g	Fat: 1 g	Carbs: 1 g
Vitamins/Minerals	Calcium: 10%	Manganese: 8%	Iron: 8%

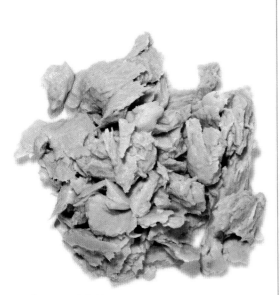

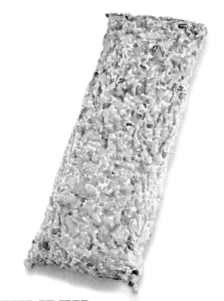

SEITAN

Seitan is another name for wheat gluten, which is a meat substitute that isn't soybean-based (like tofu). Ounce for ounce, seitan has 15 more grams of protein than a New York strip and one-fourth the fat. The only downside is that seitan carries about 40 extra calories.

TEMPEH

Tempeh is a chewy soy product that can be mixed into burgers. Made from cracked, cooked, and fermented soybeans, tempeh usually also includes another grain, such as millet, brown rice, or barley, and sometimes all three. It's sold in the refrigerated section of the supermarket and has a chewy, meaty texture. Tempeh is more protein-packed and vitamin-dense than tofu—and as a result, it's also more firm, flavorful, and meatlike. Use it in stir-fries, chili, salads, and sandwiches.

1 oz, raw (28 g)		
Calories: 104	Fiber: 0	
Protein: 21 g	Fat: 1 g	Carbs: 4 g
Selenium: 16%		

1 oz, raw (28 g)		
Calories: 54	Fiber: 0 g	
Protein: 5 g	Fat: 3 g	Carbs: 3 g
Manganese: 18%		

We probably don't have to sell you on the virtues of chicken and turkey. So let's devote our efforts to persuading you to buy free-range birds. According to a recent study in the journal *Poultry Science*, free-range chickens have significantly more omega-3s than grain-fed chickens, less harmful fat, and fewer calories.

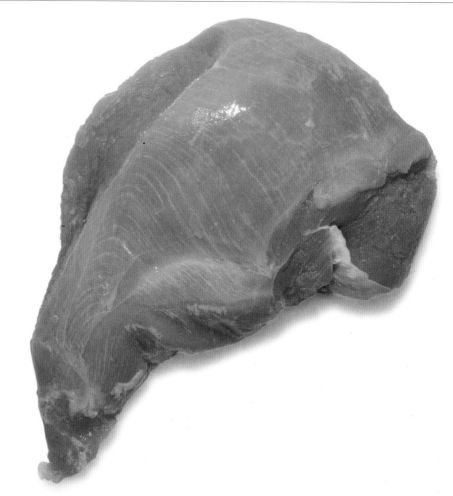

TURKEY (WHITE MEAT)

Turkey breast is nutritionally similar to chicken breast, so if you want the health benefits all it comes down to is taste and price. And if taste doesn't matter to you: What's on sale this week?

SERVING SIZE	4 oz (112 g)		
Calories/Fiber	Calories: 128		Fiber: 0 g
Macronutrients	Protein: 28 g	Fat: 1 g	Carbs: 0 g
Vitamins/Minerals	Selenium: 40%	Niacin: 32%	Vitamin B₆: 32%

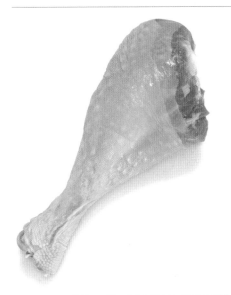

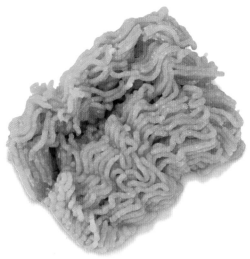

TURKEY (DARK MEAT)

Dark meat is more caloric than white meat because of its higher fat content. But only a third of the fat in a turkey drumstick is the saturated kind, according to the USDA food database. (The other two-thirds are heart-healthy unsaturated fats.) What's more, 86 percent of that saturated fat either has no impact on cholesterol, or raises HDL (good) cholesterol more than LDL (bad) cholesterol—a result that actually lowers your heart-disease risk.

TURKEY (GROUND)

Before you slap together your turkey burgers, make sure, as with ground chicken, to check what kind of meat you're buying. A mix of dark meat and white is fine—but only when you're aware that's what you're getting. If you're looking to cut calories and fat, ground dark meat isn't much of an alternative to hamburger.

PREP A BIRD LIKE A PRO

A whole chicken is cheaper than precut, so dissecting it yourself can net you more nutrients per dollar. Bill Begale, owner of Paulina Meat Market in Chicago, reveals how:

1. Remove the wings. Keep the blade flat against the chicken, and then slide it into the bird's "armpit" until you hit bone. Find the joint and cut through the cartilage.

2. Cut off the legs. Slice into the hip and bend the leg up to pop the joint. Cut through the cartilage and pull off the leg along with the backbone meat. Slice off the thighs above the drumstick.

3. Take out the backbone. From the back of the bird, cut to the neck, half an inch from each side of the spine.

4. Separate the breast. Make a shallow cut down the center of the inner chest membrane. Push the sternum up from underneath with your fingers, and pull it out completely. Cut the breast in half.

4 oz (112 g)		
Calories: 140		Fiber: 0 g
Protein: 24 g	Fat: 4 g	Carbs: 0 g
Selenium: 44%	Zinc: 24%	Vitamin B$_6$: 20%

4 oz (112 g)		
Calories: 168		Fiber: 0 g
Protein: 20 g	Fat: 8 g	Carbs: 0 g
Selenium: 32%	Phosphorus: 16%	Zinc: 16%

Poultry

BROWN EGGS VS. WHITE EGGS

No contest: They're equal. White-shelled eggs are produced by hens with white feathers and white earlobes. Brown-shelled eggs are produced by hens with red feathers and red earlobes (yes, chickens have earlobes). Generally, red hens are slightly larger and need more food, so their eggs typically cost more.

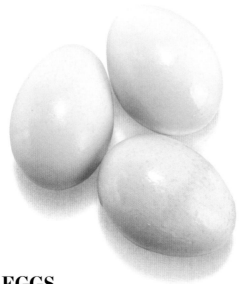

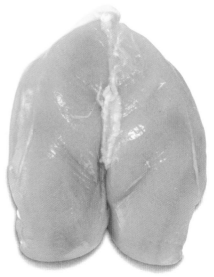

EGGS

Whole eggs contain more essential vitamins and minerals per calorie than virtually any other food. They may even be the perfect diet food: Saint Louis University scientists found that people who had eggs as part of their breakfast ate fewer calories the rest of the day than those who ate bagels instead. Even though both breakfasts contained the same number of calories, the egg eaters consumed 264 fewer calories for the entire day.

CHICKEN (WHITE MEAT)

Boneless, skinless chicken breast is a healthy go-to food. The protein isn't just vital in squashing hunger and boosting metabolism, it's also a top source of energy. University of Illinois researchers found that people who ate higher amounts of protein had higher energy and didn't feel as tired as people with proportionally higher amounts of carbs in their diet. Look for birds labeled "free range."

SERVING SIZE	1 large egg (50 g)			4 oz (112 g)		
Calories/Fiber	Calories: 71		Fiber: 0 g	Calories: 124		Fiber: 0 g
Macronutrients	Protein: 6 g	Fat: 5 g	Carbs: 0 g	Protein: 24 g	Fat: 1 g	Carbs: 0 g
Vitamins/Minerals	Selenium: 23%	Riboflavin: 14%	Vitamin B$_{12}$: 11%	Niacin: 64%	Vitamin B$_6$: 32%	Selenium: 28%

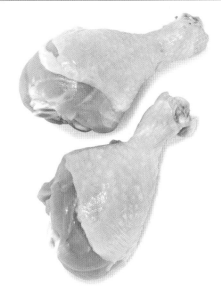

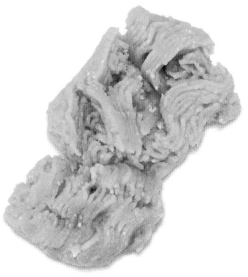

CHICKEN BREAST SALT ALERT

Why are some chicken breasts so high in salt? Plumping. Some poultry producers inject solutions into chicken breasts to make them juicier and more flavorful, says Mary Ellen Camire, PhD, a professor of food science at the University of Maine. "But the tradeoff from plumping is a huge increase in sodium content." A 4-ounce breast typically has 50 to 70 mg of sodium; a plumped piece can have 480 mg. Some enhanced breasts can be labeled "all natural," so be sure to read the ingredient list.

CHICKEN (DARK MEAT)

Research has shown that you don't need to be afraid of dark meat chicken, or even the skin. Because both are composed of animal fat, their fat composition is very similar to that of beef, meaning neither raises your risk for heart disease. Remember, eating more healthy fat—not less—is the key in helping you automatically reduce your calorie intake, without feeling deprived. How? The extra fat in dark turkey or chicken meat raises your levels of cholecystokinin, or CCK, a hormone that makes you feel full longer. The benefit: You'll be less likely to overeat in the hours that follow your meal.

CHICKEN (GROUND)

Store-bought ground chicken requires some scrutiny. Sometimes you're looking at a mixture of white and dark meat when all you want is breast. Be sure to read the label to see what you're buying.

4 oz, without skin (112 g)		
Calories: 140	Fiber: 0 g	
Protein: 24 g	Fat: 4 g	Carbs: 0 g
Niacin: 36%	Selenium: 20%	Phosphorus: 20%

4 oz (112 g)		
Calories: 160	Fiber: 0 g	
Protein: 20 g	Fat: 9 g	Carbs: 0 g
Niacin: 31%	Vitamin B₆: 29%	Phosphorus: 20%

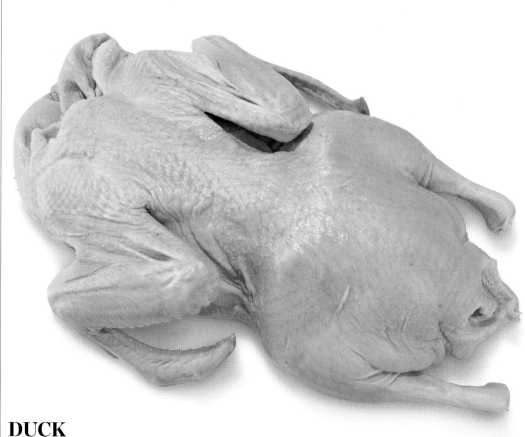

DUCK

Duck can be an acquired taste for some, but if you love it, don't think of it as a dangerous delicacy. It's loaded with protein and vitamins.

SERVING SIZE	4 oz, without skin (112 g)		
Calories/Fiber	Calories: 148		Fiber: 0 g
Macronutrients	Protein: 20 g	Fat: 4 g	Carbs: 0 g
Vitamins/Minerals	Thiamin: 28%	Riboflavin: 28%	Niacin: 28%

OSTRICH (GROUND)

A fantastic alternative when you're tired of beef burgers. One patty loads you up with double-digit recommended daily intake percentages of more than 10 nutritional markers.

Per 1 patty (109 g) serving:
180 calories, 22 g protein, 0 g carbs, 0 g fiber, 9 g fat, and RDIs of 84% vitamin B_{12}, 51% selenium, 26% vitamin B_6, and 18% iron

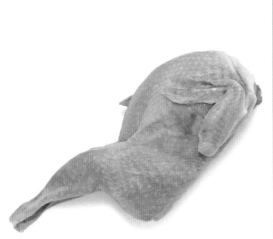

QUAIL (BREAST)

Not the protein superstar that chicken and turkey are, but quail is still high in niacin, B_6, and other vitamins. Pair it with some vegetable sides and you've got a memorable meal.

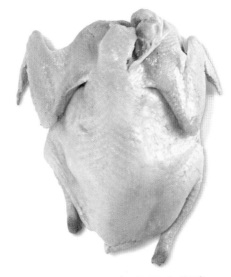

PHEASANT (BREAST)

Pheasant is a remarkably nutritious bird packed with protein, B vitamins and even a surprising 18 percent of your recommended daily intake of vitamin C.

1 breast, without skin (56 g)		
Calories: 69	Fiber: 0 g	
Protein: 13 g	Fat: 2 g	Carbs: 0 g
Niacin: 23%	Vitamin B_6: 15%	Selenium: 15%

½ breast, bone and skin removed (182 g)		
Calories: 242	Fiber: 0 g	
Protein: 44 g	Fat: 6 g	Carbs: 0 g
Niacin: 78%	Vitamin B_6: 67%	Selenium: 43%

The Spices of Life

Nutritionally, spices may not deliver a huge caloric impact to your body, nor will they affect satiety with big doses of protein and fiber. But the compounds in many spices can be deliciously healthy. For example: Nothing goes into Indian food by default. The Brahmins, mystics, and sages that historians credit with developing the Indian diet more than 7,000 years ago knew that spices, herbs, and other botanicals could have profound effects on the body. As strange as it may sound, Indians stay healthier by adding spices to their foods in the way that Americans use salt and pepper.

Here's the lowdown on some spices that may seem exotic, but are readily available in most supermarkets.

Turmeric

Curcumin, the polyphenol that gives the spice its tang and yellow hue, has antitumor, antiarthritis, and anti-inflammatory properties. Researchers at the University of California at Los Angeles have found that curcumin helps deter the accumulation of amyloid plaques in the brain, tiny blockages that may cause Alzheimer's disease. Turmeric's prevalence in India, the researchers suggest, may help explain why so few of the country's senior citizens have the disease. Add it in small doses to broths, sauces, and soups.

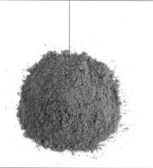

Curry Powder

Curry is a mixture of spices including coriander, cumin, turmeric, and others. While each spice has its own salutory effects, using straight tumeric as an addition to food or a rub for meat provides the best brain-protecting boost. Combine it with black pepper to enhance its bioavailability.

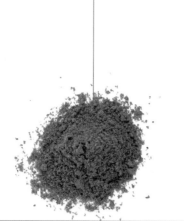

Cinnamon

Cinnamon is rich in antioxidants that inhibit blood clotting and bacterial growth (including the bad-breath variety). It also helps control your blood sugar. USDA researchers found that people with type 2 diabetes who consumed 1 gram of cinnamon a day for 6 weeks (about ¼ teaspoon each day) significantly reduced not only their blood sugar but also their triglycerides and LDL (bad) cholesterol. Credit the spice's active ingredients, methylhydroxychalcone polymers, which increase your cells' ability to metabolize sugar by up to 20 times.

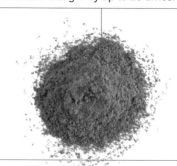

Cardamom

This spice has many varieties, each with its own distinct flavor, but Ray Sahelian, MD, a Los Angeles-based nutritionist, says they're all high in antioxidants. The spice can also help restore healthy levels of glutathione, which protects cells from toxins. Add the pods to your tea while it steeps or grind them with your coffee beans, a popular tradition in Middle Eastern countries. Or just add a pinch to coffee or cappuccino, or to a bowl of fruit and yogurt in the morning.

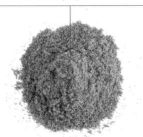

Ground Fennel

Fennel contains nearly as much potassium per cup as bananas, and upping your potassium intake is as important as decreasing salt or sodium consumption in maintaining healthy blood-pressure levels, according to researchers at the University of Texas Southwestern Medical Center.

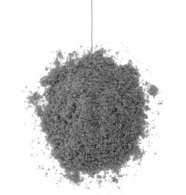

Fennel Seed

Both garlic and fennel contain active compounds that help prevent cancer, according to University of Texas researchers. In fact, these chemicals target cancer in different ways, so they complement each other. But the active compound in fennel—anethol—provides another perk: It helps neutralize garlic breath. Pour hot water over the seeds to brew a licorice-tasting tea that will open your sinuses.

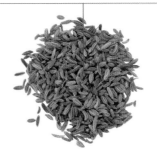

Za'atar

A spice blend from the Middle East that includes oregano, thyme, and sesame seeds, za'atar brings life to sandwiches and potato salads, and pairs great with olive oil as a dipping sauce for crusty bread. Or use it in a yogurt or fresh-herb dip.

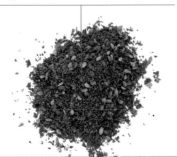

Sumac Powder

This deep-purple powder lends a tart edge to grilled beef kebabs. Or you can lightly dust grilled fish with it or sprinkle it liberally onto hummus or over a salad.

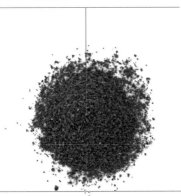

Garam Masala

This complex blend of spices, similar to curry powder, is used mostly in northern India. Sprinkle a teaspoon onto sautéed green peas, into ground beef for Indian-style meatballs, or into a pot of braised meat.

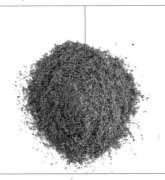

Spices | THE HEALTHIEST FOODS IN THE WORLD

Cayenne Pepper

Ground cayenne clocks in at 40,000 on the Scoville Heat Unit (SHU) scale that measures heat in peppers, which puts it about halfway between jalapeños and habaneros. That's hot. The heat-producing capsaicin in peppers has been shown to boost metabolism and calorie burn, and it's an easy way to give a no-calorie zing to boring foods.

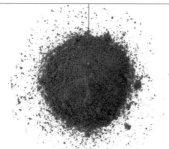

Mustard Seed

Whether brown, white, or black, mustard seeds are produced all over the world, appear in numerous cuisines, and spice up meat, fish, fowl, soups and sauces. Experiment in foods needing a flavor boost.

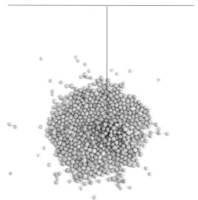

Coriander Seed

Studies suggest that coriander seeds (the fruit of the cilantro plant) could lead to treatments for diabetes and promote cardiovascular health. Chop up tomatoes, an onion, and a jalapeño, and mix with a heap of ground corriander for a versatile fresh salsa.

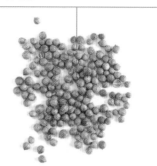

Saffron

Saffron's bright orange color comes from a natural acid called crocetin, which studies suggest may help prevent neurological disorders such as Parkinson's disease. Bold color and health benefits aside, saffron also provides a hint of honey flavor. Try adding a pinch to risotto.

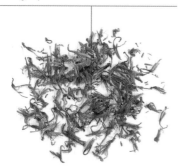

Nutmeg

The spicy scent of fresh ground nutmeg is unmistakable and beloved—it's used in Indian, Middle Eastern, European, and Carribean cuisines, and your holiday eggnog. Some research has shown it to help lower blood pressure and relieve a stomach ache.

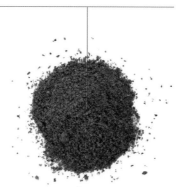

Star Anise

Anethole, the essential oil that gives this star-shaped spice its distinctive licorice flavor, helps reduce inflammation, according to a study at the University of Texas MD Anderson Cancer Center. Grind and toss a teaspoon with cauliflower or green beans, or combine them with coarse cracked pepper to rub on a meat before roasting.

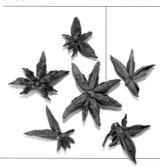

Smoked Paprika

Smoked paprika is a traditional Spanish spice that delivers savory kick to whatever you add it to—use it for a dry rub, on roasted potatoes, or in scrambled eggs (with some hot sauce).

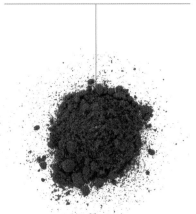

Ground Ginger

Ginger contains living compounds that improve your health. Chief among them is gingerol, a disease suppressor that studies have shown to be particularly effective against colon cancer. Grind it fresh and add it to soy-marinated fish or chicken as often as you can. The more you can handle, the better.

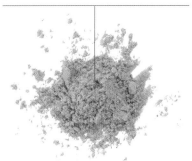

Cloves

Cloves are commonly used in sweet and spicy Indian dishes. It's also used in tea (chai teas). Research shows it may reduce blood sugar, and traditional Eastern medicines use it for everything from dental pain to curing hiccups.

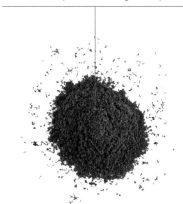

Black Pepper

Adding black pepper to turmeric or turmeric-spiced food enhances curcumin's bioavailability by 1,000 times, due to black pepper's hot property called piperine. This is one reason it's thought that curry has both turmeric (curcumin) and black pepper combined.

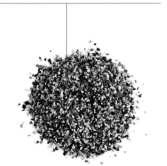

Garlic Powder

Not just a nice addition to pasta. Keith Block, MD, the medical director of the Block Center of Integrative Cancer Treatment, praises garlic's detoxifying qualities. "It will help clean your body of leftover chemical residue from drugs or pollutants, secondhand smoke, and metabolites from alcohol," he says.

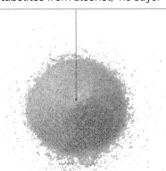

Cumin

Just half a teaspoon of these tiny seeds carries more than double the antioxidants found in half a cup of chopped tomatoes, according to the USDA, and nearly twice as much as a medium-size carrot. Sprinkle the light-brown seeds into soups and sauces to add a bittersweet peppery note.

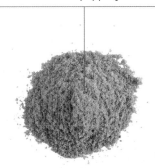

Most people think they should avoid red meat—or only choose very lean cuts—because it's high in saturated fat. But almost half of the fat in beef is a monounsaturated fat called oleic acid—the same heart-healthy fat that's found in olive oil. And most of the saturated fat in beef actually decreases your heart-disease risk—by reducing your ratio of total cholesterol to HDL (good) cholesterol.

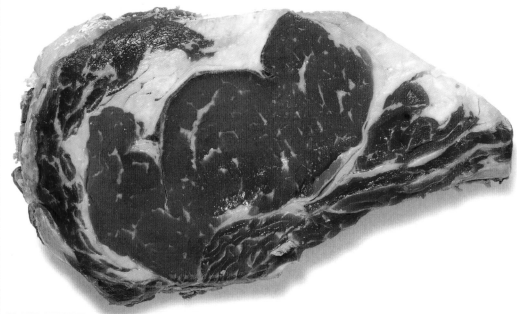

RIB EYE

Rib eye beef is from the rib section of the cow. It's fattier than other cuts (which explains why a 4-oz rib eye steak comes with 24 grams of fat, compared with 21 grams from porterhouse and 9 from top round). That said, the fat in a rib eye might add calories to your meal, but it also triggers your body to produce CCK, a satiety hormone that helps you feel full for longer.

SERVING SIZE	4 oz, 0" trim (112 g)		
Calories/Fiber	Calories: 308		Fiber: 0 g
Macronutrients	Protein: 20 g	Fat: 25 g	Carbs: 0 g
Vitamins/Minerals	Vitamin B₁₂: 60%	Zinc: 28%	Selenium: 28%

SEEK OUT GRASS-FED BEEF

Grass-fed beef is so much more nutritious than commodity (corn-fed) beef that it's almost a different food. In addition to its higher ratio of omega-3s to omega-6s, grass-fed beef contains more conjugated linoleic acid (CLA), which has been shown to reduce abdominal fat while building lean muscle. The optimal ratio of healthy omega-3 fats to less healthy omega-6 fats in our foods should be around 1:2. According to the *European Journal of Clinical Nutrition*, pasture-raised meats measure about 1:3, which is comparable to most fish. But conventionally raised, grain-fed beef? Try 1:20. This is important because omega-3s improve your mood, boost your metabolism, sharpen your brain, and help you lose weight.

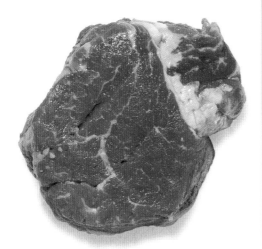

FILET MIGNON (TENDERLOIN)

Filet mignon is made from tenderloin—and it's known for its velvety tenderness. Restaurants have access to higher grades of meat than consumers do. But you can trust filets, no matter the source, because they tend to have a consistent level of quality.

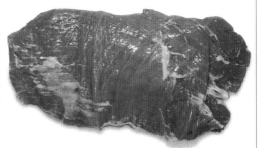

FLANK STEAK

Flank steak is made from the cow's abdominal muscles. It's one of the healthiest beef cuts—ounce for ounce, a flank steak has fewer calories and more protein than a ribeye or porterhouse. It's one of the great cuts—very lean and with a lot of flavor if you know how to cook and slice it. Namely, don't cook it past medium rare, or it'll toughen up faster than a mama's boy at military school. Then slice it across the grain.

4 oz, ⅛" trim (112 g)		
Calories: 276		Fiber: 0 g
Protein: 24 g	Fat: 20 g	Carbs: 0 g
Selenium: 36%	Niacin: 36%	Vitamin B₆: 28%

4 oz, 0" trim (112 g)		
Calories: 186		Fiber: 0 g
Protein: 24 g	Fat: 9 g	Carbs: 0 g
Niacin: 39%	Selenium: 38%	Vitamin B₆: 32%

T-BONE
(SHORT LOIN)

A T-bone is a bit of filet mignon hugging the bone, and the other side is a strip loin steak. Don't confuse it with a porterhouse, though. A porterhouse contains a full strip steak and full filet on either side of the bone.

Per 4 oz, ⅛" trim (112 g) serving: *260 calories, 20 g protein, 0 g carbs, 0 g fiber, 20 g fat, and RDIs of 52% vitamin B₁₂, 24% selenium, 24% zinc*

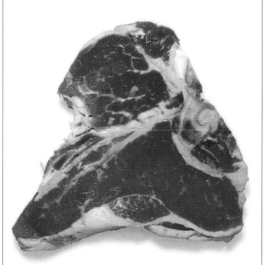

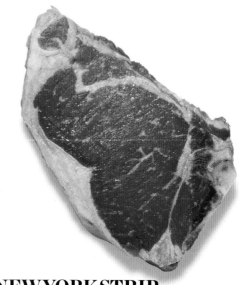

PORTERHOUSE
(SHORT LOIN)

This steak is one of the thick bone-in steaks (much like T-bone). All loins tend to run between 250 and 285 calories per 4-ounce cut, and this is on the heavier side. Doesn't have as much protein as New York Strip steak (top loin), but it still packs a good 20 grams.

NEW YORK STRIP
(TOP LOIN)

The New York Strip steak delivers an enormous 24 grams of protein per 4 ounces. It also has the least fat of any loin cut (17 grams, compared with 20 or 21 grams in other loin cuts).

SERVING SIZE	4 oz, ⅛" trim (112 g)			4 oz, ⅛" trim (112 g)		
Calories/Fiber	Calories: 288		Fiber: 0 g	Calories: 252		Fiber: 0 g
Macronutrients	Protein: 20 g	Fat: 24 g	Carbs: 0 g	Protein: 24 g	Fat: 16 g	Carbs: 0 g
Vitamins/Minerals	Vitamin B₁₂: 52%	Selenium: 28%	Zinc: 24%	Selenium: 36%	Niacin: 32%	Vitamin B₆: 32%

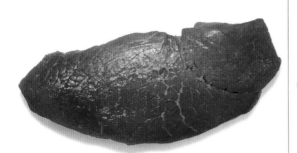

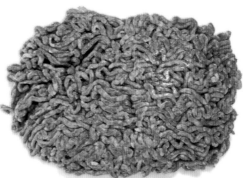

IMPORTANT NOTE:

The beef serving size for our purposes here is 4 ounces, about half of one New York Strip steak. When ordering in restaurants, beware of senseless steak-eating challenges. If you order a 48-ounce slab (4 pounds of meat!), you'll have to multiply the nutritional information found here by 12. Holy cow.

TOP ROUND (LONDON BROIL)

This is one of the lowest-calorie cuts of beef you can find. It has only 168 calories per 4 ounces, with 24 grams of protein. Compare that with the rib eye, with nearly double the calories and 4 fewer grams of belly-filling, muscle-building protein. And one of the best things about it? It's super lean, especially compared with most other cuts.

GROUND BEEF (85-15 BEEF-FAT RATIO)

The less fat you have in your ground beef, the quicker it'll dry out. Keep the meat moist with vegetables. Try onions, red peppers, and mushrooms. Add them raw or sauté them in a little bit of oil to soften them up, then cool and mix into the meat.

4 oz, 0" trim (112 g)		
Calories: 168	Fiber: 0 g	
Protein: 24 g	Fat: 8 g	Carbs: 0 g
Vitamin B$_{12}$: 88%	Selenium: 52%	Vitamin B$_6$: 40%

4 oz (112 g)		
Calories: 240	Fiber: 0 g	
Protein: 20 g	Fat: 16 g	Carbs: 0 g
Vitamin B$_{12}$: 40%	Zinc: 32%	Niacin: 28%

It's true: Pork really is the other white meat. Ounce for ounce, pork tenderloin has less fat than a chicken breast. And food scientists are finding ways to make it leaner and leaner every year. Of course, the downside to this is that fat is what makes pork taste so good—which explains why ham and bacon are far more popular than leaner cuts. But remember, when eating sensible portions there's no reason to fear fat.

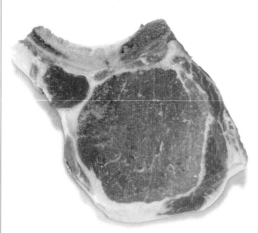

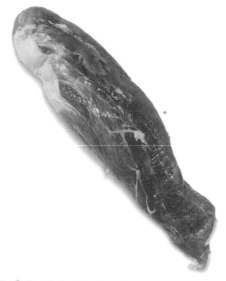

PORK CHOP (CENTER CUT)

Per gram of protein, pork chops contain twice as much selenium—an essential mineral that's linked to a lower risk of prostate cancer—as chicken. And Purdue researchers found that a 6-ounce serving daily helped people preserve their muscle while losing weight.

PORK TENDERLOIN

Though it sounds—and even looks—healthier than pork chops, pork loin is just as fatty and delivers slightly less protein.

SERVING SIZE	1 chop (158 g)			4 oz (112 g)		
Calories/Fiber	Calories: 174		Fiber: 0 g	Calories: 124		Fiber: 0 g
Macronutrients	Protein: 34 g	Fat: 4 g	Carbs: 0 g	Protein: 24 g	Fat: 4 g	Carbs: 0 g
Vitamins/Minerals	Selenium: 92%	Niacin: 69%	Vitamin B₆: 58%	Thiamin: 76%	Selenium: 48%	Vitamin B₆: 44%

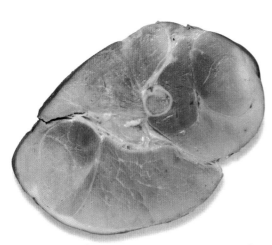

HAM (CURED, BONE IN)

Nutritionally speaking, ham is about as healthy for you as a cut of filet mignon. It has more fat than pork tenderloin, but it beats bacon or sausage every time in the battle of the breakfast sandwiches.

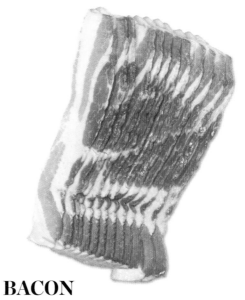

BACON

Bacon and other cured meats often contain sodium and other preservatives, such as nitrates, that may raise blood pressure or increase your risk for cancer. To limit your risk, choose fresh meats or packaged products that contain no preservatives—typically labeled "all-natural"—whenever possible.

4 oz (112 g)		
Calories: 192		Fiber: 0 g
Protein: 24 g	Fat: 12 g	Carbs: 0 g
Selenium: 36%	Thiamin: 36%	Sodium: 35%

1 oz (28 g)		
Calories: 128		Fiber: 0 g
Protein: 3 g	Fat: 13 g	Carbs: 0 g
Sodium: 110%	Selenium: 8%	

Deli lunchmeat is one of our biggest convenience foods—lining the sandwiches of brown-baggers everywhere. The protein is obvious, but you have to be careful here: The contents of some varieties are more mysterious than others, and most contain lots of salt. Your best bet is to go light on the meat and heavy on the good stuff you can pile on like veggies and mustard (easy on the mayo!).

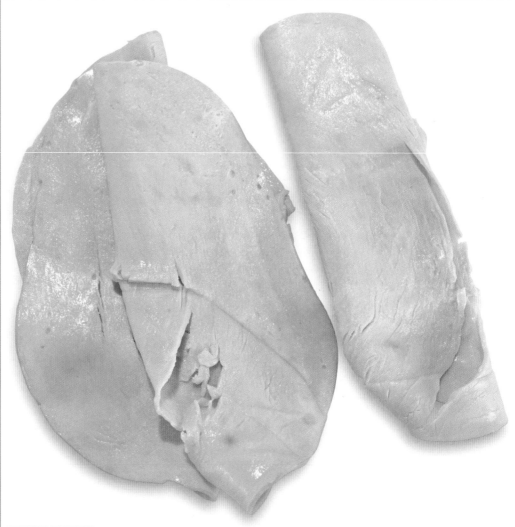

TURKEY

Pile it high. One ounce has 4 grams of protein and only 31 calories.

SERVING SIZE	1 oz (28 g)		
Calories/Fiber	Calories: 31		Fiber: 0 g
Macronutrients	Protein: 4 g	Fat: 0 g	Carbs: 2 g
Vitamins/Minerals	Sodium: 14%	Selenium: 12%	

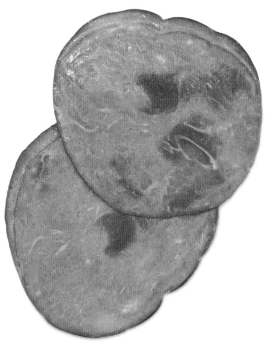

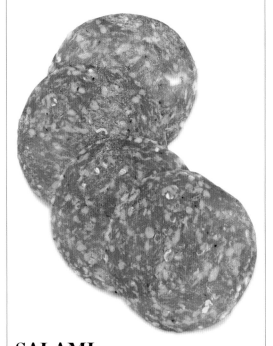

HAM

It contains only two-thirds the protein of roast beef, but it's still fairly low in fat and calories.

SALAMI

The calories stack up quickly with this lard-speckled, sodium-laden cured meat.

1 oz, extra lean (28 g)		
Calories: 29	Fiber: 0 g	
Protein: 5 g	Fat: 1 g	Carbs: 0 g
Sodium: 12%	Thiamin: 6%	

1 oz, dark, pork (28 g)		
Calories: 114	Fiber: 0 g	
Protein: 6 g	Fat: 9 g	Carbs: 0 g
Sodium: 26%	Thiamin: 17%	

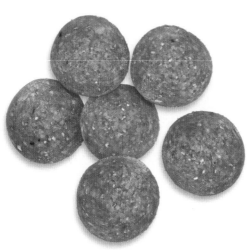

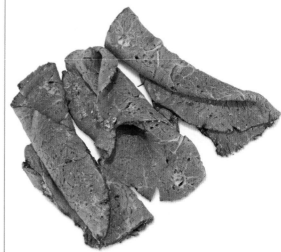

PEPPERONI

Very tasty, but with a price: At 463 milligrams, an ounce of pepperoni delivers 19 percent of your day's salt intake.

PASTRAMI

This meat has more protein, but also more fat and sodium, than ham.

SERVING SIZE	1 oz (28 g)			1 slice (1 oz, 28 g)		
Calories/Fiber	Calories: 138		Fiber 0 g	Calories: 41		Fiber: 0 g
Macronutrients	Protein: 6 g	Fat: 12 g	Carbs: 0 g	Protein: 6 g	Fat: 2 g	Carbs: 0 g
Vitamins/Minerals	Sodium: 19%	Selenium: 14%	Vitamin B₆: 8%	Sodium: 10%		

ALLIGATOR

Popular with chefs and home cooks in the Deep South, alligator has a soft, tender texture similar to veal, and a neutral flavor that takes well to big spices and sauces. It's rich in omega-3 fatty acids and packs more muscle-building protein than beef or chicken. Rub each pound of gator with 2 tablespoons of blackening seasoning. Cook over high heat on a grill or in a cast-iron skillet.

Per 4-oz serving:
260 calories, 52 g protein, 0 g carbs, 0 g fiber, 5 g fat

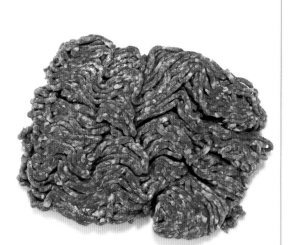

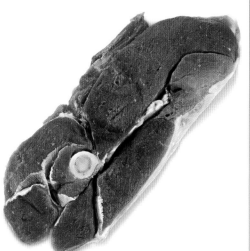

BISON (GROUND)

A tasty alternative to cow, and you don't lose any nutritional punch. Shop around for organic.

VENISON (DEER TENDERLOIN)

Four ounces of deer has more protein than an equal amount of beef. It's also very lean with comparable vitamin and mineral payoff. The only downside is having to drag it out of the woods after you shoot it (unless you pick it up at the butcher's).

4 oz (112 g)		
Calories: 248	Fiber: 0 g	
Protein: 20 g	Fat: 16 g	Carbs: 0 g
Vitamin B₁₂: 32%	Zinc: 32%	Selenium: 28%

4 oz (112 g)		
Calories: 168	Fiber: 0 g	
Protein: 32 g	Fat: 4 g	Carbs: 0 g
Vitamin B₁₂: 68%	Niacin: 48%	Vitamin B₆: 36%

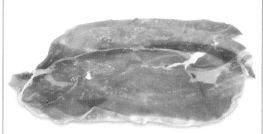

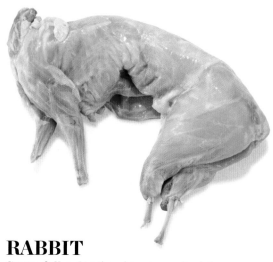

PROSCIUTTO

Prosciutto is a cured Italian ham that's usually sliced very thin and served in a variety of ways—wrapped around cantaloupe or honeydew, or even asparagus. As with all cured meats, however, watch the salt intake (685 milligrams per ounce, about a third of your recommended daily allowance).

RABBIT

Some folks don't enjoy game, but for those who do, rabbit delivers a massive dose of B_{12} along with many of the other nutrients found in meats, with a lower calorie count.

SERVING SIZE	1 oz (28 g)			4 oz (112 g)		
Calories/Fiber	Calories: 70	Fiber: 0 g		Calories: 152	Fiber: 0 g	
Macronutrients	Protein: 8 g	Fat: 4 g	Carbs: 1 g	Protein: 24 g	Fat: 8 g	Carbs: 0 g
Vitamins/Minerals	Selenium: 28%			Vitamin B_{12}: 132%	Niacin: 40%	Selenium: 36%

LIVER (BEEF)

It doesn't sound sexy, but ounce for ounce there are few better sources of fertility-boosting vitamin A than liver. Studies show that men who get plenty of A each day have higher sperm counts and perform better sexually than men who don't. Liver is also an excellent source of zinc. Your body expels 5 milligrams of zinc—a third of your daily requirement—every time you ejaculate, so a single amorous weekend could leave your body's zinc reserves running on empty.

Per 4-oz (112 g) serving:
152 calories, 24 g protein, 4 g carbs, 0 g fiber, 4 g fat, and RDIs of 1,108% vitamin B_{12} and 548% copper

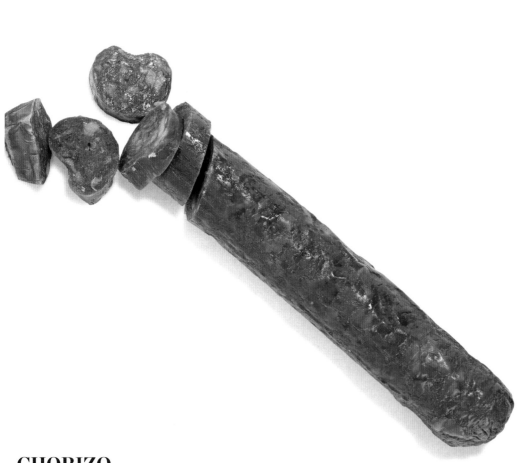

CHORIZO

This classic spicy sausage is loaded with meaty vitamins, but beware the massive salt content. Try some in scrambled eggs.

One 4" link (60 g)		
Calories: 315		Fiber: 0 g
Protein: 13 g	Fat: 29 g	Carbs: 1 g
Thiamin: 34%	Selenium: 32%	Sodium: 28%

Chapter 7:
100 of the Healthiest Meals on the Planet

BUILD A BETTER OMELET, SALAD, SANDWICH,
PIZZA, PASTA, BURRITO, SOUP, BURGER—AND MORE!—
WITH THESE GO-TO RECIPES.

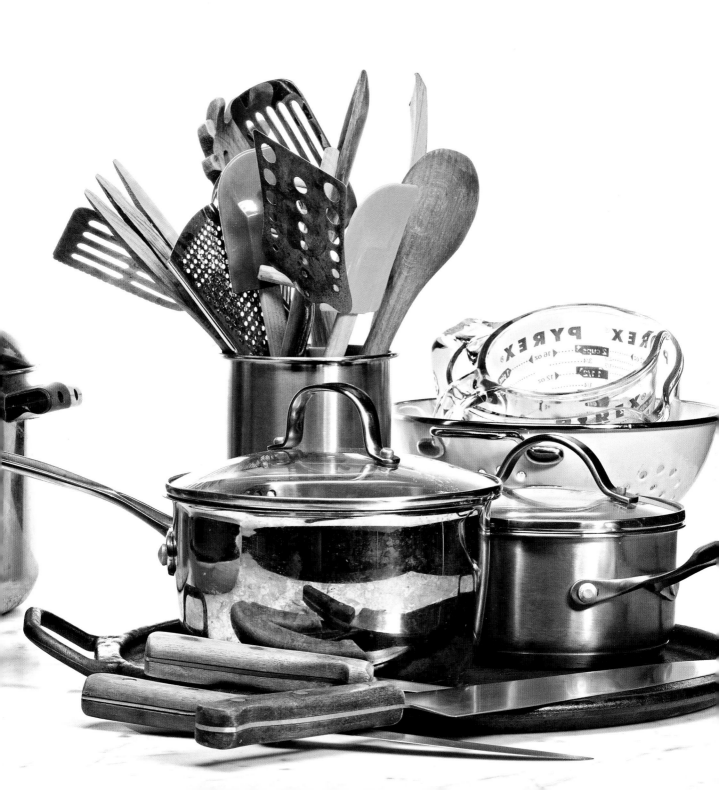

Good recipes

are easy. Great recipes are sublime because, yes, they're easy, but also because they're nutritional powerhouses and unforgettably tasty. They become part of your food vocabulary, and you return to them again and again. Every one of the 100 recipes in this chapter is designed around all the nutritional standards we've been talking about in this book—low-calorie, low-sugar, low-artificial-ingredients and high-nutrient, high-protein, high-fiber payoffs.

The recipes are grouped for easy reference: Breakfasts, Soups & Salads, Sandwiches & Burgers, Dinners, Pizzas, Snacks & Sides, and Sweet Stuff. The best part? The more you sample from this chapter, the easier it becomes to transform your entire approach to food and good health.

Your Official Chef-Lingo Cheat Sheet

Cooking is simple, really. So is food. But we make them complicated—mostly out of terror that we'll screw it all up. As you read through the recipes, remember that there's nothing to be afraid of in the kitchen. Put on some tunes. Experiment. Have fun. It's been said that once you cook a meal twice, you own it. So focus on the fundamentals. Here are five basic cooking techniques—master them and the possibilities for creating simple, delicious, healthy food become endless.

1. Roasting

Roasting employs dry, indirect heat to add a tasty crust to meat or to brown a pan of vegetables. And it's how your mom cooked all those Thanksgiving turkeys.
Chef Secret: Roasting is a great way to intensify the natural sweetness of fruits and vegetables.

2. Broiling/Grilling

Man's first cooking technique may also be his most flavorful. Whether you heat from the top, using the broiler, or underneath, on the grill, the food acquires a rapid browning. It works well with meats, of course, but also with fish, vegetables, and pizza.
Chef Secret: Always preheat a broiler for at least 5 minutes.

3. Braising

Braising is the technique responsible for the most-tender meats and the most-complex flavors. To begin, brown the meat on the stove top. Then turn down the heat and cook any additional ingredients in a small amount of liquid until very tender.
Chef Secret: Crowding the pan will cause the surface temperature to drop, and meat won't brown properly.

4. Boiling

Put food in water. Boil until done.
Chef Secret: Drain pasta as soon as it's al dente, and immediately toss with sauce and serve. Otherwise it will keep cooking itself.

5. Sautéing

Sautéing simply means cooking in a pan with butter or oil. The technique, like browning, develops and deepens flavors.
Chef Secret: Salt draws out moisture. Add it early if you want the food to simmer in its own juices; add later if you want your meal crispy and brown.

ASPARAGUS-AND-LEEK FRITTATA

1	Tbsp extra-virgin olive oil
1	medium leek, white and some green parts, halved lengthwise, rinsed, and thinly sliced
¾	lb thin asparagus, tips left whole and stems sliced ¼" thick
2	Tbsp chicken broth
¼	tsp salt
¼	tsp freshly ground black pepper
2	Tbsp flat-leaf parsley, chopped (optional)
1	Tbsp snipped fresh chives (optional)
8	eggs
½	cup milk
3	Tbsp feta cheese, crumbled (optional)

Per serving: 134.8 calories, 8.5 g fat (2.6 g saturated), 215.7 mg cholesterol, 261.9 mg sodium, 5.1 g carbohydrates, 2.3 g sugars, 1.5 g fiber, 9.7 g protein

1. Preheat the broiler to high.

2. Heat the oil in a medium cast-iron skillet over medium-high heat. Add the leek and cook, stirring often, for 3 minutes or until soft. Add the asparagus, broth, ⅛ teaspoon each of the salt and pepper, parsley, and chives. Cook, stirring often, for 3 minutes or until the asparagus is tender-crisp and the broth has evaporated. Spread the asparagus mixture evenly in the bottom of the skillet.

3. Meanwhile, in a medium bowl, whisk together the eggs, milk, and the remaining ⅛ teaspoon each of the salt and pepper. (Whisking until the eggs are especially frothy will result in a fluffier frittata.) Pour into the skillet with the asparagus.

4. Shake the skillet to evenly distribute the egg mixture. Reduce the heat to low, cover, and cook, without stirring, for 3 minutes or until the eggs begin to set at the edges. With a spatula, lift up an edge of the frittata and tilt the skillet to allow the uncooked mixture to flow to the bottom of the pan.

5. Place under the broiler. Broil for 1 to 3 minutes or until the eggs are set on the top and the frittata is lightly puffed. Cut into wedges to serve. Top with feta, if desired.

Serves six.

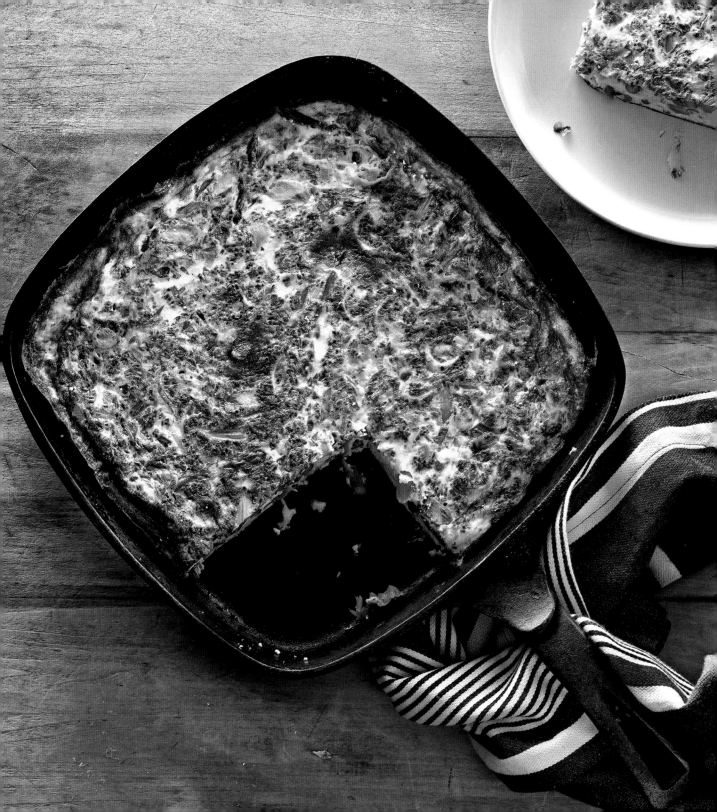

MASHED & SCRAMBLED

1	whole egg
1	egg white
1	whole-wheat English muffin, toasted
¼	cup avocado, mashed
1	slice reduced fat Cheddar cheese
2	tomato slices

Per serving: *367.5 calories, 16.8 g fat (4.2 g saturated), 217.4 mg cholesterol, 723.6 mg sodium, 34 g carbohydrates, 7.2 g sugars, 8.6 g fiber, 24 g protein*

1. Scramble the whole egg and the egg white in a small skillet coated with cooking spray.

2. Spread the mashed avocado onto the toasted English muffin.

3. Place cooked eggs on muffin and top with 1 slice reduced-fat Cheddar cheese and tomato slices.

Serves one.

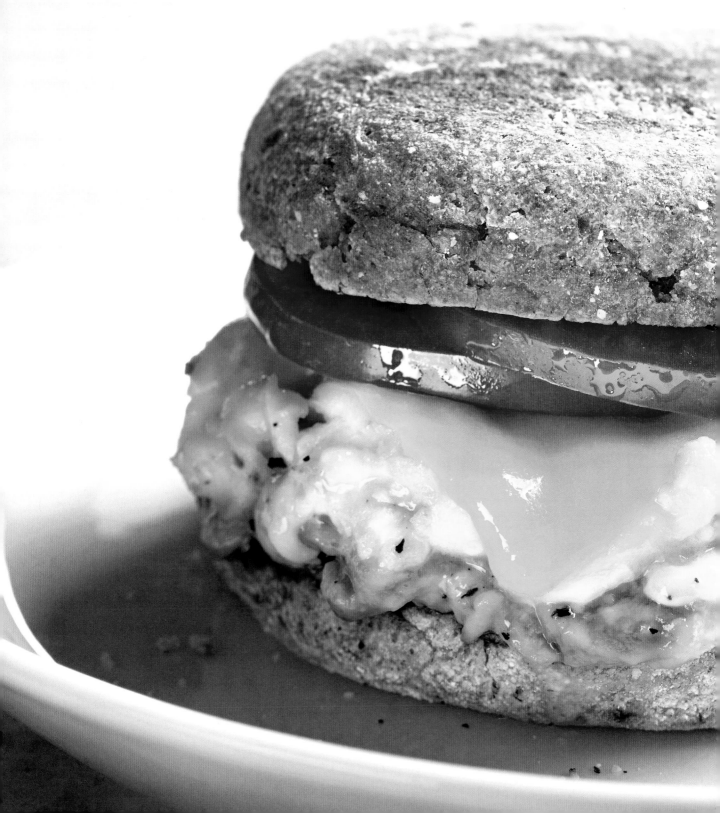

GREENS, EGGS & HAM WRAP

3	egg whites, lightly beaten
1	egg, lightly beaten
1	tsp unsalted butter
⅓	cup onion, chopped
1½	oz deli-sliced ham, such as Healthy Choice brand, chopped
¼	cup frozen peas
½	cup (1 small) plum tomato, chopped
⅛	tsp ground black pepper
1	multigrain wrap
4	tsp black-bean-and-corn salsa

1. In a small bowl, combine the egg whites and egg.

2. Melt the butter in a medium nonstick skillet over medium-high heat. Add the onion and ham; cook, stirring occasionally, until the onion starts to soften, about 2 to 3 minutes. Stir in the peas, tomato, and pepper; cook until the tomato begins to wilt, about 1 to 2 minutes. Add the egg mixture, cook for 2 minutes, flip, then cook for 2 more minutes.

3. Warm the wrap according to package directions, then place on a cutting board. Slide the egg onto the wrap, roll up jelly roll–style, then cut in half on an angle. Top each half with 2 teaspoons of the salsa.

Serves one.

Per serving: 171.4 calories, 5.6 g fat (2.4 g saturated), 118.4 mg cholesterol, 449.7 mg sodium, 18.6 g carbohydrates, 3.8 g sugars, 2.6 g fiber, 15.7 g protein

BREAKFAST IN 10 MINUTES OR LESS (PART 1)

Scramble eggs with chopped scallions and hunks of chicken sausage. Serve in warm tortillas topped with black beans, sliced avocado, and salsa.

BREAKFAST OF STEEL

4	cups filtered water
	Pinch sea salt (optional)
1	cup steel-cut oats
2	apples, skin on, cored and diced
1	tsp ground cinnamon
4	Tbsp flaxseeds, ground
⅓	cup walnuts, chopped

1. Bring the water and salt to a boil and slowly stir in the oats. Boil until the oats begin to thicken, approximately 5 minutes.

2. Reduce the heat to low, stir in the apples and cinnamon, and simmer for 30 to 40 minutes, until desired consistency.

3. Top with the flaxseeds and walnuts.

Serves four.

Per serving: 231 calories, 10.9 g fat (0.9 g saturated), 0 mg cholesterol, 70.7 mg sodium, 30 g carbohydrates, 10.2 g sugars, 7.5 g fiber, 6.7 g protein

HOLY GUACAMOLE BURRITO

2	eggs
2	slices fat-free turkey deli slices
½	avocado, sliced
2	Tbsp reduced-fat Mexican-blend cheese, shredded
1	medium whole-wheat tortilla

1. Scramble the eggs in a skillet or the microwave.

2. Place eggs, turkey, avocado, and cheese in the tortilla, fold the ends, and neatly roll.

Serves one.

Per serving: 349.1 calories, 22.3 g fat (5.1 g saturated), 229.8 mg cholesterol, 574.7 mg sodium, 29 g carbohydrates, 0.6 g sugars, 7.8 g fiber, 17.9 g protein

LONE STAR OMELET

⅓ cup scallions, chopped

¼ cup onions, chopped

¼ cup canned green chili peppers, chopped

¼ cup frozen corn kernels, thawed

½ cup tomatillos or plum tomatoes, chopped

Pinch of ground cumin

4 egg whites

2 eggs

2 Tbsp skim milk

¼ tsp ground black pepper

Pinch of salt

5½ oz reduced-fat Cheddar cheese, shredded

2 Tbsp medium-hot or hot salsa (optional)

2 Tbsp nonfat sour cream (optional)

1. Coat a medium nonstick skillet with cooking spray and place over medium heat.

2. Add the scallions, onions, chili peppers, and corn. Cook for 5 minutes or until the onions are softened.

3. Add the tomatillos (or plum tomatoes) and cumin. Cook for 3 to 4 minutes or until the tomatillos are softened. Transfer to a small bowl.

4. Wipe out the skillet, coat with cooking spray, and return to the heat.

5. In a medium bowl, whisk together the egg whites, eggs, milk, black pepper, and salt.

6. Pour half of the egg mixture into the skillet and cook, occasionally scraping the bottom of the pan, for 2 to 3 minutes.

7. Sprinkle half of the Cheddar and half of the vegetable mixture over the eggs. Cook, without stirring, for 3 to 4 minutes, or until the bottom is golden brown and the eggs are set.

8. Using a spatula, flip the omelet in half and transfer to a plate.

9. Coat the pan with cooking spray and repeat the procedure with the remaining egg mixture, Cheddar, and vegetable mixture. Serve topped with the salsa and sour cream.

Serves two.

Per serving: 209.6 calories, 7.2 g fat (2.6 g saturated), 217.6 mg cholesterol, 584.6 mg sodium, 15.5 g carbohydrates, 5.5 g sugars, 2.5 g fiber, 21.6 g protein

BREAKFAST IN 10 MINUTES OR LESS (PART 2)

Spread toasted English muffin halves with a spoonful of pesto. Top with scrambled eggs and shredded mozzarella cheese. Place under the broiler or in microwave until the cheese melts.

BANANA-BLUEBERRY SMOOTHIE

¾ cup part-skim ricotta cheese

¼ cup 1% milk

½ cup blueberries

½ banana

2 tsp vanilla whey-protein powder

6 ice cubes

1. Combine ricotta, milk, blueberries, banana, and protein powder in a blender.

2. Then add ice, and puree until smooth.

Serves one.

Per serving: *403.7 calories, 16.1 g fat (9.6 g saturated), 66.7 mg cholesterol, 272.8 mg sodium, 37.1 g carbohydrates, 18.5 g sugars, 3.3 g fiber, 31.1 g protein*

THE WHEY-TOO-GOOD SMOOTHIE

¾ cup 1% chocolate milk

2 tsp chocolate whey-protein powder

¾ cup part-skim ricotta cheese

¼ cup pecans, chopped

½ banana

2 Tbsp low-fat vanilla yogurt

2 tsp flaxseed, ground

6 ice cubes

1. Blend milk and protein powder; this will help break down the grainy powder and make sure it's evenly distributed.

2. Add ricotta, pecans, banana, yogurt, and flaxseed. Blend.

3. Then add ice, and blend. For a thicker shake, you can toss in more ice cubes; you'll add volume without the calories.

Serves two.

Per serving: *352.8 calories, 19.8 g fat (6.2 g saturated), 35.4 mg cholesterol, 189.9 mg sodium, 27 g carbohydrates, 16.1 g sugars, 3.7 g fiber, 20.1 g protein*

PASTA FAGIOLI

2	slices center-cut (30% less fat) bacon, chopped
1	cup onion, chopped
4	cloves garlic, minced
¾	cup (3 ribs) celery, chopped
½	cup carrots, chopped
4	cups low-sodium, fat-free chicken broth
1	can (14.5 oz) salt-free diced tomatoes
6	oz whole-wheat blend rotini
1	can (15 oz) dark red kidney beans, rinsed and drained
¼	cup fresh parsley, chopped
¼	cup fresh basil, chopped
⅛	tsp ground black pepper

1. Heat a large saucepan over medium-high heat.

2. Add the bacon and cook until just starting to brown, 5 to 6 minutes.

3. Add the onion, garlic, celery, and carrots and cook until just starting to soften, 2 to 3 minutes.

4. Pour in the broth, tomatoes, rotini, and beans. Cover and bring to a boil; uncover and cook until the rotini is tender, about 12 to 15 minutes.

5. Remove from the heat and stir in the parsley, basil, and pepper.

Serves six.

Per serving: 201.7 calories, 2.9 g fat (0.6 g saturated), 2.5 mg cholesterol, 502.8 mg sodium, 33.2 g carbohydrates, 6 g sugars, 8.4 g fiber, 10.2 g protein

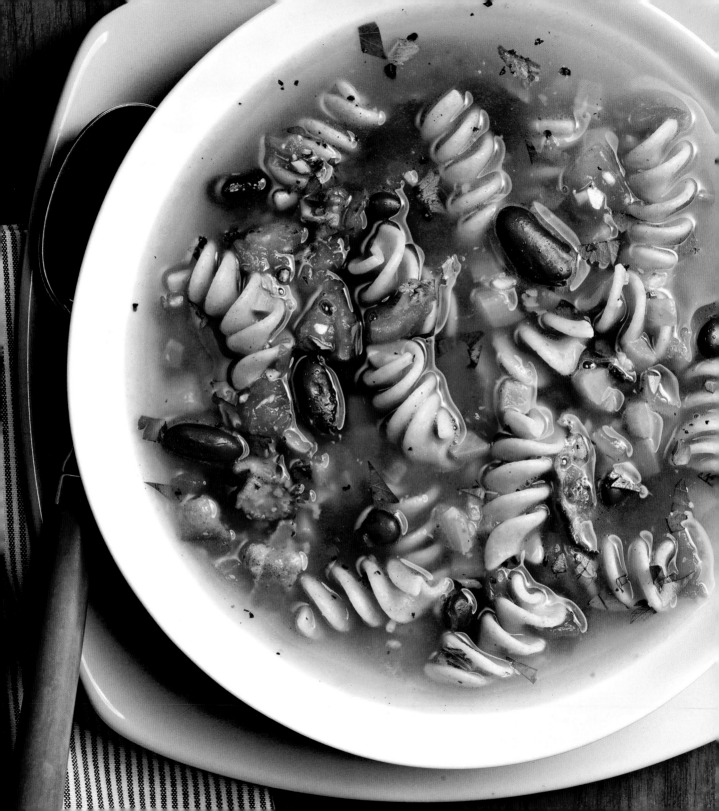

CANOODLING TURKEY SOUP

4	oz whole-wheat noodles
1	Tbsp canola oil
½	cup onion, chopped
½	cup carrot, chopped
½	cup celery, chopped
1	tsp dried sage
12	oz ground turkey breast
2	cans (14½ oz each) low-sodium, fat-free chicken broth
4	cups water
1	Tbsp balsamic vinegar
½	tsp salt
1	bag (6 oz) baby spinach leaves
	Ground black pepper

1. Cook the noodles according to the package directions. Drain and set aside.

2. Meanwhile, in a pot over medium heat, warm the oil.

3. Add the onion, carrot, celery, and sage to the pot. Cook, stirring occasionally, for 5 minutes or until the vegetables start to soften.

4. Add the turkey. Cook, breaking up the turkey with the back of a spoon, for about 4 minutes longer or until the turkey is no longer pink.

5. Add the broth, water, vinegar, and salt. Simmer for about 5 minutes or until hot. Do not boil.

6. Stir in the spinach and noodles.

7. Remove from the heat and let rest for 5 minutes. Season with pepper to taste.

Serves eight.

Per serving: *135.1 calories, 2.8 g fat (0.1 g saturated), 16.9 mg cholesterol, 447.5 mg sodium, 15.1 g carbohydrates, 1.7 g sugars, 2.3 g fiber, 13.8 g protein*

CHUNKY TILAPIA-AND-TOMATO SOUP

1	Tbsp olive oil
⅓	cup baby carrots, thinly sliced
⅓	cup red onion, slivered
½	tsp thyme
	Salt to taste
2	cups low-sodium, fat-free chicken broth
1	cup water
12	oz tilapia fillets, cut into large chunks
1½	cups broccoli florets, chopped
1	cup canned diced tomatoes, with juice
½	tsp ground black pepper

1. In a large saucepan heat oil over medium heat, combine carrots, onion, oil, thyme, and salt to taste. Cook, stirring over medium heat, until softened, about 5 minutes.

2. Add broth and water. Bring almost to boiling.

3. Add tilapia, broccoli, tomatoes, and pepper. Reduce heat and simmer until tilapia is cooked, about 8 minutes.

Serves two.

Per serving: *318.6 calories, 11.3 g fat (2.4 g saturated), 85.1 mg cholesterol, 550.1 mg sodium, 13.6 g carbohydrates, 4.9 g sugars, 3.8 g fiber, 42.1 g protein*

WHAT'S THE DIFF?

CAPPUCCINO AND LATTE

Cappuccino is espresso with foamed milk. Latte is espresso with warm milk. Pick cappucinos for fewer calories.

SUMMER CLAM CHOWDER

2   cans (6½ oz each) minced clams

2   strips bacon, chopped

1   large onion, chopped

3   ribs celery, chopped

2   cans (14½ oz each) fat-free reduced-sodium chicken broth

1   tsp dried thyme

1   bay leaf

1   lb potatoes, cut into ½" chunks

¼   cup unbleached or all-purpose flour

2   cups 2% milk

1½ cups frozen corn kernels

¼   cup fresh parsley, chopped

1. Drain the clams and reserve the juice. Set aside.

2. In a Dutch oven, cook the bacon, stirring often, over medium heat for 3 minutes. Add the onion and celery. Cook for 5 minutes or until the onion is soft. Add the broth, thyme, bay leaf, and reserved clam juice. Bring to a boil and stir well. Add the potatoes. Cook for 20 to 25 minutes, or until the potatoes are tender.

3. Meanwhile, place the flour in a small bowl. Gradually add 1½ cups milk, whisking until smooth.

4. Add the milk and flour mixture to the pot along with the corn, parsley, and reserved clams. Cook, stirring frequently, for 10 minutes or until thickened. Add up to ½ cup more milk for a thinner chowder, if desired. Remove and discard the bay leaf.

Serves eight.

Per serving: *143.6 calories, 4.1 g fat (1.7 g saturated), 17.1 mg cholesterol, 617.5 mg sodium, 18.3 g carbohydrates, 5.7 g sugars, 3.1 g fiber, 9.4 g protein*

SKINNY-BELT BORSCHT

1½ lb beets, peeled and quartered

3½ cups low-sodium vegetable broth

1   cup water

2   Tbsp lemon juice

1   Tbsp red wine vinegar

1   small cucumber, peeled and finely chopped (optional)

3   Tbsp reduced-fat sour cream

1   Tbsp snipped fresh dill

1. In a large saucepan or Dutch oven over high heat, combine the beets, broth, and water. Bring to a boil. Reduce the heat to low, cover, and simmer for 30 minutes or until the beets are very tender.

2. With a slotted spoon, place the beets in a large bowl and allow to cool to room temperature.

3. Finely chop the cooled beets and add back to the cooking liquid.

4. If serving the soup cold, cover and refrigerate until chilled. If serving the soup hot, add the lemon juice and vinegar to the soup. Use an immersion blender to smooth. Add the cucumber, if desired. Ladle the soup into bowls. In a cup, combine the sour cream and dill. Dollop onto each serving.

Serves six.

Per serving: *80 calories, 1 g fat (0.5 g saturated), 2.9 mg cholesterol, 180 mg sodium, 14 g carbohydrates, 9 g sugars, 3.4 g fiber, 2 g protein*

PINTO-SIZED SHRIMP SALAD

HOT PEPPER DRESSING

⅓   cup extra-virgin olive oil

Juice of 1 lime

2   fresh jalapeño chili peppers, minced
(wear plastic gloves when handling)

1   clove garlic, minced

SALAD

1   can (15.5 oz) pinto beans, drained and rinsed

⅓   cup red onion, chopped

1   tsp ground cumin

Salt and pepper to taste

1   lb medium shrimp, peeled and deveined

Juice of ½ lime

2   tsp extra-virgin olive oil

2   tsp chili powder

Cooked kernels from 2 ears corn,
or 2 cups frozen corn, thawed in the
microwave 1 to 2 minutes

1   red bell pepper, seeded and chopped

1   mango, cubed (nectarine or papaya can
substitute)

8   cups arugula or romaine lettuce, sliced

½   cup fresh cilantro, chopped, or 2 Tbsp dried

Per serving: *522.7 calories, 23.5g fat*
(3.4 g saturated), 174.2 mg cholesterol,
382.5 mg sodium, 49.2 g carbohydrates,
15.2 g sugars, 10.8 g fiber, 32.7 g protein

TO MAKE THE DRESSING:

1. Whisk together all of the ingredients in
a small bowl until well combined.

2. Let stand 10 minutes before using.

TO MAKE THE SALAD:

1. Combine the beans, dressing, onion, cumin,
and salt and pepper to taste in a large bowl and
let marinate while you put together the rest of
the salad.

2. Prepare a medium-hot grill or grill pan.
Toss the shrimp with the lime juice, olive oil,
chili powder, and salt and pepper to taste and let
stand while the grill heats. When the grill is hot,
grill the shrimp until opaque, about 3 minutes on
each side. (If the shrimp are small and you are
grilling outdoors, it's easier to skewer them
before grilling.)

3. Add the corn, red pepper, mango, arugula,
and cilantro to the bowl with the beans and toss.
Salt and pepper to taste.

4. Divide the salad among 4 bowls, top each
with the grilled shrimp, and serve.

Serves four.

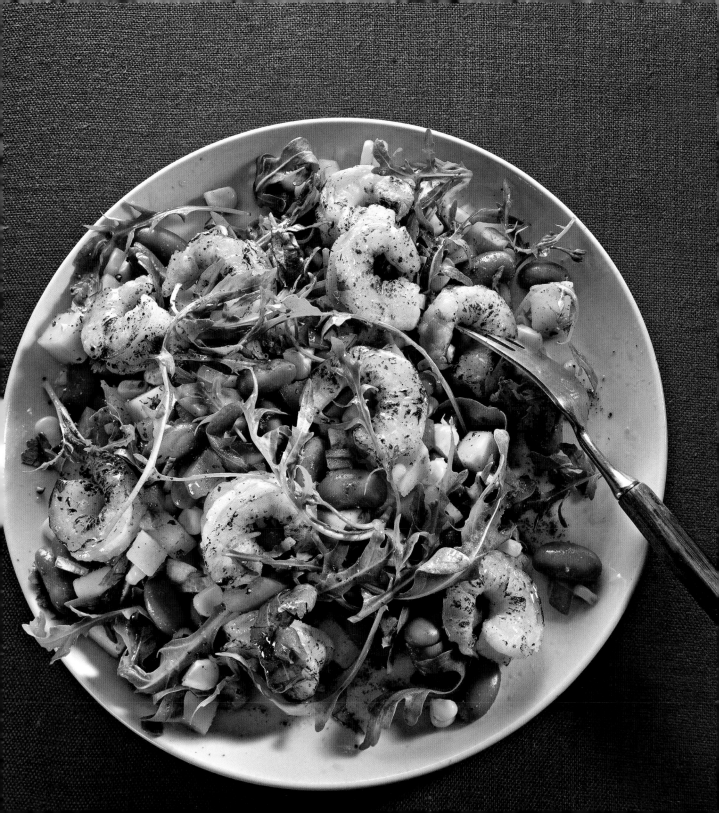

TRIPLE-THREAT BEAN SALAD

MUSTARD DRESSING

2	Tbsp Dijon mustard
2	Tbsp extra-virgin olive oil
2	Tbsp water
1	Tbsp fresh basil, chopped
¼	tsp honey
¼	cup ground black pepper

SALAD

2	cups green beans, halved
1	cup cooked or canned chickpeas
1	cup cooked or canned kidney beans
1	large tomato, seeded and diced
	Snipped fresh chives

TO MAKE THE MUSTARD DRESSING:

1. In a blender, combine the mustard, oil, water, basil, honey, and pepper.

2. Blend for 1 minute.

TO MAKE THE SALAD:

1. In a vegetable steamer, cook the green beans for 5 minutes or until crisp-tender.

2. Place the green beans in a large bowl. Add the chickpeas, kidney beans, and tomato. Mix well.

3. Pour the dressing over the salad, sprinkle with the chives, and toss well.

4. Let stand for 20 minutes before serving.

ALTERNATE VERSION

Serve the salad in lettuce cups. For variety, use colorful greens and replace the chickpeas or kidney beans with fava, pinto, or black beans.

Serves eight.

Per serving: 115 calories, 4.1 g fat (0.6 g saturated), 0 mg cholesterol, 182.9 mg sodium, 16.3 g carbohydrates, 1.8 g sugars, 4 g fiber, 4.2 g protein

SALAD BOOSTER #1: PROTEIN

Add a sliced hard-boiled egg to your salad. For a bright, creamy yolk, cook an egg in gently simmering water for 8 minutes. Want even more protein? Add ½ cup of canned chickpeas to the salad.

SPINACH SALAD WITH STRAWBERRIES AND BUTTERMILK DRESSING

DRESSING

⅓	cup buttermilk
⅓	cup reduced-fat mayonnaise
	Juice of ½ lemon
1	Tbsp sugar
	Pinch cayenne pepper
	Salt and pepper to taste
2	scallions (white and green parts), chopped

SALAD

4	cups baby spinach
3	cups strawberries, quartered and hulled (Feel free to add or substitute your favorite summer fruit, such as peaches, nectarines, plums, or raspberries.)
12	fresh mint leaves, coarsely chopped
⅓	cup almonds, sliced

TO MAKE THE DRESSING:

1. Combine the buttermilk, mayonnaise, lemon juice, sugar, cayenne, salt, and black pepper in a bowl and whisk until well combined.

2. Stir in the scallions.

TO MAKE THE SALAD:

1. Divide the spinach among four plates.

2. Add the strawberries and sprinkle with the mint.

3. Drizzle the dressing over, garnish with the almonds, and serve.

Serves four.

Per serving: 150 calories, 7.2 g fat (1.1 g saturated), 0.8 mg cholesterol, 308.6 mg sodium, 20.6 g carbohydrates, 11.7 g sugars, 4.6 g fiber, 3.9 g protein

FRUIT SALAD DAZE

HONEY-LIME DRESSING

1   cup plain yogurt

½   cup red raspberries

¼   cup fresh lime juice

4   Tbsp honey or other sweetener

1   tsp vanilla extract

FRUIT SALAD

2   peaches or nectarines, sliced

1   cup green or red grapes

1   cup honeydew chunks

1   cup pineapple chunks

1   cup red raspberries

1   cup blackberries

    Mint leaves, for garnish

TO MAKE THE DRESSING:

1. Place the yogurt, raspberries, lime juice, honey, and vanilla extract in a blender.

2. Process until smooth.

TO MAKE THE FRUIT SALAD:

1. In a large bowl, combine all the fruit.

2. Add the dressing and toss well.

3. Allow to sit for 30 minutes, covered, at room temperature.

4. Garnish with mint leaves just before serving.

ALTERNATE VERSION

Substitute other fruits that look good in the supermarket. Try strawberries, kiwi, cantaloupe, watermelon, papaya, or apricots.
In the winter, use apples and pears and top with a sprinkling of pomegranate seeds.

Serves six.

Per serving: 150.9 calories, 0.6 g fat (0.1 g saturated), 0.8 mg cholesterol, 29.8 mg sodium, 37.1 g carbohydrates, 29.3 g sugars, 4.8 g fiber, 3.4 g protein

ROASTED BUTTERNUT-AND-SPINACH SALAD

2   cups (¾ lb) precut butternut squash cubes (¾") or ½ medium butternut squash, peeled, seeded, and cubed

1   large red bell pepper, cut into ¾" pieces

2   Tbsp extra-virgin olive oil

1   tsp fresh thyme, chopped, or ½ tsp dried thyme

½   tsp salt

¼   tsp freshly ground black pepper

2   Tbsp freshly squeezed lemon juice

2   tsp honey

¼   cup small red onion, chopped

4   oz (4 cups) loosely packed baby spinach

1   small Gala or Golden Delicious apple, cored and thinly sliced

1   cup thinly sliced radicchio

½   cup unsalted sunflower seeds

1. Preheat oven to 425°F.

2. Coat rimmed baking sheet with olive oil spray.

3. Toss the squash and bell pepper with 2 teaspoons of the oil, thyme, ¼ teaspoon of the salt, and ⅛ teaspoon of the black pepper in a medium bowl. Arrange in a single layer on a prepared baking sheet. Roast 25 to 30 minutes, stirring occasionally to prevent sticking, until tender and lightly browned. Let cool for 10 minutes.

4. While the squash roasts, whisk the lemon juice, honey, and remaining 4 teaspoons oil, ¼ teaspoon salt, and ⅛ teaspoon black pepper in a large salad bowl. Stir in onion. Add spinach, apple, radicchio, sunflower seeds, and squash mixture and toss to combine.

Serves four.

Per serving: 244.3 calories, 15.3 g fat (1.9 g saturated), 0 mg cholesterol, 337.3 mg sodium, 28.2 g carbohydrates, 10.7 g sugars, 6.9 g fiber, 5.1 g protein

SALAD BOOSTER #2: CRUNCH

Croutons lend texture but do nothing for your body. Opt for thinly sliced red or yellow bell peppers for more vitamin C, and a deep crunch.

THE MUSCLE-BUILDING SALAD

9	oz flank steak
	Salt and pepper to taste
2	plum tomatoes, cut into eighths
⅓	cup onion, sliced
1	small clove garlic, crushed
5	cups, romaine lettuce, chopped
4	Tbsp balsamic vinaigrette (see page 279)
3	Tbsp blue cheese, crumbled

Per serving: 307.4 calories, 14.8 g fat (6.5 g saturated), 54.1 mg cholesterol, 627.8 mg sodium, 15.4 g carbohydrates, 5.8 g sugars, 4.1 g fiber, 32.4 g protein

1. Preheat a grill pan on medium-high.

2. Season both sides of the steak with salt and pepper, and cook it about 6 minutes on each side. Remove the steak, let it rest for 3 to 5 minutes, and then slice it diagonally across the grain into thin strips.

3. In a large bowl, mix the tomatoes, onion and garlic. Add the meat and lettuce, pour on the vinaigrette, and toss well to completely coat everything. Top with the cheese.

Serves two.

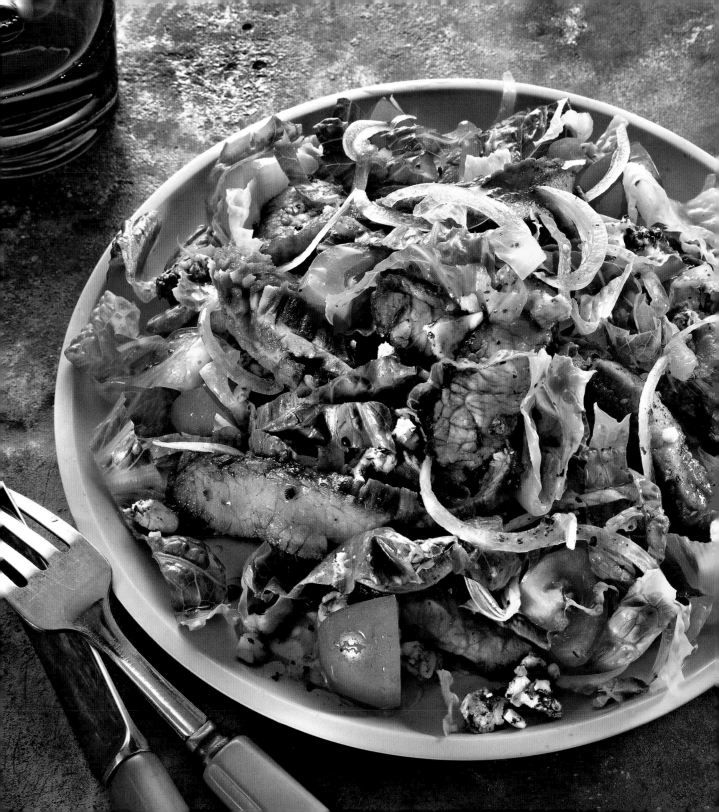

A VERY CORNY SALAD

1	can (15 oz) corn, drained
1	large cucumber, peeled and diced
½	cup red onion, finely chopped
1	medium-size red bell pepper, diced finely
1	medium-size tomato, seeded and diced
½	cup fresh cilantro, chopped (optional)
2	Tbsp seasoned rice vinegar
2	Tbsp apple cider or distilled vinegar
1	Tbsp lemon juice (optional)
1	clove garlic, minced
1	tsp ground coriander
⅛	tsp cayenne pepper

1. In a large salad bowl, combine corn, cucumber, onion, red pepper, tomato, and cilantro.

2. In a small bowl, combine vinegars, lemon juice, garlic, coriander, and cayenne. Pour over the salad and toss gently to mix.

Serves six.

Per serving: 81.5 calories, 1 g fat (0.1 g saturated), 0 mg cholesterol, 233.9 mg sodium, 18 g carbohydrates, 4.3 g sugars, 2.8 g fiber, 2.8 g protein

SALAD BOOSTER #3: SERVE ON A PLATE

Yes, even the serving dish matters. A Cornell University study found that a salad heaped on a plate creates the perception of a more substantial meal than one hidden deep in a bowl.

GRANNY'S TURKEY SALAD

DRESSING

½	cup buttermilk
2	Tbsp reduced-calorie mayonnaise
1	Tbsp cider vinegar
1½	tsp grainy Dijon mustard
½	tsp coarse-ground black pepper
	Pinch of salt

SALAD

1	package (6 oz) prewashed baby spinach
1	large Granny Smith apple, quartered, cored, and thinly sliced crosswise
1	large ripe pear, quartered, cored, and thinly sliced crosswise
4	oz sliced smoked turkey or lean ham, cut into 2" x ½" strips
¼	cup red onion, thinly sliced
2	Tbsp pumpkin seeds
2	Tbsp golden raisins
2	Tbsp walnuts, coarsely chopped and toasted

TO MAKE THE DRESSING:

1. In a salad bowl, whisk together the buttermilk, mayonnaise, vinegar, mustard, pepper, and salt.

TO MAKE THE SALAD:

1. Add the spinach, apple, pear, ham or turkey, onion, pumpkin seeds, raisins, and walnuts to the salad bowl.

2. Toss until well coated with the dressing.

Serves four.

Per serving: 195.4 calories, 5.7 g fat (1 g saturated), 22.1 mg cholesterol, 565 mg sodium, 30.1 g carbohydrates, 16.1 g sugars, 5.5 g fiber, 9.2 g protein

ROOTIN' TOOTIN' SALAD

1 can (15 oz) diced beets, drained

1 small jicama, peeled and cut into thin strips or diced

2 medium-size carrots, peeled and cut into thin strips or diced

3 Tbsp lemon juice (optional)

2 Tbsp seasoned rice vinegar

2 Tbsp stone-ground mustard

½ tsp dried dill weed

1. Place beet cubes in a large salad bowl along with jicama and carrot pieces.

2. In another small bowl, mix lemon juice, vinegar, mustard, and dill.

3. Pour the dressing mixture over the salad. Toss to combine. Serve warm or chilled.

Serves six.

Per serving: 63.8 calories, 0.2 g fat (0 g saturated), 0 mg cholesterol, 93.7 mg sodium, 14.8 g carbohydrates, 7 g sugars, 5.6 g fiber, 1.8 g protein

AVOCADO, TOMATO, AND ARUGULA SALAD

DRESSING

2 Tbsp extra-virgin olive oil

1 Tbsp balsamic vinegar

1 small clove garlic, crushed

¼ tsp salt

¼ tsp ground black pepper

SALAD

4 cups baby arugula

4 ripe medium tomatoes (about 12 oz total), cored and cut into wedges

1 large ripe avocado, halved, pitted, peeled, quartered, and sliced crosswise

¼ cup red onion, thinly sliced

1 Tbsp toasted sunflower seeds (substitute with slivered almonds or pumpkin seeds)

1. In a salad bowl, use a fork to mix the oil, vinegar, garlic, salt, and pepper.

2. Add the arugula, tomatoes, avocado, and onion. Toss gently to mix.

3. Sprinkle with the sunflower seeds.

Serves four.

Per serving: 216.5 calories, 6.9 g fat (0.9 g saturated), 0 mg cholesterol, 250.6 mg sodium, 33 g carbohydrates, 1.8 g sugars, 9.3 g fiber, 8.3 g protein

SALAD BOOSTER #4: DRESSING

Try this healthy vinaigrette: In a jar, combine ⅓ cup extra-virgin olive oil with ¼ cup red-wine vinegar, 2 tablespoons minced onion, 1 tablespoon Dijon mustard, and a bit of cracked black pepper. Screw on the top and shake.

MEDITERRANEAN VEGGIE BURGER

2   large red leaf lettuce leaves

2   grilled-vegetable soy burgers

2   Tbsp goat cheese

1   jarred roasted red pepper, halved

½   cup BroccoSprouts or other types of sprouts

½   cup baby spinach leaves

1. Place the lettuce leaves onto a work surface, with the long sides facing you.

2. With your fingers, press lightly to flatten the center of each.

3. Prepare the burgers per the package directions.

4. Place one on the center of each lettuce leaf. Top each with half of the cheese, red pepper, sprouts, and spinach. Fold up the bottom and sides of each lettuce leaf to enclose the burgers. Serve immediately.

NOTE:

BroccoSprouts is a brand of sprouted broccoli seeds, created by scientists at Johns Hopkins University School of Medicine, that provide high levels of antioxidants. They are available in many supermarkets.

Serves two.

Per serving: 180.9 calories, 6.7 g fat (2.1 g saturated), 6.5 mg cholesterol, 444.4 mg sodium, 13.7 g carbohydrates, 4.7 g sugars, 7.6 g fiber, 16.6 g protein

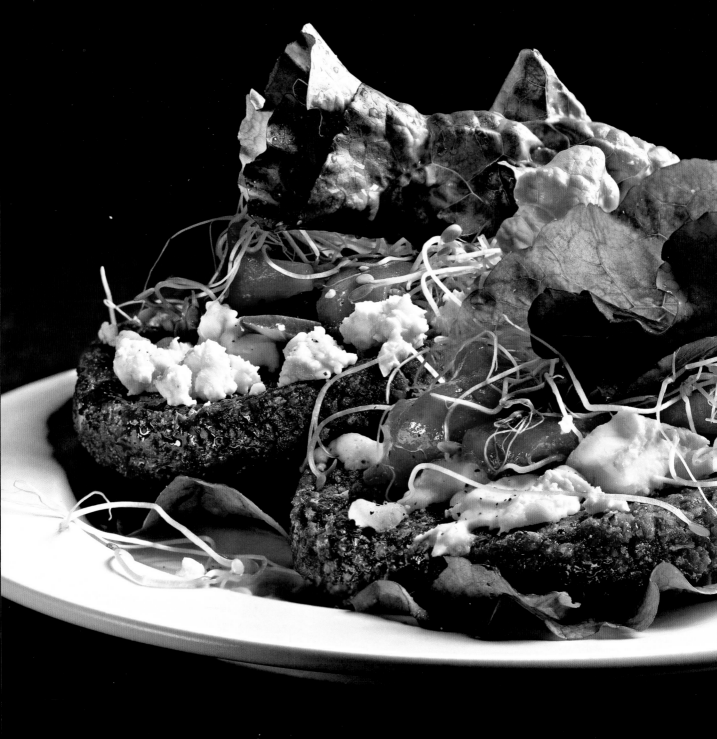

PB AND B SANDWICH

1	toasted whole-wheat English muffin
2	Tbsp peanut butter
½	cup banana, sliced
½	cup blueberries

1. Toast a split English muffin.

2. Onto each half, spread peanut butter and top with banana.

3. Eat as an open-faced sandwich with a side of blueberries.

Serves one.

Per serving: 405.2 calories, 17.9 g fat (3.7 g saturated), 0 mg cholesterol, 570 mg sodium, 54.2 g carbohydrates, 20.2 g sugars, 9 g fiber, 14.9 g protein

THAI-DYED TURKEY BURGER

1½	pounds ground turkey
3	scallions, thinly sliced
4	mushrooms, finely chopped
¼	cup carrots, chopped
1	Tbsp garlic paste (ask your grocer if they stock pastes, or make your own with a food processor)
1	Tbsp ginger paste
2	Tbsp cilantro paste
3	Tbsp soy sauce
1	Tbsp ground black pepper
	Salt to taste
6	ciabatta rolls, split
1	Tbsp extra-virgin olive oil
¼	cup Thai satay sauce
6	tomato slices
½	head napa cabbage, shredded

1. Preheat the grill.

2. Stir together the turkey, scallions, mushrooms, carrots, pastes, soy sauce, pepper, and salt. Shape into 6 burgers.

3. Grill the burgers for 10 to 12 minutes, turning once, until no longer pink.

4. Brush the rolls with the oil and place on the grill 1 minute before the burgers are done.

5. Divide the rolls among 6 plates. Spread 1 tablespoon satay sauce on each roll. Top each with a burger, tomato slice, and cabbage.

Serves six.

Per serving: 325.1 calories, 13.9 g fat (3.8 g saturated), 74.7 mg cholesterol, 947.4 mg sodium, 26.7 g carbohydrates, 4.7 g sugars, 2.8 g fiber, 24.8 g protein

WHAT'S THE DIFF?

TEQUILA AND MEZCAL

Both are distilled from the agave plant. But the agave for tequila is usually roasted in an oven whereas the agave for mezcal is roasted in earthen pits, which gives it its distinctive smokey flavor. By law, tequila only has to be 51% agave, and mezcal is usually 100%.

ROASTED VEGGIE SANDWICH

ARTICHOKE TAPENADE

1	cup canned (in water) artichoke hearts, drained
	Juice of ½ lemon
1	Tbsp extra-virgin olive oil
1	tsp minced garlic
1	tsp white wine vinegar
¼	tsp salt
	Ground black pepper

SANDWICH

2	portobello mushroom caps
1	zucchini, cut in 3" segments, then sliced lengthwise
1	medium tomato, sliced
2	crusty multigrain rolls (4 oz each), insides scooped out, or 2 slices whole-grain bread
2	oz fresh goat cheese

TO MAKE THE TAPENADE:

1. In the bowl of a food processor fitted with a metal blade, combine the artichokes, lemon juice, oil, garlic, vinegar, and salt.

2. Pulse about eight times, scraping down the sides of the bowl as needed, or until the mixture is spreadable. Season to taste with pepper.

TO MAKE THE SANDWICH:

1. Preheat the oven to 400°F.

2. Arrange the mushrooms and zucchini on a nonstick baking sheet. Roast for 10 minutes.

3. Arrange the tomato slices on the same baking sheet and continue roasting, flipping the vegetables halfway through cooking, for 20 minutes or until sizzling and any liquid is cooked away.

4. Divide the sandwich fillings between the rolls, layering the mushrooms, then zucchini, cheese, tomato, and tapenade.

Serves two.

Per serving: *231.9 calories, 10.7 g fat (6.1 g saturated), 22.4 mg cholesterol, 300.9 mg sodium, 26.7 g carbohydrates, 6.8 g sugars, 9.3 g fiber, 12.4 g protein*

PORTOBELLO SANDWICH

1	tsp olive oil
1	onion slice, ¼" thick
¼	red bell pepper, cut into thick strips
1	medium portobello mushroom cap
	Salt to taste
1	slice reduced-fat provolone cheese
1	tsp prepared pesto
1	focaccia roll or one 2" slice focaccia bread (2 oz)
1	lettuce leaf
1	tomato slice

1. Preheat the oven to 400°F.

2. In a nonstick skillet over medium heat, warm the oil. Add the onion and bell pepper. Cook, tossing occasionally, for about 5 minutes or until softened. Scrape the vegetables to the side.

3. Place the mushroom in the pan, top side up. Cook for about 2 minutes. Turn over and cook for 2 minutes more or until softened. Season the mushroom cap and vegetables lightly with salt.

4. Transfer the mushroom to a baking pan or piece of heavy aluminum foil. Top with the onion, pepper, and cheese. Bake for 5 minutes, or until the cheese bubbles.

5. Meanwhile, spread the pesto on both sides of the roll or bread.

6. Transfer the mushroom, onion, pepper, and cheese to the bottom bun. Top with lettuce, tomato, and top bun. Slice in half and serve.

Serves one.

Per serving: 302.2 calories, 12.1 g fat (3.3 g saturated), 11.7 mg cholesterol, 649.8 mg sodium, 39.1 g carbohydrates, 6 g sugars, 3.3 g fiber, 11.6 g protein

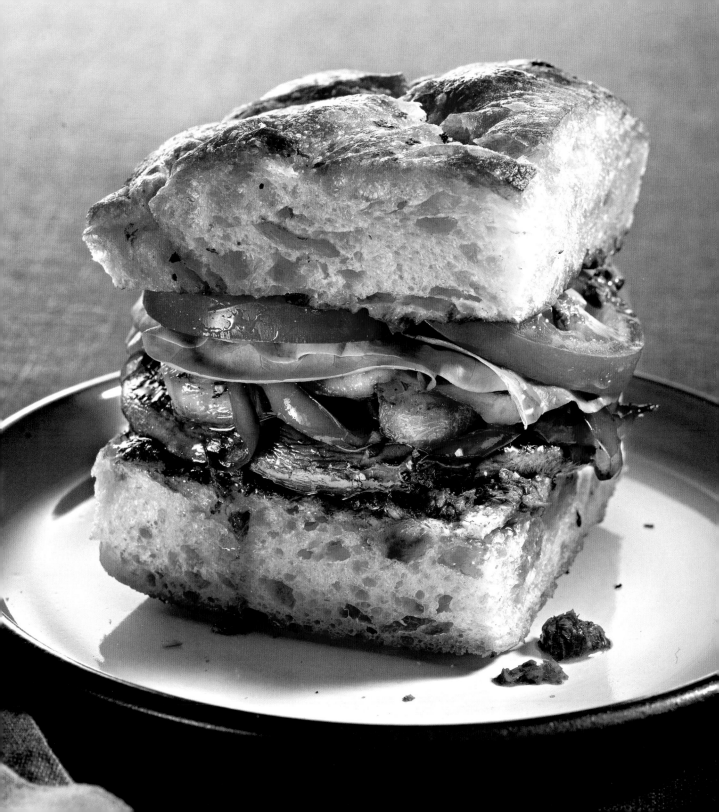

CALIFORNIA CLUB SANDWICH

4	slices country-style multigrain bread
1½	tsp Dijon mustard
½	cup cucumber, thinly sliced
3	oz (⅛) avocado, sliced
½	jarred roasted red pepper, drained and halved
1	oz soft goat cheese, crumbled
¼	cup alfalfa sprouts

1. Place 2 slices of the bread on a work surface. Spread one side of each with the mustard.

2. Top each with half of the cucumber, half of the avocado, half of the roasted pepper, ½ ounce goat cheese, 2 tablespoons of the sprouts, and 1 of the remaining bread slices. Cut each in half.

Serves two.

Per serving: 200.1 calories, 9.4 g fat (3 g saturated), 11.1 mg cholesterol, 382.6 mg sodium, 26.1 g carbohydrates, 1.1 g sugars, 8.4 g fiber, 7.9 g protein

AHI-AHA! BURGER

10	oz ahi tuna, divided into two portions
	Olive oil
	Salt and pepper to taste
2	ciabatta or focaccia rolls, toasted
2	Tbsp prepared pesto
2	Tbsp mayonnaise
1	tomato, sliced
¼	red onion, thinly sliced
2	cups mixed greens

1. Coat the tuna with olive oil and season with salt and pepper.

2. Grill on high heat for 2 minutes per side until the outside is lightly charred but the interior is still pink and cool.

3. Serve on a toasted bun slathered with the pesto and mayo and dressed with the vegetables.

Serves two.

Per serving: 483.5 calories, 17.4 g fat (3.3 g saturated), 72.6 mg cholesterol, 759 mg sodium, 40.9 g carbohydrates, 5.5 g sugars, 3.6 g fiber, 41.7 g protein

WHAT'S THE DIFF?

GRILLING AND BARBECUING

You're grilling when you cook a steak on your (you guessed it) grill. You're barbecuing when you get up at 5 a.m. to start a smoldering fire in a pit and turn slabs of ribs or a brisket into falling-apart wonderfulness by dinnertime.

RED ONION TURKEY BURGER WITH PEACH-GINGER TERIYAKI RELISH

RELISH

1	Tbsp olive or canola oil
3	peaches, peeled, pitted, and chopped
1	tsp fresh ginger, minced
1	Tbsp teriyaki sauce
1	cup light or fat-free mayonnaise

BURGER

2	lb ground turkey breast
1	Tbsp teriyaki sauce
½	small red onion, chopped
½	tsp salt
½	tsp ground black pepper
6	whole-grain or whole-wheat kaiser rolls, split

TO MAKE THE RELISH:

1. Heat the oil in a medium skillet over medium-high heat.

2. Add the peaches and ginger. Cook, stirring, for 5 minutes.

3. Stir in the teriyaki sauce. Cook for 1 minute.

4. Transfer to a bowl. Let cool for a minute or two. Stir in the mayonnaise.

TO MAKE THE BURGER:

1. Preheat the grill.

2. Stir together the turkey, teriyaki sauce, onion, salt, and pepper in a large bowl.

3. Shape into 6 burgers. Grill the burgers for 10 to 12 minutes, turning once, until no longer pink.

4. Coat the rolls with cooking spray and place on the grill 1 minute before the burgers are done.

5. Divide the rolls among 6 plates. Top each with a burger and the relish.

Serves six.

Per serving: *414.5 calories, 8.1 g fat (0.9 g saturated), 64.3 mg cholesterol, 1,140.9 mg sodium, 44.1 g carbohydrates, 11.1 g sugars, 3.4 g fiber, 44.2 g protein*

VINEGAR: THE UNSUNG HEALTH FOOD

To cut calories and fat, swap in vinegar for mayo:

1. Douse thick-cut oven fries with malt vinegar.

2. Marinate sliced tomatoes and onions in red-wine vinegar; layer on a sandwich.

TURKEY SLIDERS

1	egg white, beaten
½	small red onion, minced
¼	cup fresh cilantro, minced
½	tsp ground cumin
¼	tsp salt
1	lb extra-lean ground turkey breast (99% fat-free)
8	whole-wheat dinner rolls, cut in half
4	leaves lettuce, halved
2	plum tomatoes, each cut into 4 slices
1	avocado, sliced
	(Also add sliced onion or pickled hot peppers as toppings if you like)

1. Whisk together the egg white, onion, cilantro, cumin, and salt in a medium bowl.

2. Add the turkey and mix until just blended.

3. Shape into 8 burgers, about 3" thick each.

4. Heat a skillet coated with cooking spray over medium heat. Cook the burgers, turning once, for 6 minutes or until well browned and a thermometer inserted in the thickest portion registers 165°F.

5. Place the bottoms of 2 dinner rolls on 4 plates. Top with 1 piece of lettuce and 1 tomato slice. Place 1 burger on each and top with the avocado and the top of the roll.

Serves four.

Per serving: 347.7 calories, 9.8 g fat (1.3 g saturated), 45 mg cholesterol, 502.2 mg sodium, 34.9 g carbohydrates, 6.6 g sugars, 7.6 g fiber, 35.2 g protein

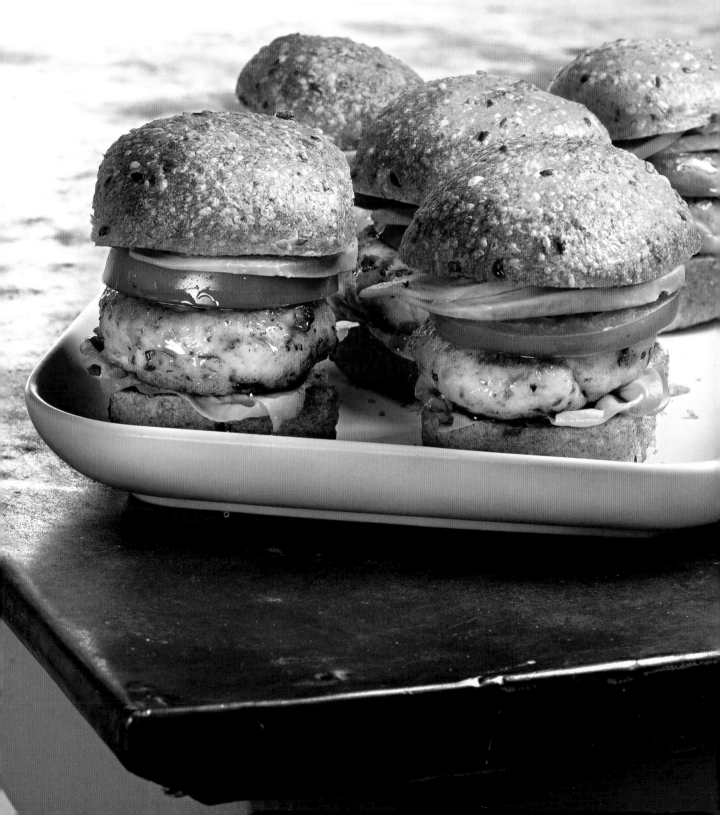

THE BEST SUMMER BURGER

1	egg
1	lb lean ground beef
½	cup oats
⅓	cup onion, diced
½	cup spinach, chopped
2	Tbsp reduced-fat Mexican-blend cheese, shredded
	Salt and black pepper to taste
4	whole-grain buns

1. In a large bowl, whisk the egg.

2. Add beef, oats, onion, spinach, cheese, salt, and pepper and mix (your hands are the best tool) until well blended.

3. Form the meat into four patties.

4. Place the burgers on a grill pan or nonstick skillet that's heated over medium-high. Cook for 6 minutes per side or to the desired level of doneness.

Serves four.

Per serving: 320.1 calories, 9.3 g fat (2.6 g saturated), 115.4 mg cholesterol, 316.5 mg sodium, 30.8 g carbohydrates, 4.7 g sugars, 4.7 g fiber, 30.1 g protein

TUNED-UP TUNA SANDWICH

1	can chunk light tuna, drained
⅓	fresh avocado
	Salt and pepper to taste (salt in tuna may be enough for some)
2	slices whole-grain bread

1. In a small bowl, mix tuna, avocado, salt, and pepper.

2. Spread on bread. (Also try with a slice of tomato.)

Serves one.

Per serving: 375 calories, 10.3 g fat (1.7 g saturated), 41.7 mg cholesterol, 982.3 mg sodium, 26.5 g carbohydrates, 3.5 g sugars, 7 g fiber, 43.3 g protein

WHAT'S THE DIFF?

LAGERS AND ALES

Lagers, which are cold-stored for 2 to 4 weeks after fermentation, have a smoother, cleaner taste than ales, which are bottled quickly and tend to be hearty and robust. They'll both get you drunk in the same amount of time.

SOUTHWEST BEAN BURGERS WITH LIME CREAM

BURGER

2	dried chipotle peppers (wash your hands thoroughly after)
1	cup red onion, chopped
½	cup carrots, chopped
1	cup mushrooms, chopped
1	cup frozen corn kernels, thawed
¼	cup fresh Italian parsley, chopped
1	tsp ground cumin
¼	tsp cider vinegar
1	can (19 oz) black beans, rinsed and drained
¼	cup blue or yellow cornmeal
⅓	cup unseasoned dry bread crumbs

LIME CREAM (to save time, you can substitute jarred salsa for Lime Cream)

⅓	cup fat-free sour cream
1	Tbsp lime juice
¼	tsp chili powder
	Dash of hot-pepper sauce

TO MAKE THE BURGERS:

1. Place the peppers in a small bowl and cover with boiling water. Let soak for 10 minutes or until softened.

2. Drain, pat dry, and remove and discard the stems and seeds. Chop the flesh.

3. Coat a large nonstick skillet with cooking spray. Add the onions and carrots. Cook over medium heat for 2 to 3 minutes or until softened.

4. Stir in the peppers, mushrooms, corn, parsley, cumin, and vinegar. Cook for 5 minutes or until the vegetables are tender. Remove from the heat.

5. Place the beans in a large bowl. Use the back of a wooden spoon to mash about half of the beans. Stir in the cornmeal and the vegetable mixture until well combined. Form into four 1"-thick patties. Roll in the bread crumbs to coat.

6. Wipe out the skillet and coat with nonstick spray. Place over medium heat until hot. Add the burgers and cook for 5 minutes per side or until browned and hot throughout.

TO MAKE THE LIME CREAM:

1. In a cup, combine the sour cream, lime juice, chili powder, and hot-pepper sauce. Serve on the burgers.

Serves four.

Per serving: *260.2 calories, 2.2 g fat (0.4 g saturated), 1.9 mg cholesterol, 586.8 mg sodium, 53.2 g carbohydrates, 8.1 g sugars, 11.1 g fiber, 12.8 g protein*

SPICE UP BORING BEER

1	bottle regular or light domestic beer
	Dash of hot sauce
	Dash of Worcestershire sauce
½	oz lime juice
1	lime slice

1. Fill a pint beer glass with ice. Add hot sauce and Worcestershire.

2. Fill glass with beer, then top with lime juice and lime slice. (Optional: Rim the glass with salt, before adding ice.)

GRILLED CHICKEN-AND-PINEAPPLE SANDWICHES

4	boneless, skinless chicken breasts
	Teriyaki sauce
4	slices Swiss cheese
4	slices pineapple (½" thick)
4	whole-wheat kaiser rolls
½	medium red onion, thinly sliced
¼	cup pickled jalapeño slices or 1 fresh jalapeño, thinly sliced

1. Place the chicken in a resealable plastic bag, and add enough teriyaki sauce to cover. Let it marinate in the refrigerator for at least 30 minutes (or up to 12 hours).

2. Heat a grill; it's ready when you can't hold your hand above the grate for longer than 3 seconds.

3. Remove the chicken from the marinade and place it on the grill. (Discard any remaining marinade.) Grill for 4 to 5 minutes, flip, and immediately add the cheese to each breast.

4. Continue cooking until the cheese is melted and the chicken is lightly charred and feels firm to the touch. Remove and set aside.

5. While the chicken is resting, place the pineapple slices and rolls on the grill. Toast the rolls lightly and cook the pineapple until it's soft and caramelized, about 2 minutes on each side.

6. Top each roll with chicken and, if you like, drizzle on a bit of teriyaki sauce from the bottle. Top the sandwiches with pineapple, onion, and jalapeño.

Serves four.

Per serving: 461.5 calories, 11.7 g fat (5.8 g saturated), 108 mg cholesterol, 793.4 mg sodium, 44.8 g carbohydrates, 19.7 g sugars, 5.4 g fiber, 45.5 g protein

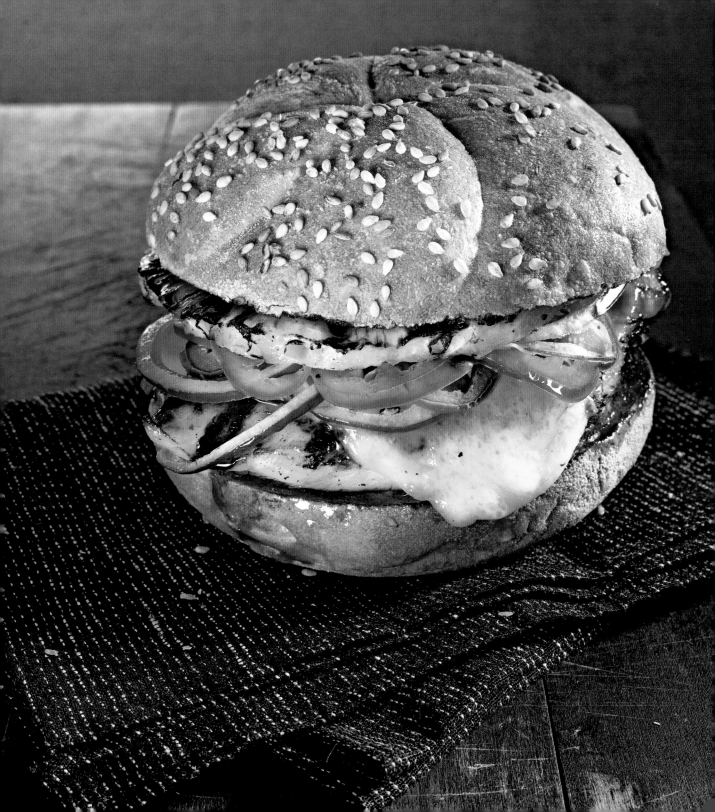

EGG SALAD SANDWICH

2	hard-boiled eggs
4	hard-cooked egg whites
2	Tbsp fat-free sour cream
2	Tbsp onion, finely chopped
1	heaping Tbsp brown mustard
¼	tsp dried dill
	Dash of ground black pepper
4	slices whole-grain bread, toasted

1. In a bowl, use a potato masher to mash the eggs and egg whites into small pieces.

2. Add the sour cream, onion, mustard, dill, and pepper. Stir until well mixed.

3. Spread half the egg salad on 2 slices of the toast.

4. Complete each sandwich with another slice of toast.

Serves two.

Per serving: 263.3 calories, 7.3 g fat (2.1 g saturated), 212.9 mg cholesterol, 447.5 mg sodium, 30 g carbohydrates, 7.7 g sugars, 3.4 g fiber, 19.7 g protein

ALASKAN BURGER

1	egg (use omega-3 eggs to up the good-fat count)
1	can salmon, drained
2	pieces of whole-wheat toast, diced
1	Tbsp ground flaxseeds
	Salt and pepper to taste
4	whole-grain rolls

1. Preheat oven to 375°F.

2. In a large bowl, break open the egg and whisk.

3. Add the salmon, diced toast, flaxseed, salt, and pepper, mixing with your hands until well blended.

4. Form into four patties. Bake for 20 minutes, turning once. Serve on whole-grain rolls.

Serves four.

Per serving: 327.6 calories, 17.8 g fat (0.5 g saturated), 52.9 mg cholesterol, 235.7 mg sodium, 7.5 g carbohydrates, 0.8 g sugars, 1.9 g fiber, 34.6 g protein

WHAT'S THE DIFF?

NUTRITIONIST AND DIETITIAN

A nutritionist can work under that title with no formal training; when Dave in the pub says the deep-fried cheese you're always chomping on will clog your arteries, he's being a nutritionist. But state-registered dietitians (RD) must be qualified in dietetics and nutrition before a doctor can refer you and your cheese addiction to them.

POWER BURGER

1   lb extra-lean ground beef (hormone-, pesticide-, and antibiotic-free)

1   Tbsp sunflower seeds, shelled

1   Tbsp onion, finely chopped

1   Tbsp red bell pepper, finely chopped

¼   tsp fresh-ground black pepper

    Toasted wheat germ

4   whole-grain buns

    Lettuce and tomato slices as topping

    Honey mustard

1   apple, sliced

1. Place the ground beef, sunflower seeds, onion, bell pepper, and black pepper in a large mixing bowl and knead with your hands until it's well mixed.

2. Make four thin patties, then roll them in the wheat germ until they're covered.

3. Grill or panfry the burgers.

4. Place the cooked burgers on the buns, and top with lettuce, tomato, and honey mustard. Serve with sliced apple as a side dish.

Serves four.

Per serving: *354.6 calories, 10.8 g fat (3.3 g saturated), 70.5 mg cholesterol, 325.2 mg sodium, 33.2 g carbohydrates, 7.2 g sugars, 6.2 g fiber, 33.2 g protein*

PREWORKOUT TURKEY SANDWICH

1   tsp honey mustard (use the lowest-sodium brand you can find)

2   slices whole-grain bread

2   oz low-sodium turkey breast, thinly sliced

2   tomato slices

1   small handful alfalfa sprouts or shredded lettuce

1. Spread the mustard onto the bread slices.

2. On one of the slices, stack the turkey, tomato, and sprouts or lettuce.

3. Top with the second bread slice. Eat 1 hour before workout.

Serves one.

Per serving: *159.2 calories, 1.9 g fat (0.3 g saturated), 24.4 mg cholesterol, 878.8 mg sodium, 24.1 g carbohydrates, 6.8 g sugars, 9.1 g fiber, 15 g protein*

YOUR HEALTH OUTLOOK: CLOUDY

Is your apple juice cloudy? Drink up. In a recent study, Polish scientists determined that unfiltered apple juice contains four times more disease-fighting antioxidants than the clear, purified kind does. Look for brands with 100 percent apple juice that you can't see through, such as Odwalla or R.W. Knudsen.

UNCLE ALFALFA SANDWICH

2	slices 7-grain sandwich bread, toasted
2	tsp stone-ground mustard
2	oz (2 slices) sharp Cheddar cheese
¼	cup cucumber, thinly sliced
2	Tbsp carrots, shredded
¼	cup alfalfa sprouts

1. Place the bread on a work surface.

2. Spread the mustard on the top sides.

3. On top of 1 slice, layer the cheese, cucumber, carrots, sprouts, and the other bread slice.

4. Cut diagonally.

Serves one.

Per serving: *347.4 calories, 21.5 g fat (14.4 g saturated), 65.4 mg cholesterol, 739.7 mg sodium, 22.6 g carbohydrates, 1.1 g sugars, 6.3 g fiber, 16.9 g protein*

ULTIMATE GRILLED CHEESE

8	slices multigrain bread
8	slices low-fat Jarlsberg or Cheddar cheese
1	large tomato, cut into 8 slices
2	roasted red peppers, halved
12	large leaves fresh basil

1. Coat both sides of the bread with olive oil-flavored cooking spray.

2. In a large nonstick skillet over medium heat, cook the bread on 1 side for 2 minutes or until lightly toasted. Do this in batches, if necessary. Remove from the pan.

3. Arrange four of the bread slices, toasted side up, on a work surface. Top with the cheese, tomato, peppers, and basil. Top with the remaining bread slices, toasted sided down.

4. Carefully place the sandwiches in the skillet. Cook for 2 minutes per side, or until toasted and the cheese melts.

Serves four.

Per serving: *302.2 calories, 8.3 g fat (2.5 g saturated), 11.9 mg cholesterol, 651.7 mg sodium, 36.5 g carbohydrates, 7.9 g sugars, 7.8 g fiber, 22.8 g protein*

HEALTHY HOME-MADE CHIP DIP

Mix a little avocado, some lime juice, half a jalapeño, and a few sprinkles of salt and you have instant guacamole— and a delivery system for fiber, vitamins and minerals, and heart-healthy monounsaturated fat. Low-cal, high-in-vitamins salsa and fiber-rich bean dips are also smart choices.

PORTOBELLO BURGERS WITH ROASTED PEPPERS, SWISS, AND CARAMELIZED ONIONS

3	tsp extra-virgin olive oil
1	cup onion, thinly sliced
1	tsp sugar
1	Tbsp balsamic vinegar
4	portobello mushroom caps, about 3½–4 oz each
¼	tsp salt
¼	tsp ground black pepper
2	oz (4 slices) reduced-fat Swiss cheese
4	light (100-calorie) multigrain English muffins, split
2	jarred roasted red peppers, drained and cut into strips

1. Preheat the grill.

2. Heat 1 teaspoon of the oil in a small nonstick skillet over medium-high heat.

3. Add the onion and sugar and cook, stirring occasionally, until lightly browned, about 5 to 6 minutes. Remove from the heat.

4. Combine the remaining 2 teaspoons oil and the vinegar in a small bowl.

5. Brush the mixture over the mushroom caps and sprinkle with the salt and pepper. Grill, covered, turning occasionally, until tender, 9 to 11 minutes.

6. Top each with 1 slice of the cheese and continue to grill until the cheese melts, about 1 to 2 minutes longer. Transfer to a plate and keep warm.

7. Toast the English muffins.

8. Place the bottom half of each muffin on a plate and top with 1 portobello cap, ¼ of the roasted peppers, and ¼ of the onion. Top with the remaining muffin halves.

Serves four.

Per serving: 228.8 calories, 7.6 g fat (1.9 g saturated), 6.8 mg cholesterol, 441.8 mg sodium, 33.7 g carbohydrates, 8.5 g sugars, 4.9 g fiber, 11.4 g protein

GRILL THE PERFECT BURGER

High heat is critical. "You want to develop charred, carmelized flavors on the surface before the interior is done," says chef Jamie Purviance, the author of *Weber's Way to Grill.*

1. Front-load the flavor: Use hardwood charcoal or, if you have a gas grill, add a smoker box, which burns wood chips. "Wood smoke can do as much for the taste as a glaze, seasoning, or topping can," says Purviance.

2. Bring the heat: The grill is ready when you can't hold your hand 5 inches above the grate for 3 seconds. Add the patties and close the lid. After 4 minutes, ease your spatula under each burger. If it gives, flip it. If the burger sticks, leave it on for another minute, and then flip the patty and grill it for 4 more minutes. Add cheese when there's a minute to go.

SAUSAGE AND BROCCOLI RABE PASTA

1	lb broccoli rabe, 2" trimmed from ends, cut into 2" segments
8	oz whole-wheat fusilli pasta*
1	Tbsp olive oil
6	oz chicken sausage, cut into ½" slices
4	dry-packed sun-dried tomatoes, roughly chopped
3	cloves garlic, minced or put through garlic press

*Other shapes of dried pasta, such as rotini, bow ties, penne, or shells, can replace the fusilli.

1. Bring a large pot of water to a boil. Add the broccoli rabe and blanch for 2 minutes.

2. Remove from the pot and plunge into a bowl of cold water (save the pot of hot water for the pasta). Drain and set aside.

3. Add the pasta to the boiling water. Stir and cook for 10 minutes or until al dente.

4. Meanwhile, heat the oil in a large skillet over medium-high heat. Add the sausage and cook, turning occasionally, for 5 minutes or until browned. Add the tomatoes, garlic, and broccoli rabe to the pan. Cook for 2 minutes or until the sausage is no longer pink.

5. Drain the pasta, reserving 2 tablespoons of the cooking water.

6. Add the pasta and reserved water to the skillet. Toss with the sausage mixture.

Serves four.

Per serving: 362.7 calories, 9.4 g fat (3.2 g saturated), 30.2 mg cholesterol, 145.2 mg sodium, 50.5 g carbohydrates, 4.7 g sugars, 5.5 g fiber, 20 g protein

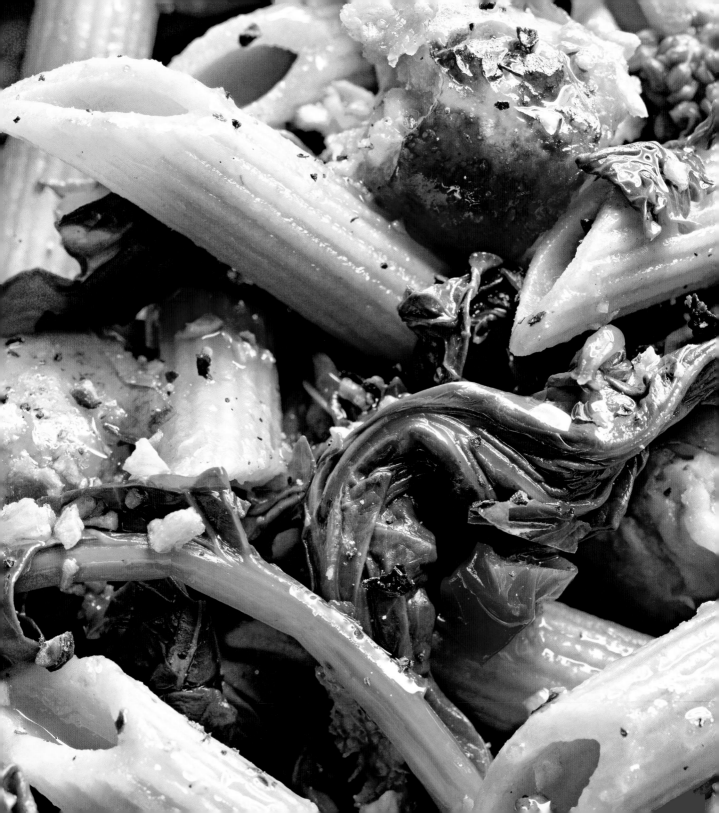

OPEN-FACED CHICKEN QUESADILLA

4   flour tortillas (10" diameter)
½   cup low-fat mayonnaise
1   Tbsp roasted-garlic-and-red-pepper spice blend
2   cups chicken, cooked and shredded
1   cup (4 oz) shredded Monterey Jack cheese
2   medium tomatoes, seeded and chopped
2   cups romaine lettuce, shredded

1. Preheat the oven to 350°F. Place the tortillas on baking sheets and toast for 5 minutes.

2. In a small bowl, combine the mayonnaise and the spice blend. Spread 2 tablespoons of the mixture over each tortilla.
Evenly top the center of each tortilla with chicken, then sprinkle with cheese.
Arrange the tomatoes around the chicken.

3. Bake for 10 minutes or until heated through. Sprinkle the lettuce around the tomato.

Serves four.

Per serving: 580.4 calories, 26.7 g fat (8.9 g saturated), 92.3 mg cholesterol, 881.2 mg sodium, 48.5 g carbohydrates, 5.8 g sugar, 3.8 g fiber, 36 g protein

JAMMIN' JAMBALAYA

1   large onion, peeled and diced
3   cloves garlic, peeled and minced
2   stalks celery, diced
2   carrots, diced
2   medium-sized sweet red peppers, diced
1   can (15 oz) crushed tomatoes
1   cup long-grain brown rice
1   package (12 oz) andouille turkey or chicken sausage, cut into ½-inch-thick rounds
1   tsp hot sauce
2   Tbsp fresh thyme, minced, or 2 tsp dried
1   tsp sea salt
½   tsp ground black pepper
2   cups water
3   Tbsp fresh parsley, minced
1   lb shrimp, peeled and deveined

1. Place onion, garlic, celery, carrots, peppers, tomatoes, rice, and sausage in a slow cooker in that order.
Add hot sauce, thyme, salt, pepper, and water.
Cover and cook on low for 7 to 8 hours.

2. Toss in parsley and shrimp. Stir until well combined, adding more water if needed.
Cook for 1 hour longer.

Serves six.

Per serving: 316.2 calories, 5.7 g fat (2 g saturated), 128.9 mg cholesterol, 939.2 mg sodium, 40 g carbohydrates, 5.6 g sugar, 5.2 g fiber, 29.4 g protein

HOW TO "SEASON TO TASTE"

The biggest mistake many home cooks make is not tasting the food until it's at the table, which is why it often ends up bland or, worse, overseasoned. Most chefs don't follow recipes; instead of using teaspoons and tablespoons, they use their hands to season and their tastebuds to adjust. Next time you make a tomato sauce or stir-fry, taste it first and then add small amounts of salt and pepper until your tastebuds begin to jump. (If you actually taste salt, it's probably too salty.)

COQ AU VIN

1	cup dry red wine
½	cup tomato paste
3	Tbsp flour
1½	tsp herbes de Provence
1½	tsp salt
1½	tsp ground black pepper
3	lb boneless, skinless chicken thighs
1	lb (2 cups) frozen pearl onions
8	oz (2 cups) small cremini mushrooms
6	precooked bacon slices, coarsely chopped
1	Tbsp preminced oil-packed garlic

1. Coat the inside of a 5- to 6-quart slow cooker with cooking spray.

2. In the pot, combine the wine, tomato paste, flour, herbes, salt, and pepper.
Whisk until smooth. Add the chicken, onions, mushrooms, bacon, and garlic.

3. Stir to coat the chicken with the sauce.
Cover and cook on the low-heat setting for 5 to 6 hours, or on high for 2½ to 3 hours.

Serves six.

Per serving: 479.1 calories, 19.8 g fat (5.5 g saturated), 158 mg cholesterol, 1,047.3 mg sodium, 18.1 g carbohydrates, 6.4 g sugars, 2.4 g fiber, 47.5 g protein

DILL-STUFFED GRILLED TROUT

1	trout (3 to 4 lb), gutted
	Salt and pepper to taste
1	bunch dill
1	bunch thyme
1	lemon
30	inches butcher's twine, cut into thirds
1	Tbsp canola or olive oil

1. Heat a grill to medium high.

2. Season the fish inside and out with salt and pepper. Stuff the cavity with dill and/or thyme and top with the juice of half a lemon.
Cut the other half into several slices and place them inside the cavity.

3. Tie the fish with twine and rub it with the oil to make the skin crisp and prevent sticking.
Rub the grill grates with oil, too.

4. Cook the fish until the flesh flakes fairly easy, about 6 to 8 minutes a side.

ALTERNATE VERSION

Wrap the trout in bacon or prosciutto before tying the fish with twine to add flavor and help prevent it from sticking to the grates.

Serves one to two.

Per serving: 170 calories, 11 g fat (1.5 g saturated), 35 mg cholesterol, 40 mg sodium, 7 g carbohydrates, 1 g sugars, 3 g fiber, 13 g protein

IS IT BETTER TO COOK WITH CHEAP WINE?

Whether cooking or sipping, price doesn't matter, says *Men's Health* Wine Guy Gary Vaynerchuk. The best rule is to cook with what you drink. If you like $8 chardonnay, cook with it. Then pour it at the table and you've created a quick harmony of the palate.

CHICKEN-SPINACH PARM

1   Tbsp olive oil

1   boneless, skinless chicken breast

1   Tbsp Italian-seasoned bread crumbs

1   tsp Parmesan, grated
    Salt and pepper to taste

1   small clove garlic, crushed

¼   cup marinara sauce

3   handfuls baby spinach leaves

Per serving: 366 calories, 17.4 g fat (2.9 g saturated), 70 mg cholesterol, 806.3 mg sodium, 21 g carbohydrates, 6 g sugar, 4.1 g fiber, 32.1 g protein

1. Heat the oil in a nonstick skillet over medium heat.

2. As the oil is heating, pound the chicken to ¼" thickness, then sprinkle with bread crumbs, cheese, salt, and pepper, pressing so the crumbs stick.
Place in the pan with the garlic and sauté for 2 to 3 minutes per side.

3. Top with hot marinara. Add the spinach, turning frequently with tongs until it wilts (about 6 minutes).

Serves one.

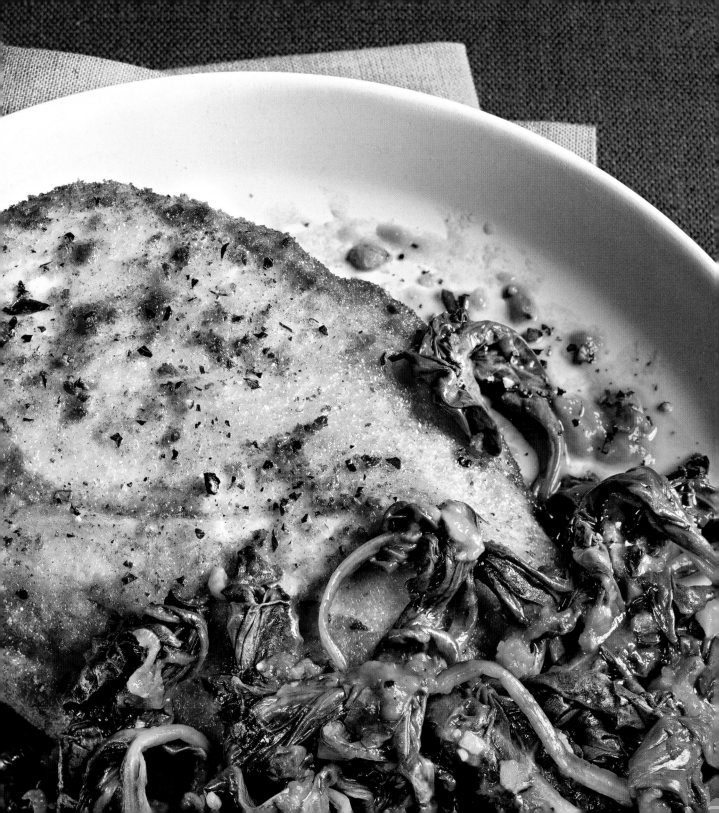

MOM'S MEATLOAF

½   cup ketchup

¼   cup packed dark brown sugar

4   Tbsp lemon juice, divided

1   tsp mustard powder

2   lb lean ground beef

4   slices whole-grain bread or higher-fiber white bread, broken up into small pieces (about 2 cups of soft cubes)

⅔   cup onion, finely chopped

1   egg

1   tsp low-sodium beef-broth powder or granules

1. Preheat the oven to 350°F.

2. Coat a 9" x 5" loaf pan with canola oil cooking spray.

3. In a small bowl, mix together the ketchup, brown sugar, 1 tablespoon of the lemon juice, and the mustard powder. Set aside.

4. In a bowl, mix together the ground beef, bread, onion, egg, beef-broth powder, remaining 3 tablespoons of lemon juice, and one-third of the ketchup mixture. Press the mixture into the prepared loaf pan. Bake for 1 hour.

5. Coat the top with the remaining ketchup mixture and bake for 10 additional minutes.

Serves eight.

Per serving: 245.1 calories, 6.3 g fat (2.1 g saturated), 53.4 mg cholesterol, 379.2 mg sodium, 18.3 g carbohydrates, 11.8 g sugars, 1.3 g fiber, 28.1 g protein

CEDAR PLANK SALMON

1   large, untreated cedar plank

2   salmon fillets (6 oz each)

    Salt and pepper to taste

    Canola or olive oil

1. Soak the cedar plank in water for at least 2 hours.

2. Clean a grill or grill pan thoroughly. Rub the grates with an oil-soaked paper towel. Preheat over high heat.

3. Lay the cedar plank on the grill. Season the salmon with salt and pepper. When the plank begins to smoke, lay the fillets on it, skin side down.

4. Close the top and grill for 10 to 12 minutes, until the salmon flakes with light pressure from your finger.

ALTERNATE VERSION

Combine 1 seeded and sliced cucumber, 2 tablespoons rice wine vinegar, red-pepper flakes, sesame seeds, and 2 tablespoons fresh, chopped mint or cilantro in a mixing bowl. Season to taste with salt and pepper. Top the cooked salmon with the cucumbers and garnish with a sprinkling of sesame seeds.

Serves two.

Per serving: 281.6 calories, 12.6 g fat (1.7 g saturated), 93.6 mg cholesterol, 156.6 mg sodium, 4.2 g carbohydrates, 2 g sugars, 1.3 g fiber, 35.2 g protein

SERVING SIZE, MADE SIMPLE:

MASHED POTATOES
½ cup at 112 calories

Same size as:
Half an apple

GRILLED FLANK STEAK WITH CHIMICHURRI SAUCE

CHIMICHURRI

3 Tbsp red wine vinegar

2 Tbsp water

3 cloves garlic, minced

½ tsp salt

½ tsp dried red-pepper flakes

½ tsp coarsely ground black pepper

¼ cup olive oil

½ cup fresh flat-leaf parsley, finely chopped

STEAK

12 oz flank, skirt, or sirloin steak

Salt and pepper to taste

1 bunch scallions

1. Make the chimichurri sauce by mixing the vinegar, water, garlic, salt, pepper flakes, and black pepper. Whisk in the oil. When everything's blended, whisk in the parsley. Set aside.

2. Preheat a grill or grill pan on high. Season the steak with salt and pepper and place it on the hot grill. For medium-rare, cook until a thermometer inserted into the thickest part reads 140°F.

3. Trim the roots from the scallions and add the entire bunch to the grill just after you've flipped the steak. Cook the scallions until they're lightly charred, about 4 to 5 minutes.

4. Drizzle the steak with the chimichurri and serve it with the grilled scallions.

Serves two.

Per serving: 562.5 calories, 41.5 g fat (9.7 g saturated), 69.7 mg cholesterol, 697.1 mg sodium, 8.6 g carbohydrates, 2 g sugars, 2.8 g fiber, 38.3 g protein

CHICKEN ENCHILADAS

1 pound boneless, skinless chicken breasts, cubed

1 whole bell pepper, chopped

½ tsp cumin

½ tsp mild chili powder

1 jar (16 oz) fat-free refried beans

6 medium whole-wheat flour tortillas

1 can (10 oz) spicy salsa

3 oz reduced-fat Cheddar cheese, shredded

Sour cream (optional)

1. Cook the chicken, pepper, and spices in a nonstick pan coated with cooking spray over medium-high heat for 4 minutes. Remove from heat and add the beans.

2. Add ¾ cup chicken filling to each tortilla, roll up, and place seam-side down in a nonstick baking dish. Top with the salsa. Cover and bake at 350°F for 40 minutes.

3. Right out of oven, sprinkle with cheese and allow to melt. To serve, garnish with more salsa and sour cream (optional).

Serves six.

Per serving: 520 calories, 9 g fat (1.5 g saturated), 65 mg cholesterol, 1,700 mg sodium, 65g carbohydrates, 7 g sugars, 13 g fiber, 41 g protein

WHAT'S THE DIFF?

JELLY, JAM, AND PRESERVES

Jelly is fruit juice with gelatin, so it jiggles. Jam has bits of fruit. Preserves have chunks. And yes, jiggles, bits, and chunks are formal FDA terminology.

CRAB CAKES

1	can (16 oz) jumbo lump crab meat
2	Tbsp jalapeño, minced
2	scallions, chopped
½	cup red bell pepper, minced
1	egg, lightly beaten
2	tsp Dijon mustard
	Juice of 1 lemon
¼	tsp Old Bay seasoning
½	tsp salt
¾	cup bread crumbs

Per serving: *207.5 calories, 3.5 g fat (0.8 g saturated), 120.4 mg cholesterol, 859 mg sodium, 17.9 g carbohydrates, 2.4 g sugars, 1.6 g fiber, 24.4 g protein*

1. Preheat the oven to 425°F.

2. Gently mix everything except ½ cup of the bread crumbs. Using your hands, loosely form the crab mixture into eight patties.

3. Spread the remaining bread crumbs on a plate and roll each patty over the crumbs to lightly and evenly coat it. Shape the crab cakes, using the palm of your hand to press each one into an evenly shaped disc the size of a small hockey puck.

4. Place them on a nonstick baking sheet or in a baking dish that you've coated with nonstick cooking spray. Bake until golden brown on the outside, 12 to 15 minutes.

Serves eight.

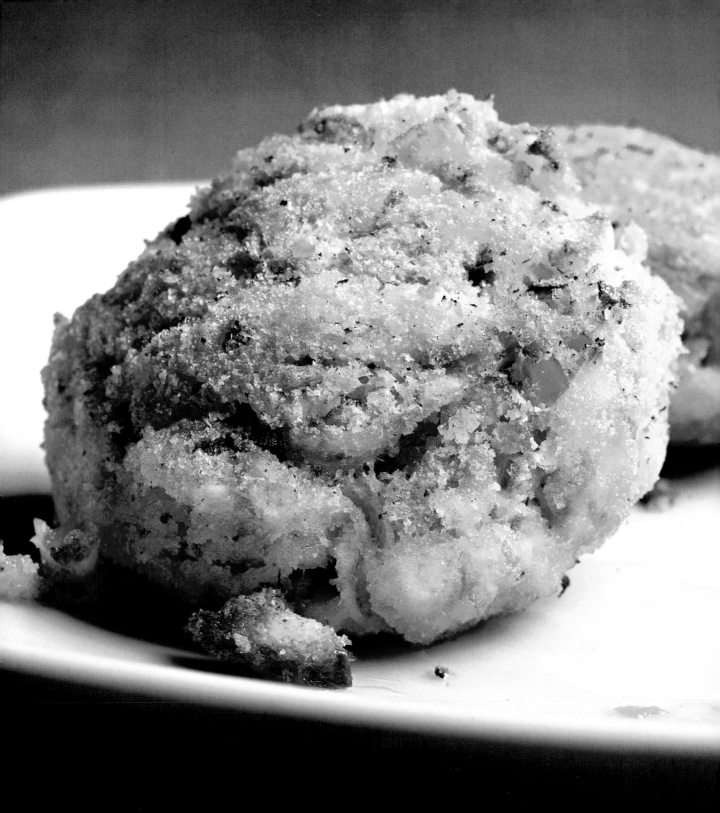

SPRING RISOTTO

1	Tbsp butter
1	Tbsp olive oil
½	cup onion, chopped
½	tsp salt
1½	cup arborio rice
3	cups reduced-sodium chicken or vegetable broth, heated, divided
¾	lb fresh in-the-pod peas, shelled, or 1 cup frozen
1	Tbsp lemon juice
¼	cup Parmesan cheese, freshly grated
	Salt and pepper to taste

1. Melt butter with oil in medium saucepan over medium-low heat. Add onion and salt. Cover and cook, stirring occasionally, until onion is translucent, about 3 minutes.

2. Add rice and stir.

3. Add about 1½ cups of the broth and adjust heat to maintain a good simmer. Stir occasionally until most of the liquid has been absorbed.

4. Add 1 cup of the remaining broth and continue simmering and stirring until absorbed.

5. Add remaining ½ cup broth and peas and continue to simmer and stir until rice is just done, about 4 minutes. If you run out of broth before the rice is cooked through, use water.

6. Stir in lemon juice and cheese. Taste and season as needed with salt and freshly ground pepper.

Serves four.

Per serving: 424.3 calories, 9.6 g fat (3.9 g saturated), 12 mg cholesterol, 770.8 mg sodium, 72.8 g carbohydrates, 3.4 g sugars, 3.1 g fiber, 13.3 g protein

THAI BEEF LETTUCE WRAPS

12	oz flank, skirt, or sirloin steak
	Salt and pepper to taste
1	Tbsp chili sauce, such as sriracha
2	Tbsp fish sauce
	Limes, cut into wedges
1	jalapeño pepper, thinly sliced
½	red onion, thinly sliced
½	cup fresh cilantro, chopped
1	carrot, peeled and grated
1	head Bibb lettuce, washed and dried, leaves separated

1. Heat the grill or grill pan over high heat for at least 5 minutes.

2. Season the steak with salt and pepper and toss it on the grill. Cook for about 4 minutes on each side, until it's firm but yielding to the touch. Let it rest for 5 minutes.

3. Combine the chili sauce, fish sauce, and juice of one lime in a small saucepan over low heat.

4. Slice the steak thinly (if it's skirt or flank steak, be sure to cut against the grain) and drizzle half of the warm sauce over it.

5. Set out the jalapeño and onion slices, cilantro, carrot, lettuce, and remaining lime wedges and sauce. Use the leaves like tortillas to wrap up the steak slices with the other ingredients. Save some lime and sauce to use on your wrap as you eat.

Serves two.

Per serving: 290 calories, 8 g fat (3g saturated), 79.9 mg cholesterol, 1,520 mg sodium, 14 g carbohydrates, 5.4 g sugars, 4 g fiber, 40 g protein

GIVE IT A REST!

Nothing is more tempting than fresh meat hot off the grill. But meat needs time to rest before you go cutting into it; otherwise, the meat's juices will run off onto the cutting board instead of staying where you want them. Thick steaks, roasts, and whole birds should rest 10 minutes; thinner cuts of meat, such as chicken breast, are ready to eat after 5 minutes.

RICE AND BEANS WITH GREENS

BEANS

1½   cups dry pinto beans

6   cups cold water

4   cups water

4   large cloves garlic, minced

1½   tsp cumin seed

¾   tsp salt

RICE

4   cups water

1   cup brown rice

½   tsp salt

GREENS

6–8   cups chopped (1 medium-size bunch)
      kale or collard greens

½   cup water

2   tsp balsamic vinegar

¼   tsp salt

3   medium-size cloves garlic, minced

TO MAKE THE BEANS:

1. Rinse the beans and soak them overnight in a large pot filled 6 cups cold water.

2. Drain and rinse the beans.

3. Place them in a large pot with 4 cups water and the garlic and cumin seed.

4. Simmer for about 1 hour or until tender. Add salt.

TO MAKE THE RICE:

1. In a large pot, bring the water to a boil.

2. Lower the heat to a bare simmer, and add rice and salt. Cover loosely and simmer for about 40 minutes or until tender. Pour off excess water.

TO MAKE THE GREENS:

1. Wash greens, remove the stems, and chop the leaves into ½"-wide strips.

2. In a large pot, bring water to a boil.

3. Add vinegar, salt, and garlic. Cook for 1 minute.

4. Stir in greens. Cover and cook over medium heat for 3 to 5 minutes, or until tender. Drain.

5. To serve, place a generous portion of rice on each plate, then top with some beans with their liquid. Serve kale on top of beans or to the side.

Serves eight.

Per serving: *242.8 calories, 1.7 g fat (0.3 g saturated), 0 mg cholesterol, 478 mg sodium, 47.2 g carbohydrates, 0.7 g sugars, 9.7 g fiber, 11.7 g protein*

WHAT'S THE DIFF?

BAKING SODA AND BAKING POWDER

Baking soda is sodium bicarbonate. It soaks up bad fridge odors, doubles as toothpaste, and makes a cool home volcano when an acid—like vinegar—is added. Oh yeah, and it's ideal for making batter. Baking powder is baking soda with an acid already mixed in—so it's ready to go to work when a liquid is added—and used to bake banana bread and other tasty things.

STEAK FA-HEAT-AS

6	oz flank steak
1	small onion, cut into eighths
1	green or red bell pepper, cut lengthwise into strips
1	small jalapeño pepper, cut into rings
1	tsp olive oil
1	Tbsp cilantro, chopped
⅛	tsp cinnamon
¼	tsp cumin
	Salt and pepper to taste
4	whole-wheat tortillas
	Salsa or diced fresh tomatoes

1. Preheat a skillet to medium-high heat.

2. Cut meat diagonally and across the grain into thin strips. Place in a large zip-top plastic bag with all other ingredients except tortillas and salsa. Shake well to combine.

3. Place the mixture in the skillet. Cook for 5 to 6 minutes or until meat reaches desired doneness, turning frequently. Serve with tortillas and salsa or tomatoes.

Serves two.

Per serving: *449.4 calories, 13.2 g fat (2.1 g saturated), 28.1 mg cholesterol, 390.8 mg sodium, 50.7 g carbohydrates, 5.2 g sugars, 6 g fiber, 27.4 g protein*

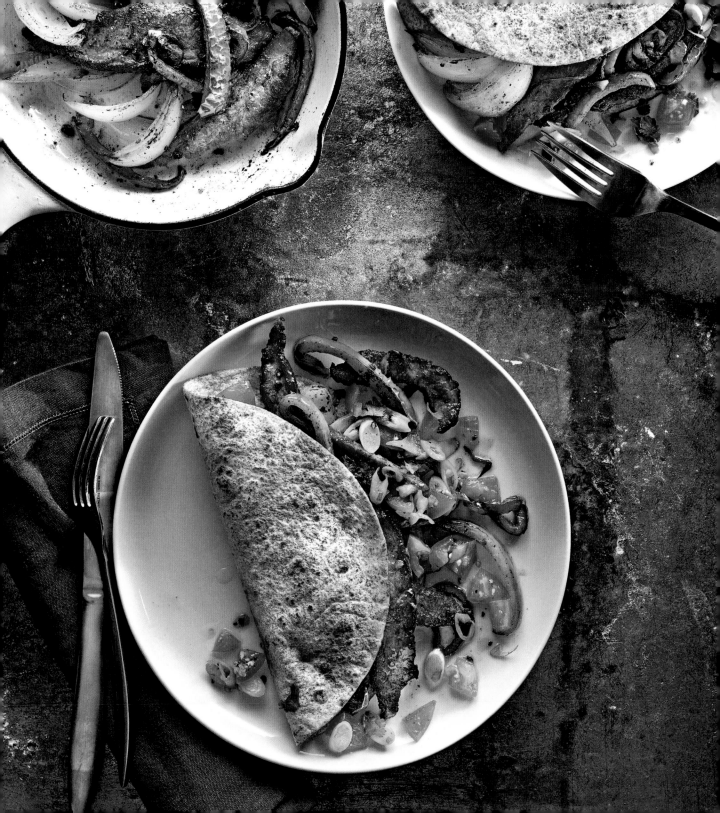

ULTIMATE GAME-DAY CHILI

1	lb ground beef
1	onion, diced
3	cloves garlic, crushed
2	cans (15 oz each) kidney beans, rinsed and drained
2	cans (8 oz each) diced tomatoes
2	cans (10.75 oz each) chicken broth
½	tsp salt
½	tsp pepper
1	tsp chili powder
½	tsp cumin
⅛	tsp cayenne
⅛	tsp cinnamon
1	oz dark chocolate

1. Brown the beef in a nonstick skillet over medium-high heat. Remove it with a slotted spoon and set it aside, leaving some of the fat in the skillet.

2. Sauté the onion and garlic in the fat until soft (about 6 minutes).

3. In a large stockpot, combine the browned beef, sautéed onion and garlic, beans, tomatoes, broth, spices, and chocolate. Simmer on low heat for 1 hour.

Serves six.

Per serving: *311 calories, 10 g fat (4 g saturated), 40 mg cholesterol, 631 mg sodium, 29 g carbohydrates, 5.9 g sugars, 7 g fiber, 26 g protein*

BLACK BEAN, VEGETABLE, AND NOODLE STIR-FRY

2	tsp olive oil
¾	cup (1 medium) red bell pepper, chopped
¾	cup (1 medium) green bell pepper, chopped
½	cup (1 small) onion, chopped
1	cup (1 small) zucchini, halved and cut into chunks
2	cloves garlic, minced
1	bag (16 oz) shirataki noodles, drained and rinsed in hot water
1	cup (about half of a 15–16 oz can) canned black beans, drained and rinsed
2	Tbsp reduced-sodium soy sauce
1½	tsp sodium-free seasoning mix
2	Tbsp fresh cilantro or parsley, chopped
	Hot-pepper sauce

1. In a wok or large nonstick skillet over high heat, warm the oil.

2. Add the bell peppers, onion, zucchini, and garlic. Reduce the heat to medium-high and cook, stirring frequently, for 4 minutes or until the vegetables start to soften.

3. Add the noodles, beans, soy sauce, and seasoning mix. Reduce the heat to medium. Cook, stirring frequently, for 3 to 4 minutes longer or until the mixture is hot.

4. Add the cilantro or parsley. Toss to mix. Pass around the hot-pepper sauce at the table.

Serves four.

Per serving: *106.5 calories, 2.7 g fat (0.4 g saturated), 0 mg cholesterol, 538.5 mg sodium, 18.1 g carbohydrates, 3.7 g sugars, 5.3 g fiber, 5.2g protein*

SERVING SIZE, MADE SIMPLE:

BUTTER
1 tsp, 34 calories

Same size as:
Tip of thumb

GREEK GRILLED CHICKEN BREAST

CHICKEN

4	boneless, skinless chicken breast halves (6 oz each)
1	Tbsp olive oil
1	Tbsp lemon juice, freshly squeezed
1	tsp dried oregano
1	clove garlic, minced
½	tsp salt
¼	tsp freshly ground black pepper

YOGURT CHEESE

1¼	cups fat-free Greek-style yogurt
½	cup cucumber, shredded
1	tsp fresh dill, chopped
2	cloves garlic, minced
½	cup shelled pistachios, coarsely chopped, divided

TO MAKE THE CHICKEN:

1. Butterfly the chicken breasts or just pound them with a meat mallet or the bottom of a heavy pot until thin.

2. Combine the chicken, oil, lemon juice, oregano, and garlic in a bowl and refrigerate for 1 to 2 hours, turning occasionally. Meanwhile, make yogurt cheese (below).

3. Heat the grill to medium-hot.

4. Remove the chicken from the marinade. Sprinkle with the salt and pepper and grill for 2 to 3 minutes per side or until the chicken is well marked and cooked through.

TO MAKE THE YOGURT CHEESE:

1. Place the yogurt in a coffee filter over a bowl and set in the refrigerator for 1 to 2 hours.

2. Combine the drained yogurt with cucumber, dill, garlic, and ¼ cup of the pistachios.

3. Place each breast on a serving plate, top with the yogurt cheese, and sprinkle with the remaining ¼ cup pistachios.

Serves four.

Per serving: 314.2 calories, 12.2 g fat (1.8 g saturated), 78.9 mg cholesterol, 406.1 mg sodium, 9.1 g carbohydrates, 4.4 g sugars, 2 g fiber, 41.5 g protein

BEST TIP FOR FRESH MEAT

People say you should always know a good lawyer or bartender, but it's also wise to make friends with a local butcher. If you're a friendly, regular customer, there's no better way to ensure that you'll always get a better quality cut of meat, and he or she will always be able to tell you what's good that week. They'll also prep the meat like the pro that they are, whether you need it specially cut or wrapped for freezing.

ROASTED HALIBUT

Aluminum foil

2   fillets of halibut or other firm white fish
     (5 oz each)

8   oz jar marinated artichoke hearts

1   cup cherry tomatoes

½   medium onion, thinly sliced

1   lemon, cut into fourths

2   Tbsp olive oil

Salt and pepper to taste

Per serving: *400 calories, 23 g fat
(2.5 g saturated), 510 mg sodium,
18 g carbohydrates, 3 g sugars, 5 g fiber,
35 g protein*

1. Preheat the oven to 400°F.

2. Take two large sheets of foil, place a fillet
in the center of each, and top equally with the
artichokes, tomatoes, and onion.
Squeeze a lemon quarter onto each fillet.
Drizzle with olive oil and top with salt
and pepper, then fold the foil and seal to
create a secure pouch.

3. Place the pouches on a baking sheet in the
center of the oven and bake for 12 to 15 minutes,
depending on how thick the fish is.
Serve with the remaining lemon wedges.

Serves two.

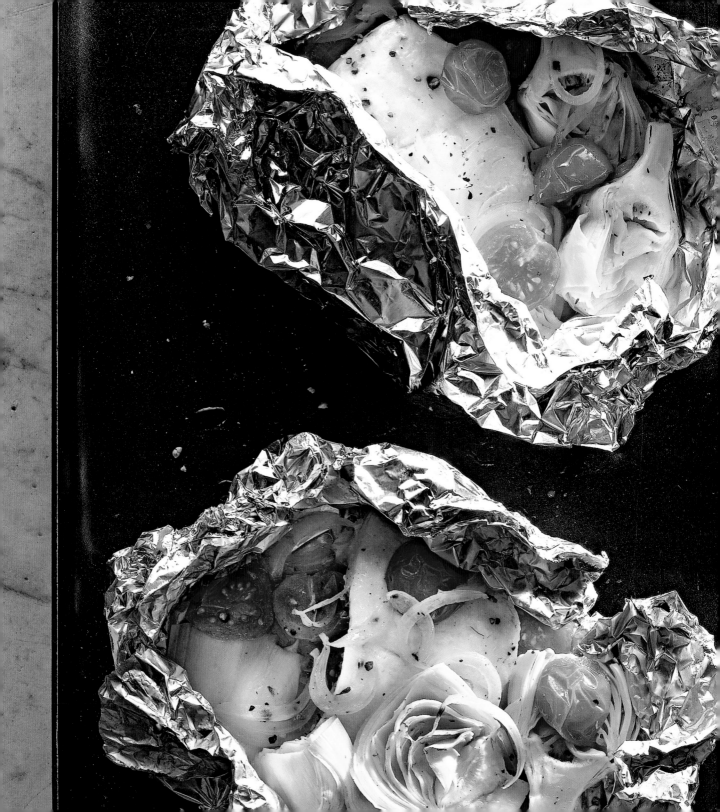

FISH STEW AND COUSCOUS

1	onion, halved lengthwise, quartered, and thinly sliced
2	cloves garlic, minced
1	tsp ground cumin
¼	tsp ground cinnamon
1	can (15 oz) chopped tomatoes
1	can (15 oz) chickpeas, rinsed and drained
1	cup fat-free reduced-sodium chicken broth
⅓	cup dates, chopped
¼	cup kalamata olives, pitted and halved
4	orange roughy or halibut fillets (4 oz each)
1	box (10 oz) couscous

1. Coat a large nonstick skillet with nonstick spray.

2. Add the onion, garlic, cumin, and cinnamon. Set over medium heat. Cook, stirring, for 7 to 8 minutes or until soft.

3. Add the tomatoes, chickpeas, broth, dates, and olives. Cook, stirring occasionally, for 5 minutes.

4. Push the mixture to the edges of the skillet. Add the fish. Spoon the chickpea mixture over the fish. Cover the pan. Reduce the heat to low. Cook for 10 minutes or until the fish flakes easily.

5. Meanwhile, cook the couscous according to package directions.

6. Fluff the couscous with a fork, then divide among four plates. Top with the fish and the chickpea mixture.

Serves four.

Per serving: 557.9 calories, 6.7 g fat (0.6 g saturated), 68 mg cholesterol, 707.7 mg sodium, 89.7 g carbohydrates, 16.5 g sugars, 10.5 g fiber, 34.8 g protein

PASTA SALAD WITH CUCUMBER, RED PEPPER, AND FETA

6	oz multigrain chiocciole, elbow macaroni, shells, or other pasta shape
½	cup fat-free sour cream
½	cup reduced-fat mayonnaise
¼	cup (1 oz) feta cheese, crumbled
3	Tbsp fresh mint leaves, chopped
3	Tbsp 2 percent milk
1	Tbsp Dijon mustard
1	tsp lemon juice, freshly squeezed
¼	tsp salt
¼	tsp freshly ground black pepper
1	cup (½ medium) cucumber, chopped
½	cup (½ medium) red bell pepper, chopped
	Salt and pepper to taste

1. Prepare pasta per package directions. Rinse.

2. Combine sour cream, mayonnaise, cheese, mint, milk, mustard, lemon juice, salt, and pepper in large bowl. Add pasta, cucumber, and red pepper, and mix. Add salt and pepper to taste, if needed.

Serves four.

Per serving: 323.3 calories, 13.4 g fat (3.4 g saturated), 22.6 mg cholesterol, 590.5 mg sodium, 40 g carbohydrates, 6.3 g sugars, 4.1 g fiber, 11.8 g protein

WHAT'S THE DIFF?

SPARKLING, SELTZER, AND TONIC WATER

Sparkling water is H_2O with CO_2 in it, meaning carbon dioxide, hence the term "carbonated," or the technical term, "fizzy." Seltzer water is water that is filtered and carbonated and sprayed liberally down the Three Stooges' shorts. Tonic water, which makes your gin and vodka go down so easily, has a touch of lemon, lime, and quinine, which is known for its anti-malarial properties. Self-medication with style.

STIR-FRY WITH TOFU AND VEGETABLES

1	lb firm tofu, drained
2	Tbsp reduced-sodium soy sauce + additional to taste
1½	tsp peanut or canola oil
2	Tbsp fresh ginger, minced
1	Tbsp garlic, minced
½	tsp crushed red-pepper flakes
6	oz mushrooms, sliced
1	large sweet red pepper, seeded and cut into thin strips
6	scallions, cut into 1½"-wide diagonal slices
1	lb bok choy, coarsely chopped
1	can (15 oz) baby corn, drained
1½	tsp toasted sesame oil
3	cups white or brown rice, cooked

1. Set the tofu between two plates and place a heavy pot on top. Set aside for 10 minutes to release excess water.

2. Cut the tofu into ½" cubes and place in an airtight container or plastic bag. Add the soy sauce and marinate, shaking occasionally, for 10 minutes.

3. Warm a wok or large nonstick skillet over medium-high heat. Add the oil and tilt the pan in all directions to coat it. Add the ginger and garlic. Stir-fry for 10 seconds. Add the red-pepper flakes, mushrooms, and red pepper strips. Stir-fry for 2 to 3 minutes or until the mushrooms release their liquid and the liquid has evaporated. Stir in the scallions, bok choy, tofu, and tofu marinade. Cover and cook for 1 to 2 minutes, or until the bok choy is crisp-tender. Stir in the baby corn, sesame oil, and additional soy sauce to taste. Serve over the rice.

Serves four.

Per serving: 513 calories, 16.1 g fat (2.4 g saturated), 0 mg cholesterol, 382.5 mg sodium, 73.2 g carbohydrates, 7.5 g sugars, 9.1 g fiber, 28.8 g protein

EASY ROASTED SALMON

4	salmon fillets (6 oz each)
1	tsp balsamic vinegar
¼	cup plain bread crumbs
2	lemons
¼	tsp ground black pepper
2	Tbsp dried or fresh parsley, chopped
4	small yellow squash, halved lengthwise
1	Tbsp Parmesan cheese, grated

1. Preheat the oven to 400°F.

2. Place the salmon on a broiling rack. Drizzle with the balsamic vinegar. Sprinkle 2 tablespoons of the bread crumbs over the fillets. Squeeze the juice of 1 lemon over the top. Sprinkle with half the pepper and 1 tablespoon of the parsley. Thinly slice the remaining lemon into four pieces and place a slice on top of each fillet. Lay the squash halves cut-sides up around the salmon.

3. In a small bowl, mix the cheese with the remaining bread crumbs, pepper, and parsley. Sprinkle the crumb mixture over the squash. Bake for 15 to 20 minutes or until the salmon is opaque and the squash is slightly tender.

Serves four.

Per serving: 364.9 calories, 19.1 g fat (4 g saturated), 101.5 mg cholesterol, 124.7 mg sodium, 8.4 g carbohydrates, 3.8 g sugars, 2.8 g fiber, 39.2 g protein

PERFECT FISH EVERY TIME

Perfectly cooked fish should be slightly springy to the touch and flake gently with pressure. Or try this: Insert a metal skewer into the center of the fish, and leave it in for 5 seconds. The fish is done when the skewer feels warm when touched to the back of your hand.

JERK PORK KEBABS

4   wooden skewers, presoaked in cold water
     for 30 minutes

12   oz pork tenderloin, cut into 1" cubes

2   cups fresh pineapple or mango chunks

1   red bell pepper, cut into 1" pieces

1   large onion, cut into 1" slices

½   cup of your favorite prepared jerk sauce
     (try Walker's Wood)

Per serving: *370 calories, 9 g fat
(1.5 g saturated), 110 mg cholesterol,
520 mg sodium, 35 g carbohydrates,
22 g sugar, 6 g fiber, 38 g protein*

1. Preheat a grill or grill pan over high heat.

2. Assemble the kebabs by skewering pieces
of pork, pineapple or mango, pepper, and onion,
alternating as you go.

3. Brush with half of the jerk sauce and place
on the hot grill. Grill for 4 minutes on each side,
basting with the rest of the jerk sauce.
The kebabs are done when the vegetables are
lightly charred and the pork is firm to the touch.

Serves two.

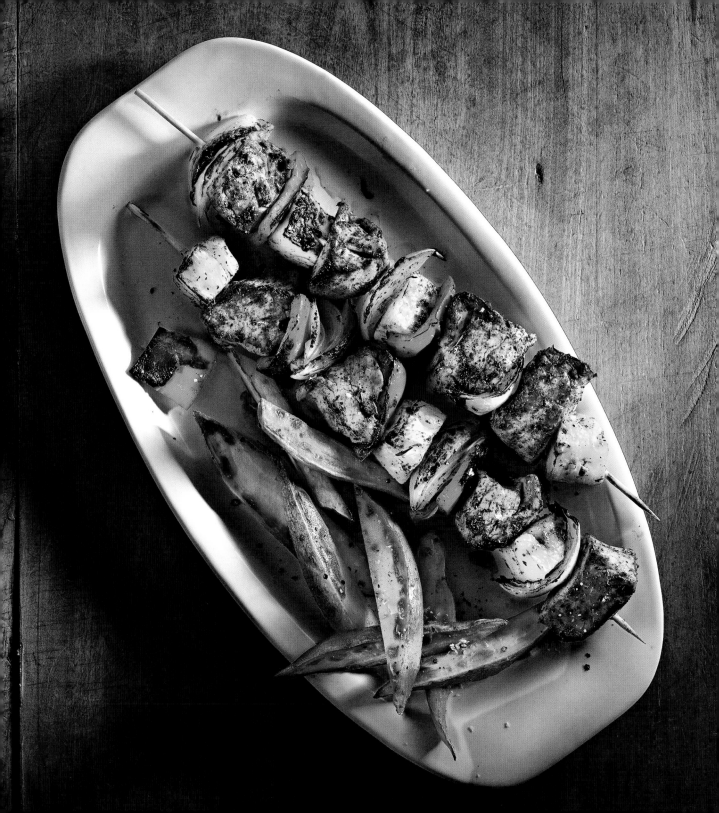

TUSCAN-STYLE CHICKEN PASTA

2　oz penne pasta (use enriched pasta for a bump in fiber and omega-3 fatty acids)

2　chicken breasts (4–5 oz each), pounded to an even ¼" thickness

　　Salt and pepper to taste

4　cups baby spinach leaves

1　cup cannellini beans, rinsed

1　tsp olive oil

1　clove garlic, crushed

½　tsp dried rosemary, finely chopped

2　Tbsp roasted red bell pepper, diced

2　Tbsp grated Parmesan cheese

1. Boil 1½ quarts water, drop in the penne, stir, and cook until the pasta is al dente (about 9 to 11 minutes).

2. While the pasta cooks, sear the chicken in a skillet coated with cooking spray on medium-high heat (about 4 to 5 minutes per side), seasoning each side with a pinch of salt and pepper as the other side cooks.
Remove the chicken from the skillet and set it aside.

3. Reduce skillet heat to medium.
Add the spinach, beans, oil, garlic, rosemary, and bell pepper. Turn frequently until the spinach wilts, about 1 to 2 minutes.

4. Slice the chicken and toss it with drained pasta and the spinach and bean mixture.
Top each serving with 1 tablespoon of the cheese.

Serves two.

Per serving: 405.2 calories, 6.3 g fat (1.7 g saturated), 72.8 mg cholesterol, 633 mg sodium, 46.4 g carbohydrates, 1.7 g sugars, 8.9 g fiber, 39.5 g protein

ITALIAN PASTA SALAD

8　oz whole-grain spiral pasta

½　cup broccoli, chopped

½　cup carrot, chopped

½　cup tomato, chopped

½　cup red bell pepper, chopped

½　cup onion, chopped

½　cup low-fat sharp Cheddar cheese, shredded

1　cup reduced-fat Italian dressing

1. Prepare the pasta according to the package directions, omitting any salt.
Drain, rinse under cold water, and drain.

2. Stir together the broccoli, carrot, tomato, pepper, onion, and cheese in a large bowl.
Stir in the pasta and dressing, tossing to coat well.

Serves eight.

Per serving: 184.7 calories, 5.8 g fat (0.7 g saturated), 1.8 mg cholesterol, 284.5 mg sodium, 28.8 g carbohydrates, 4 g sugars, 3.8 g fiber, 6.1 g protein

WHAT'S THE DIFF?

PENNE, RIGATONI, AND ZITI

They're all tube-shaped pasta, but size matters. Penne is the smallest and best for lighter sauces. Rigatoni is the biggest and can handle something heavy. Ziti is the middle one—and regularly over-eaten when baked at grandma's house.

SPAGHETTI WITH MEAT SAUCE

2   tsp olive oil

1   onion, chopped

1   rib celery, minced

1   carrot, chopped

2   cloves garlic, minced

¾   lb extra-lean ground round beef

1   cup dry red wine or nonalcoholic red wine

1½   Tbsp unbleached or all-purpose flour

1½   cups fat-free milk

1   can (28 oz) crushed tomatoes

1   can (8 oz) tomato sauce

2   Tbsp parsley, chopped

1   tsp dried basil or oregano

12   oz spaghetti

1. Warm the oil in a large nonstick skillet set over medium-high heat. Add the onion, celery, carrot, and garlic. Cook, stirring often, for 7 to 10 minutes or until tender. Add the beef. Cook for 3 minutes or until no longer pink. Add the wine. Cook for 2 minutes or until the wine is almost evaporated.

2. Place the flour in a small bowl. Gradually add the milk, whisking constantly, until blended. Add to the skillet. Cook, stirring constantly, for 2 minutes or until the sauce is thickened and reduced by one-third. Add the crushed tomatoes, tomato sauce, parsley, and basil or oregano. Simmer for 15 minutes.

3. Meanwhile, cook the pasta according to package directions. Place in a serving bowl. Top with the sauce.

Serves six.

Per serving: *392.7 calories, 5.1 g fat (1 g saturated), 31.2 mg cholesterol, 148.7 mg sodium, 56.6 g carbo-hydrates, 12 g sugars, 12.2 g fiber, 24.8 g protein*

FARMER'S MARKET PASTA SALAD

1   package (9 oz) refrigerated tricolor cheese tortellini

2   cups sugar snap peas, trimmed

2   Tbsp homemade or store-bought pesto

1   cup cherry tomatoes, halved

¼   tsp ground black pepper

    Fresh basil (optional)

1. Place the tortellini into a large pot of boiling water. Cook for 5 minutes, stirring occasionally.

2. Add the sugar snap peas and cook for 3 minutes or until tender but still crisp.

3. Drain the pasta and peas and rinse with cold water. Place into a large bowl and toss with the pesto. Gently fold in the tomatoes and pepper. Garnish with basil, if using.

Serves four.

Per serving: *279.6 calories, 8.2 g fat (3.3 g saturated), 29.3 mg cholesterol, 352.8 mg sodium, 39.6 g carbo-hydrates, 5.4 g sugars, 4.2 g fiber, 12.6 g protein*

SERVING SIZE, MADE SIMPLE:

COOKED SPAGHETTI
½ cup, 99 calories

Same size as:
Your fist

HERB-CRUSTED PORK TENDERLOIN

1	lb pork tenderloin
2	tsp canola or olive oil
1	tsp sage
1	tsp thyme
½	tsp garlic, minced
	Salt to taste
¼	tsp ground black pepper

1. Preheat oven to 375°F.

2. Cover a small baking sheet with aluminum foil. Place pork on pan.

3. Drizzle oil over pork; sprinkle with sage, thyme, garlic, salt, and pepper. Rub to coat evenly with seasonings.

4. Roast until instant-read thermometer inserted in center registers 155°F and the juices run clear, about 30 to 35 minutes. Let stand for 10 minutes before slicing.

ALTERNATE VERSION

For spice-rubbed pork tenderloin, substitute 1 tsp curry powder for sage and a pinch of cayenne pepper for thyme. Omit black pepper.

Serves four.

Per serving: 160.1 calories, 6.2 g fat (1.7 g saturated), 73.7 mg cholesterol, 56.9 mg sodium, 0.6 g carbohydrates, 0 g sugars, 0.3 g fiber, 23.9 g protein

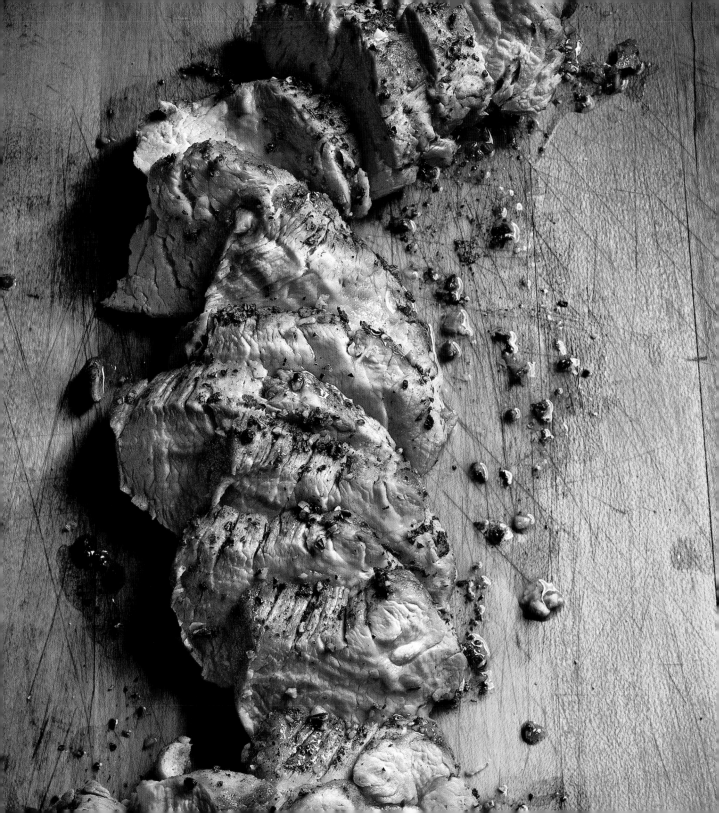

LINGUINE WITH CLAMS

12	oz spinach linguine
1	Tbsp olive oil
2	shallots, chopped
1	clove garlic, minced
1	cup plum tomatoes, chopped
1	cup dry white wine or nonalcoholic wine
1½	cups chicken broth
¼	cup Italian parsley, chopped
3	dozen littleneck clams, scrubbed

1. Prepare the linguine according to package directions.

2. Meanwhile, heat the oil in a large saucepot or Dutch oven over medium-high heat. Add the shallots and garlic and cook, stirring often, for 4 minutes or until soft.

3. Add the tomatoes and cook for 1 minute.

4. Add the wine and bring to a boil. Cook for 2 minutes.

5. Add the broth and parsley. Bring to a boil.

6. Add the clams, cover, and cook for 5 minutes or until the clams open. (Discard any unopened clams.) Using a slotted spoon, remove the clams and set aside.

7. Return the broth mixture to the heat and bring to a boil. Boil for 4 minutes or until reduced by one-third.

8. Remove 24 of the clams from their shells and mince; discard those shells. Keep the remaining 12 clams in their shells.

9. Add the minced clams and pasta to the pot. Toss to combine. Add the clams in the shells.

Serves four.

Per serving: 471.8 calories, 6.7 g fat (1 g saturated), 27.5 mg cholesterol, 431.6 mg sodium, 70.9 g carbo-hydrates, 6.1 g sugars, 4.5 g fiber, 24.2 g protein

SHRIMP FRA DIAVOLO

2	tsp red-pepper flakes
½	Tbsp extra-virgin olive oil
1	medium yellow onion, chopped
2	cloves garlic, minced
¼	tsp dried oregano or thyme
14	oz crushed tomatoes
4	oz dried spaghetti
12	oz shrimp, peeled and deveined
	Salt and pepper to taste
2	Tbsp chopped flat-leaf parsley

1. Boil a large pot of salted water for the pasta.

2. Heat a large sauté pan over medium heat. Add the red-pepper flakes, olive oil, onion, garlic, and oregano or thyme, and cook until the onions are soft. Add the tomatoes.

3. Drop the pasta into the boiling water and cook according to the package directions.

4. Add the shrimp to the sauce and season with salt and pepper. Cook for 3 to 4 minutes.

5. Drain the pasta, toss with as much of the sauce as you like, and garnish with parsley.

Serves two.

Per serving: 518.3 calories, 8.2 g fat (1.4 g saturated), 258.5 mg cholesterol, 813.3 mg sodium, 65.9 g carbo-hydrates, 4.1 g sugars, 7.3 g fiber, 46.4 g protein

SMART ALTERNATIVES TO SALT

All you need are a few diversionary tactics to keep your tastebuds distracted. Herbs like rosemary and thyme and assertive spices like cayenne and cumin are healthy ways of imparting big flavors to your dishes. Skip subtle forms of cooking like steaming and poaching in favor of high-heat techniques like grilling, roasting, and pan searing, which bring out the natural sugars and salts in foods. Before serving, add a few grinds of black pepper and a squeeze of lemon juice. With this flavor smokescreen, your palate won't know what it's missing.

GRILLED SPICY FISH TACOS

1	mango, peeled, pitted, and cubed
1	avocado, peeled, pitted, and cubed
½	medium red onion, diced
1	handful cilantro, chopped
2	limes
	Salt and pepper to taste
	Canola oil
12	oz mahimahi
½	Tbsp blackening spice
4	corn tortillas
1	cup red cabbage, finely shredded
1	cup black beans, plain or spiked with dash of cumin

1. Clean and oil a grill or grill pan thoroughly. Preheat to medium-high.

2. Make the mango salsa by combining the mango, avocado, red onion, cilantro, and the juice of one lime. Season to taste with salt and pepper.

3. Drizzle a light coating of oil over the fish, and rub on the blackening spice.
Place the fish on the grill and cook, undisturbed, for 4 minutes. Carefully flip with a spatula and cook for another 4 minutes. Remove.

4. Before turning off the grill, warm the tortillas directly on the surface for 1 to 2 minutes.

5. Divide the fish evenly among the warm tortillas, add a bit of cabbage, and spoon the salsa on top. Serve each taco with a wedge of lime and half of the black beans.

Serves two.

Per serving: *650 calories, 18 g fat (2 g saturated), 125 mg cholesterol, 240 mg sodium, 82 g carbohydrates, 19 g sugars, 18 g fiber, 44 g protein*

CHILI-GLAZED PORK CHOPS

½	Tbsp chipotle sauce
½	Tbsp Dijon mustard
½	Tbsp honey
½	Tbsp olive oil
2	pork chops (6 oz each)
	Salt and pepper to taste
1	apple, peeled, cored, and sliced into thick wedges
½	cup apple juice
1	Tbsp butter

1. Mix the chipotle sauce, mustard, and honey. Divide in half, and set aside.

2. Heat oil in a skillet over medium heat. Sprinkle the chops with salt and pepper and cook on the skillet, undisturbed, until a crust forms.

3. Before flipping the chops, brush the uncooked side with half of the chipotle glaze.
Once flipped, use a clean brush to add the other half of the reserved glaze to the cooked side.

4. Add the apple pieces to the pan; cook 3 or 4 more minutes.

5. Lower the heat and add the juice. Simmer for 4 to 5 minutes until the chops are cooked all the way through.

6. Remove them, season the apple mix with more salt and pepper, and add the butter. Pour the apple mix over the pork chops.

Serves two.

Per serving: *380 calories, 16 g fat (6 g saturated), 135 cholesterol, 340 mg sodium, 21 g carbohydrates, 18 sugars, 1 g fiber, 38 g protein*

HOW TO GRILL A FISH

First, clean the grill beforehand: As soon as the grate is hot, scrub off the gunk with a wire brush. Next, apply some cooking oil directly to the grate with a brush or paper towel. Cook skinless fillets, as skin tends to stick. Once it's on the grill, don't touch it: Those nice caramelized grill marks will make it easier to pull off. In general, cook the fish on one side for 70 percent of its total cooking time before you flip it. Then slip a thin metal spatula under the fillet, scraping if you must to free the flesh from the grate.

ULTIMATE POWER PASTA

4	qt water
1	cup frozen shelled edamame
2	tsp extra-virgin olive oil
1	Tbsp dried oregano
1	Tbsp dried basil
1	tsp red-pepper flakes
2	cups whole-wheat ziti, bow ties, wheels, or penne pasta
2	cups broccoli florets
2	yellow squash, sliced
2	zucchini, sliced
½	cup (3.5 oz) reduced-fat feta cheese, crumbled
4	Tbsp grated Parmesan cheese (optional)

Per serving: 377.9 calories, 9.8 g fat (3 g saturated), 13.2 mg cholesterol, 475 mg sodium, 54.2 g carbohydrates, 6.3 g sugars, 10.5 g fiber, 21.3 g protein

1. In a large pot, combine the water, edamame, oil, oregano, basil, and red-pepper flakes. Bring to a boil over high heat. Add the pasta. Cook for 4 minutes.

2. Add the broccoli, squash, and zucchini. Cook for 5 to 7 minutes, or until the pasta is al dente.

3. Drain the pasta and vegetables until dripping but not dry. Add the feta and toss until completely mixed. Sprinkle on the Parmesan (if using).

ALTERNATE VERSION

You can mix and match just about any vegetables in this dish. Make it colorful with one of the following blends: yellow squash, asparagus, and red bell pepper; zucchini, mushrooms, yellow squash, and no-salt sun-dried tomatoes; yellow squash, peas, mushrooms, and tomatoes.

Serves four.

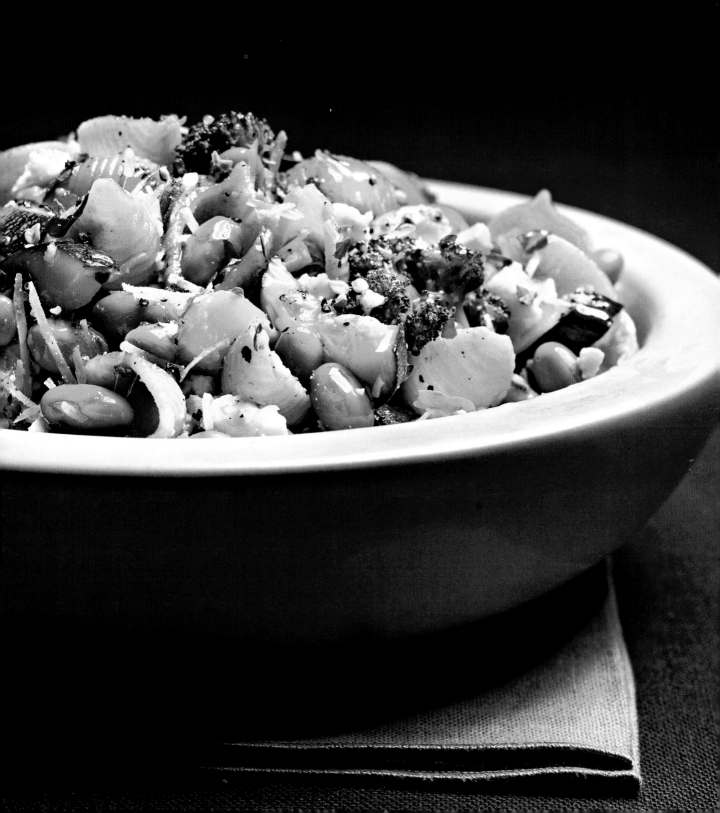

QUINOA-STUFFED BELL PEPPERS

⅓ cup almonds, slivered

1½ cups water

¼ tsp salt

¾ cup quinoa

4 large red, orange, or yellow bell peppers

1 tsp olive oil

1 medium onion, chopped

2 large cloves garlic, minced

1 package (10 oz) fresh spinach, tough stems removed, torn into large pieces

½ cup feta cheese, crumbled

¼ cup dried currants or raisins

1 can (14½ oz) diced tomatoes

2 Tbsp tomato paste

¼ tsp dried Italian seasoning

Per serving: *326.3 calories, 10.6 g fat (2.3 g saturated), 7.5 mg cholesterol, 701.4 mg sodium, 49.6 g carbohydrates, 16.3 g sugars, 8.9 g fiber, 13.8 g protein*

1. Preheat the oven to 375°F.

2. Cook the slivered almonds in a small nonstick skillet over medium heat, stirring often, for 3 to 4 minutes or until lightly toasted. Pour onto a plate and let cool.

3. In a saucepan, bring the water and salt to a boil. Place the quinoa in a fine-mesh strainer and rinse under cold running water for 2 minutes. Stir into the boiling water. Reduce the heat, cover, and simmer for 20 minutes or until the water is absorbed and the quinoa is tender. Uncover and set aside.

4. Bring a large pot of water to a boil. Cut off and reserve the tops of the peppers. Remove the seeds and ribs. Add the peppers and tops to the boiling water and cook for 5 minutes. Drain.

5. In the same pot, heat the oil over medium heat. Add the onion and cook, stirring occasionally, for 6 minutes or until golden brown. Stir in the garlic. Remove 2 tablespoons of the onion mixture and set aside. Add the spinach to the pot and cook, stirring frequently, for 5 minutes or until wilted and any water evaporates. Remove the pot from the heat. Add the feta, currants or raisins, almonds, and quinoa to the spinach mixture. Stir to combine.

6. Arrange the peppers in a shallow baking dish. Spoon in the stuffing, mounding to fill, and replace the tops. Add ½" of water to the baking dish. Cover loosely with foil and bake for 40 to 45 minutes or until the peppers are tender.

7. Meanwhile, in a saucepan, combine the tomatoes (with juice), tomato paste, Italian seasoning, and the reserved 2 tablespoons of the onion mixture. Bring to a boil. Reduce the heat, cover, and simmer for 30 minutes or until thickened. Spoon the sauce onto plates and top with the peppers.

Serves four.

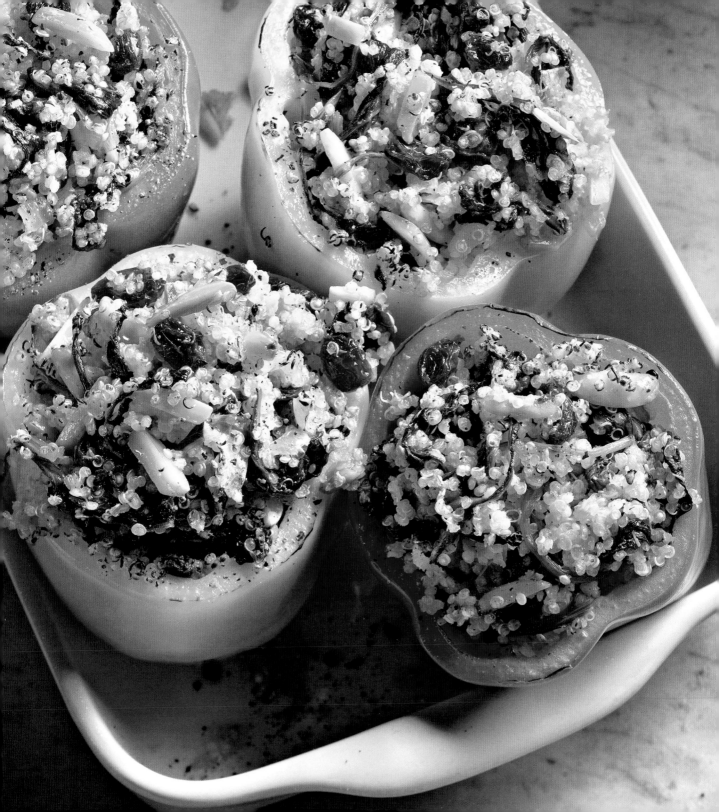

SOPPRESSATA PICANTE

1	lb. pizza dough, store-bought or homemade (page 332)
⅓	cup crushed San Marzano tomatoes
2	oz fresh Fior di latte mozzarella, cut into medium-sized cubes
1	clove garlic, thinly sliced
1	fresh jalapeño (preferably red), sliced
1	Tbsp fresh oregano
10	small slices soppressata picante sausage
1	Tbsp Pecorino Romano cheese, grated
1	Tbsp extra-virgin olive oil
½	tsp sea salt

Per serving: *220 calories, 10 g fat (3.5 g saturated), 15 mg cholesterol, 595 mg sodium, 23 g carbohydrates, 0 g sugars, 2 g fiber, 8 g protein*

Spread the tomatoes, mozzarella, garlic, jalapeño, oregano, and soppressata on the dough. Top with Pecorino Romano, oil, and salt. Bake at 400°F until the cheese is bubbly and the crust is crisp, about 10 minutes.

Serves four.

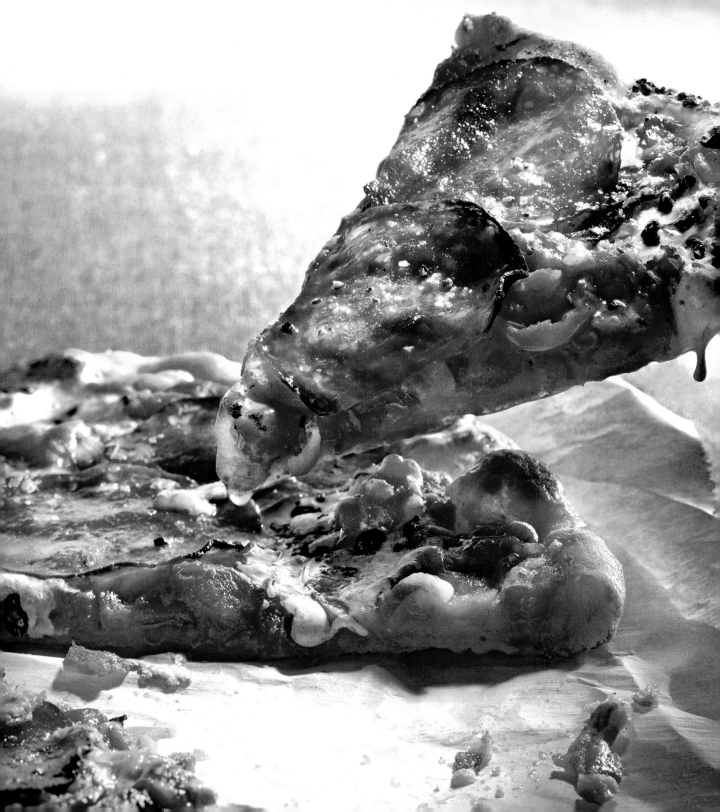

PIZZA DOUGH

1½ cups lukewarm water

1 packet active dry yeast

3½ cups unbleached or all-purpose flour

1 tsp fine-ground, non-iodized salt
(preferably sea salt)

1 Tbsp extra-virgin olive oil

1. Lightly coat a large bowl with nonstick spray.

2. Combine the water and yeast.
Let stand for 5 minutes or until foamy.

3. In the bowl of an electric mixer fitted
with a dough hook, combine 3¼ cups of the flour
and the salt. With the machine running, add the
yeast mixture and oil. Process just until the dough
comes together in a slightly sticky mass.

4. Turn the dough onto a lightly floured
work surface. Knead for 4 to 7 minutes,
adding the remaining ¼ cup flour if necessary,
to prevent sticking, until smooth and elastic.
Shape into a ball. Place in the prepared bowl.
Cover tightly with plastic wrap.
Let rise in a warm place for 1 hour or until doubled.

5. Punch the dough down, and shape it into
four balls. Store in the refrigerator—extras will
keep for 2 to 3 days.

6. With floured hands or a rolling pin, pat or roll
balls into 12-inch circles.

Makes four 12-inch thin pizza crusts.

*Per serving: 430 calories, 4.5 g fat (0.5 g saturated),
0 mg cholesterol, 700 mg sodium, 84 g carbohydrates,
0 g total sugar, 3 g fiber, 12 g protein*

PIZZA DOUGH TIP:

Nervous about making
your own dough?
Call around to your
local pizza shops to
see who sells pre-made
dough balls.

PIZZA MARGHERITA

Pizza dough (page 332)

1 tomato, thinly sliced

3 oz fresh mozzarella, thinly sliced

¼ cup fresh basil, slivered

1 Tbsp extra-virgin olive oil

1. Pat dry the tomatoes and mozzarella.

2. Arrange the tomatoes on the dough. Sprinkle with the basil. Cover with the mozzarella, then drizzle with the oil. Bake at 400°F until the cheese is bubbly and the crust is crisp, about 10 minutes.

Serves four.

Per serving: 190 calories, 8 g fat (3 g saturated), 10 mg cholesterol, 145 mg sodium, 22 g carbohydrates, 1 g sugars, 1g fiber, 8 g protein

PINEAPPLE-HAM PIZZA

1 flat Thomas multigrain pita

1 Tbsp extra-virgin olive oil

¼ cup marinara pasta sauce

¼ cup pineapple tidbits, drained

¼ cup fresh red bell peppers, chopped

2 oz uncured black forest ham, chopped

2 Tbsp Gorgonzola cheese, crumbled

Brush one side of the pita with olive oil, then top with marinara sauce, pineapple, peppers, and ham. Sprinkle with cheese.
Bake at 400°F until the cheese is bubbly and the crust is crisp, about 10 minutes.

Serves one.

Per serving: 456 calories, 22 g fat (6 g saturated), 38 mg cholesterol, 1,390 mg sodium, 46 g carbohydrates, 5 g sugars, 7 g fiber, 21 g protein

GRILLED FAVA BEAN AND PANCETTA PIZZA

Pizza dough (page 332)

¼ lb fava beans or peas, podded

3 oz fresh Fior di latte or fresh mozzarella, cut into medium-sized cubes

2 oz pancetta or bacon

½ large garlic clove, cut into slivers

1 Tbsp extra-virgin olive oil

1 Tbsp Grana Padano or Parmesan cheese, grated

1. Blanch the fava beans by boiling them in salted water for about 1 minute. Let them cool and then pinch the beans to remove their skins. Transfer them to ice water to cool.

2. If you're using peas, blanch them for 1 minute.

3. Lay the mozzarella on the dough first, followed by the fava beans and pancetta or bacon. Top with garlic, olive oil, and cheese.
Bake at 400°F until the cheese is bubbly and the crust is crisp, about 10 minutes.

Serves four.

Per serving: 260 calories, 13 g fat (4 g saturated), 10 mg cholesterol, 435 mg sodium, 24 g carbohydrates, 2 g fiber, 12 g protein

SERVING SIZE, MADE SIMPLE:

SAUSAGE
1 ounce, 54 calories

Same size as:
A shotgun shell

THE WORKS

Pizza dough (page 332)

¼ cup sun-dried tomato pesto

1 small zucchini, sliced

1 cup orange and yellow bell peppers, thinly sliced

1 cup fresh mushrooms, sliced

½ cup red onion, thinly sliced

2 tsp olive oil

2 oz fresh mozzarella cheese, thinly sliced

2 Tbsp grated Parmesan cheese

¾ cup sun-dried tomatoes

½ cup fresh basil leaves, thinly sliced

Per serving: *330 calories, 7 g fat (2 g saturated), 10 mg cholesterol, 555 mg sodium, 34 g carbohydrates, 8 g sugars, 4 g fiber, 10 g protein*

1. Spread the pesto on the dough.

2. Toss the zucchini, peppers, mushrooms, and onion with oil. Place the vegetables in a medium skillet over medium-high heat and sauté in the oil until the vegetables are soft and any excess liquid has evaporated, about 6 to 8 minutes.

3. Top the dough evenly with the cheeses. Arrange the sautéed vegetables over the cheese and top with the sun-dried tomatoes. Bake at 400°F until the cheese is bubbly and the crust is crisp, about 10 minutes.

4. Sprinkle with the basil leaves. Let stand a few minutes before cutting into quarters.

Serves four.

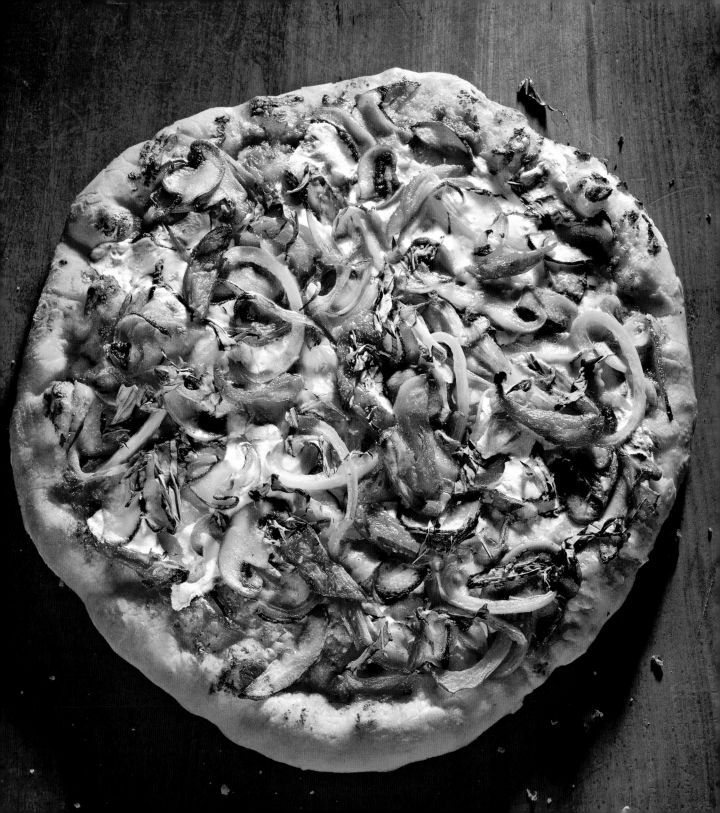

SPICY CHICKEN BBQ PIZZA

Pizza dough (page 332)

1   Tbsp olive or vegetable oil
1   red bell pepper, cut into strips
1   red onion, thinly sliced
2   cups chicken, cooked and shredded
½   cup barbecue sauce
½   cup (2 oz) Monterey Jack cheese, shredded
½   cup (2 oz) sharp Cheddar cheese, shredded
    Grated Parmesan cheese (to taste)

1. Heat the oil in a large skillet over medium-high heat. Add the pepper and onion and cook, stirring occasionally, for 5 minutes or until tender-crisp.

2. In a medium bowl, combine the chicken and ¼ cup of the barbecue sauce.

3. Spread the remaining ¼ cup barbecue sauce over the dough. Top with the chicken and vegetables. Sprinkle with the cheeses. Bake at 400°F until the cheese is bubbly and the crust is crisp, about 10 minutes. Top with grated Parmesan cheese.

Serves four.

Per serving: *440 calories, 16 g fat (7 g saturated), 85 mg cholesterol, 735 mg sodium, 39 g carbohydrates, 12 g sugars, 2 g fiber, 32 g protein*

MEXICAN PIZZA

2   multigrain wraps
1½   cups (1 large) tomato, chopped
¼   cup (1 small) onion, chopped
2   Tbsp fresh cilantro, chopped
1   Tbsp lime juice
½   jalapeño chili pepper, finely chopped
1   cup canned black beans, rinsed and drained
⅔   cup reduced-fat Cheddar cheese, shredded

1. In a small bowl, combine the tomato, onion, cilantro, lime juice, and pepper.

2. Sprinkle the wraps each with ½ cup of the beans and ⅓ cup of the cheese. Top with tomato mixture. Bake at 400°F until the cheese is bubbly and the crust is crisp, about 10 minutes.

Serves four.

Per serving: *154 calories, 5 g fat (2 g saturated), 13 mg cholesterol, 472 mg sodium, 24 g carbohydrates, 2 g sugars, 5 g fiber, 10 g protein*

RED PEPPER PESTO PIZZA

1   ready-made flatbread
3   Tbsp reduced-fat ricotta cheese
1   tsp roasted garlic
1   Tbsp pesto
2   Tbsp roasted red peppers
3   Tbsp reduced-fat mozzarella cheese, grated
1   tsp ground black pepper

1. Mix the ricotta and roasted garlic, blending well.

2. Spread the mixture on the flatbread. Top with dollops of pesto, peppers, and mozzarella. Season with pepper. Bake at 400°F until the cheese is bubbly and the crust is crisp, about 10 minutes.

Serves one.

Per serving: *306 calories, 16 g fat (6 g saturated), 27.5 mg cholesterol, 768 mg sodium, 25 g carbohydrates, 3.7 g sugars, 2 g fiber, 15 g protein*

PIZZA PREP TIP:

Slice toppings thin to help them cook faster—this is especially important for vegetables.

GREEK PIZZA

Pizza dough (page 332)
½   cup dry sun-dried tomatoes, packed
1   Tbsp lemon juice, freshly squeezed
2   cup garlicky sautéed greens (see page 341)
5   kalamata olives, pitted and chopped
3   oz mild feta cheese, crumbled
2   tsp fresh oregano leaves

1. Soak the tomatoes in hot water for 10 minutes or until soft. Drain and chop.

2. Squeeze the lemon juice onto the greens and then scatter the greens onto the dough. Top with tomatoes and olives, crumble feta on top, and sprinkle with oregano. Bake at 400°F until the cheese is bubbly and the crust is crisp, about 10 minutes.

Serves four.

Per serving: 330 calories, 10 g fat (3.5 g saturated), 20 mg cholesterol, 775 mg sodium, 29 g carbohydrates, 4 g sugars, 3 g fiber, 8 g protein

WILD MUSHROOM PIZZA

Pizza dough (page 332)
1   Tbsp canola or olive oil
1   cup red onions, thinly sliced
4   oz shiitake mushrooms, thinly sliced
4   oz portobello mushrooms, thinly sliced
3   oz goat cheese, crumbled
1   Tbsp fresh rosemary, chopped
1   oz Parmesan cheese

1. Coat a large nonstick skillet with canola or olive oil and place over medium heat.

2. Add the onions, shiitake mushrooms, and portobello mushrooms. Cook, stirring often, for 8 to 10 minutes or until browned.

3. Spread the mixture on top of the dough. Sprinkle with the goat cheese and rosemary. Bake at 400°F until the cheese is bubbly and the crust is crisp, about 10 minutes. Top with grated Parmesan.

Serves four.

Per serving: 270 calories, 11 g fat (4.5 g saturated), 15 mg cholesterol, 315 mg sodium, 31 g carbohydrates, 3 g sugars, 3 g fiber, 11 g protein

HOW TO BEST USE HERBS

There is no comparison between fresh and dried herbs. Fresh herbs work best on fully cooked dishes, providing a nice hit of flavor and visual appeal to a finished product. Dried herbs perform better in slow-cooked dishes like pasta sauces, chili, and stewed beans. Herbes de Provence, a dried mix of rosemary, thyme, and bay, is a must for your pantry.

CAJUN CHICKEN FINGERS WITH COOL-HAND CUKE DIP

DIP

½   cup fat-free sour cream

½   cup hot-house cucumbers, coarsely shredded

1   Tbsp scallions, minced

1   tsp lemon juice

⅛   tsp salt

⅛   tsp ground black pepper

CHICKEN

1   lb chicken breast tenders

2   tsp olive oil

2   tsp Cajun seasoning rub

  Hot-pepper sauce to taste (optional)

*Per serving: 160.6 calories, 3.2 g fat
(0.6 g saturated), 69.6 mg cholesterol,
548.7 mg sodium, 6.2 g carbohydrates,
3.1 g sugars, 0.4 g fiber, 27.7 g protein*

TO PREPARE THE DIP:

1. In a bowl, combine the sour cream, cucumbers, scallions, lemon juice, salt, and pepper. Stir to mix.
Cover and refrigerate for at least 1 hour.

TO PREPARE THE CHICKEN:

1. Place the chicken, oil, and seasoning rub in a resealable plastic storage bag.
Seal the bag and massage to coat the chicken evenly. Refrigerate for 1 hour.

2. Preheat a grill or stove-top griddle pan.

3. Cook the chicken on the grill or pan for 2 to 3 minutes on each side or until no longer pink and the juices run clear.

4. Serve with the dip and hot-pepper sauce, if using.

Serves four.

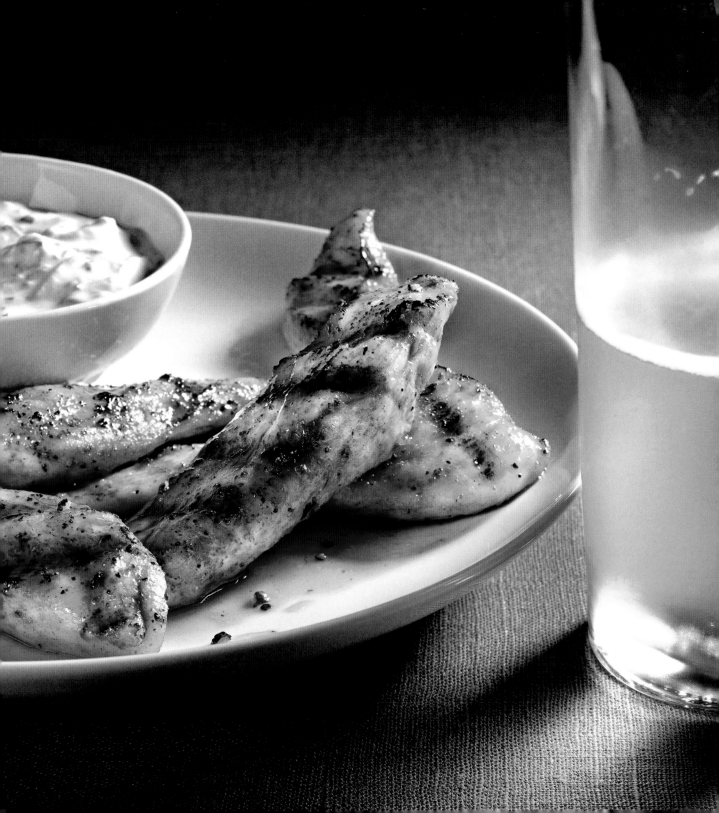

GRILLED SWEET POTATO ROUNDS

2   medium sweet potatoes, sliced
     into ¼"-thick rounds
1½   tsp extra-virgin olive oil
     Ground black pepper to taste

1. Coat a grill rack with cooking spray.
Preheat the grill to medium.

2. Boil a large pot of water over high heat.
Add the sweet potatoes. Cook for 6 to 8 minutes
or until tender but not soft.
Drain and rinse with cold water to stop
further cooking.

3. Lightly brush the potatoes with the olive oil.
Sprinkle generously with the pepper.
Grill for 3 to 5 minutes per side or until
slightly charred.

Serves four.

Per serving: *85 calories, 1.7 g fat (0.2 g saturated),
0 mg cholesterol, 22.5 mg sodium, 16 g carbohydrates,
3.5 g sugars, 2 g fiber, 1 g protein*

SAUTÉED BRUSSELS SPROUTS

1½   lb brussels sprouts
2   Tbsp canola or olive oil
3–4 cloves garlic, diced
     Salt and freshly ground pepper to taste

1. Clean the brussels sprouts by removing
the outer layer of leaves (including any visible
blemishes) and trimming the stems.
Cut each sprout into ¼"-thick slices.

2. Heat the oil over medium-high heat in
a large nonstick pan. Add the garlic and cook
until softened. Add the sprouts.
Cook for 2 to 3 minutes until the oil is absorbed.

3. During this time the sprouts will begin to
brown. Turn the heat down slightly and cook for
about another 5 minutes, stirring occasionally,
until the sprouts become browned and slightly
crispy. Season with salt and pepper.

ALTERNATE VERSION

Add diced chorizo and onion while sautéing
the garlic.

Serves four.

Per serving: *140 calories, 8 g fat (0.5 g saturated),
0 mg cholesterol, 45 mg sodium, 16 g carbohydrates,
4 g sugars, 7 g fiber, 6 g protein*

COOK-WARE: NONSTICK VS. STAINLESS

Stainless steel
holds heat well and
distributes it evenly,
a necessity for browning
food at high tempera-
tures and building
sauces in the pan. Use
nonstick pans for more
delicate tasks; try an
8-inch pan for cooking
eggs and a 12-inch
one for sautéing fish.

ROASTED ROOT VEGETABLES

8   oz (1) onion, cut into walnut-size chunks

8   oz (1) sweet potato, cut into walnut-size chunks

6   oz (1) turnip, cut into walnut-size chunks

6   oz (1) russet potato, cut into walnut-size chunks

2   Tbsp olive oil, preferably extra-virgin

2   tsp herbes de Provence

¼   tsp salt

1. Preheat the oven to 375°F.

2. In a 13" x 9" baking dish, combine the onion, sweet potato, turnip, russet potato, olive oil, herbes de Provence, and salt. Toss to coat the vegetables with the seasoning. Roast, stirring occasionally, for about 45 minutes or until golden and tender.

ALTERNATE VERSIONS

Go for more of a kitchen-sink strategy by adding more root vegetables, such as golden beets and celeriac.

Toss the vegetables with maple syrup or honey in addition to the olive oil and herbes de Provence.

For a quick and satisfying roasted vegetable soup, reheat 1 serving of the vegetables with 1 cup of chicken or vegetable broth.

Serves eight.

Per serving: *88.3 calories, 3.5 g fat, 0.5 g saturated), 0 mg cholesterol, 184.8 mg sodium, 13.6 g carbohydrates, 3.3 g sugars, 2 g fiber, 1.4 g protein*

GARLICKY SAUTÉED GREENS

3   cloves garlic, sliced

1   Tbsp extra virgin olive oil

8   cups (packed) stemmed and roughly chopped Swiss chard (can also substitute spinach)

¼   tsp red pepper flakes

¼   tsp kosher salt

1. Heat garlic and oil in large skillet over medium low heat until garlic begins to turn golden, about 3 minutes. Transfer mixture to small bowl and set aside.

2. Add greens, red pepper flakes, and salt to skillet. Using tongs, turn greens until wilted enough to fit in pan. Raise heat to medium, cover, and cook 7 to 10 minutes, tossing. Transfer greens to a colander to drain. Return greens to pan and toss with reserved garlic and oil mixture.

NOTE:

Refrigerate leftover greens in an airtight container for up to 3 days.

Per serving: *188 calories, 14 g fat (2 g saturated), 715 mg sodium, 11 g carbohydrates, 8 g fiber, 9 g protein*

RESCUE OVER-COOKED VEGGIES

It's almost as easy to revive a lifeless vegetable as it is to overcook it. Offset the loss of texture by making a warm salad with a snappy vinaigrette: Mix a bit of Dijon mustard and chopped shallot with one part sherry vinegar and three parts extra-virgin olive oil or argan oil— a Moroccan oil that works wonderfully with vegetables. Arrange the overcooked vegetables on a plate and drizzle with the vinaigrette.

GRILLED MEXICAN CORN

½   cup sour cream

½   tsp ground cumin

½   tsp salt

¼   tsp garlic powder

⅛   tsp freshly ground black pepper

4   ears corn, husked

¼   cup cilantro, chopped

1   tsp chili powder

Per serving: *126.6 calories, 4.9 g fat (2.5 g saturated), 15.5 mg cholesterol, 323.5 mg sodium, 19.4 g carbohydrates, 4.9 g sugars, 2.6 g fiber, 4.4 g protein*

1. Coat a grill rack with cooking spray. Preheat the grill to high.

2. In a large, shallow dish, stir together the sour cream, cumin, salt, garlic powder, and pepper.

3. Grill the corn until browned in spots, 8 to 10 minutes, turning occasionally. Coat with sour cream mixture. Sprinkle with cilantro and chili powder.

Serves four.

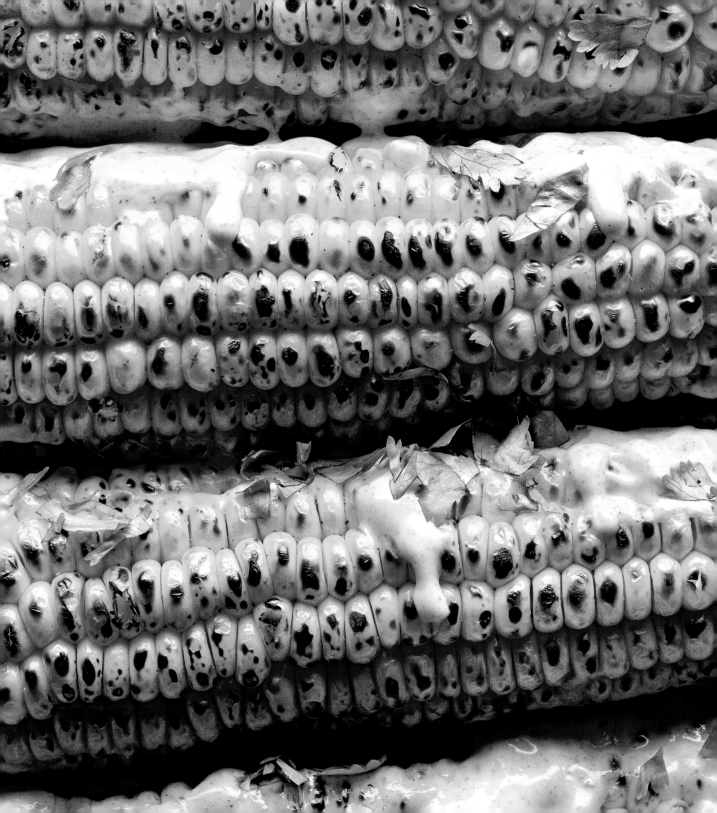

BROCCOLI WITH ANCHOVIES

3–4 heads of broccoli, chopped into bite-size florets

3 oz oil-packed anchovies

Juice of one lemon

Olive oil (optional)

Salt to taste

1. Steam the broccoli florets until bright green, about 3 to 4 minutes.

2. Combine the anchovies and lemon juice. Mash with a wooden spoon until the mixture resembles a paste. Add a splash of olive oil or more lemon juice, as desired. Add the broccoli florets, and toss to coat.

Serves four.

Per serving: *240 calories, 4 g fat (0.5 g saturated), 15 mg cholesterol, 820 mg sodium, 41 g carbohydrates, 11 g sugars, 16 g fiber, 22 g protein*

SAUTÉED YELLOW SQUASH, ZUCCHINI, AND ONIONS

2 Tbsp olive oil

2 onions, cut into ¼" slices

2 zucchini, cut in half lengthwise, then cut into ¼" slices

2 yellow squash, cut in half lengthwise, then cut into ¼" slices

3 cloves garlic, finely chopped

½ cup white wine

Salt and ground black pepper to taste

¼ tsp Italian seasoning

1. Place the oil in a large saucepan over medium-high heat.

2. Add the onions and cook for 3 to 5 minutes or until translucent.

3. Add the zucchini and the yellow squash, and cook for 4 to 5 minutes, stirring occasionally.

4. Add the garlic, and cook for 30 seconds.

5. Add the wine, salt and pepper to taste, and Italian seasoning. Cook for 2 to 3 minutes or until the liquid has reduced by half.

Serves four.

Per serving: *153.8 calories, 7 g fat, 1 g saturated), 0 mg cholesterol, 56.9 mg sodium, 15.9 g carbohydrates, 8.5 g sugars, 4.6 g fiber, 3.4 g protein*

WHAT'S THE DIFF?

BRANDY AND COGNAC

Brandy is the general name for an after-dinner drink made from distilled grapes; it should be sipped slowly while canoodling. Cognac is brandy from a specific place in France called, of all things, Cognac; it should be sipped slowly while canoodling while on an expense account.

SAUTÉED BROCCOLI RABE

1   lb broccoli rabe

1   Tbsp balsamic vinegar

1   Tbsp Parmesan cheese, grated

2   tsp extra-virgin olive oil

1   tsp fresh thyme, minced

1. Rinse the broccoli rabe in cold water and shake off the excess water.

2. Cut the thick stems into 1" pieces.

3. Cut the leafy tops into 3" pieces.

4. Place the stems and tops in a large, heavy saucepan or Dutch oven with just a little water left clinging to the pieces. Cover the pan and cook the broccoli rabe over medium heat for 5 minutes or until softened.

5. Drain and transfer to a serving platter. Sprinkle with the vinegar, Parmesan, oil, and thyme. Toss to coat.

ALTERNATE VERSION

Cut the broccoli rabe as directed, sauté in canola or olive oil with garlic for 5–10 minutes, and season with red-pepper flakes and salt.

Serves four.

Per serving: *63.4 calories, 2.7 g fat (0.5 g saturated), 1.1 mg cholesterol, 53.4 mg sodium, 6.1 g carbohydrates, 1.9 g sugars, 0 g fiber, 4.5 g protein*

SERVING SIZE, MADE SIMPLE:

BEEF
3 ounces, 219 calories

Same size as:
A deck of cards

ANTIOXIDANT PARFAIT

¼ cup cashews, crushed

2 cups low-fat vanilla yogurt

1 cup graham crackers, crushed

½ cup strawberries or tropical fruit, diced

2 cups blackberries, raspberries, or blueberries

Per serving: 220 calories, 7 g fat (2 g saturated), 5 mg cholesterol, 125 mg sodium, 34 g carbohydrates, 24 g sugars, 4 g fiber, 9 g protein

1. Coat a skillet with cooking spray, add the cashews, and stir over medium heat for 2 minutes.

2. Making thin layers, divide the yogurt, graham crackers, strawberries, and blackberries among four martini glasses, ending with yogurt.

3. Top with large blackberries, raspberries, or blueberries and the warm cashews.

Serves four.

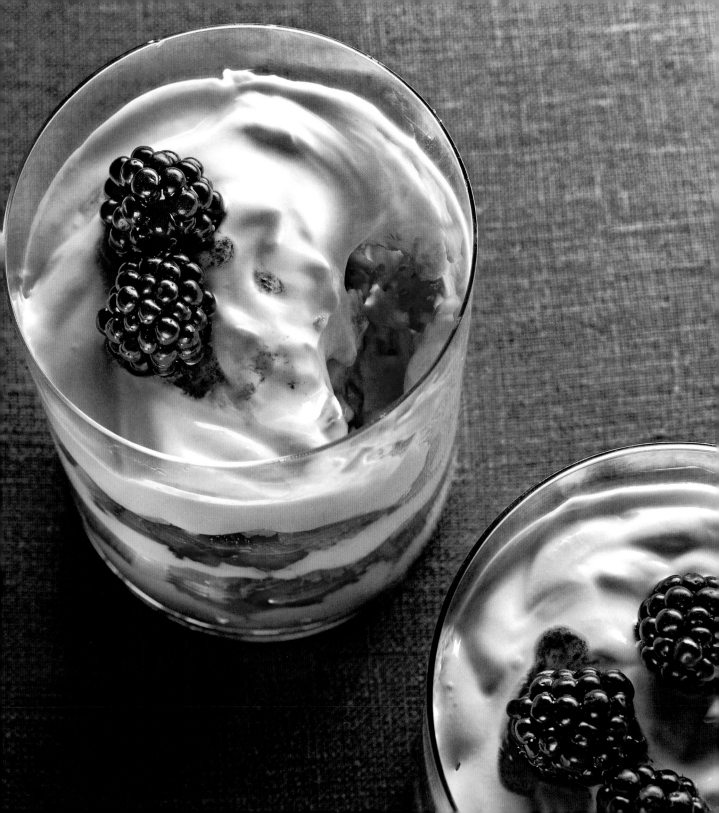

APPLE PIE PITA

1	apple, sliced
1	tsp pecans, finely chopped
1	tsp brown sugar or Splenda
¼	tsp ground cinnamon
	Pinch of ground nutmeg
½	small pita bread
2	Tbsp light whipped cream

1. Place the apple slices on a microwaveable plate.

2. Lightly coat the apples with butter-flavored cooking spray.

3. Sprinkle on the pecans, sugar or Splenda, cinnamon, and nutmeg.

4. Microwave on high power, tossing occasionally, for 3 to 4 minutes or until soft.

5. Toast the pita.

6. Spoon the apple mixture onto the pita and top with a dollop of the whipped cream.

Serves one.

Per serving: 188.3 calories, 7.6 g fat (3.2 g saturated), 16.7 mg cholesterol, 82.3 mg sodium, 31 g carbo-hydrates, 17.5 g sugars, 4.9 g fiber, 2.3 g protein

CRUNCHY BANANA POPS

4	popsicle sticks
2	bananas, peeled and cut in half crosswise
½	cup chocolate sauce (the kind that forms a shell)
4	Tbsp unsalted peanuts, diced

1. Insert a popsicle stick into the cut end of each banana piece so that the banana can be held like a popsicle.

2. Pour chocolate sauce over the bananas until they're completely coated.

3. Roll chocolate-coated bananas in peanuts.

4. Freeze.

Serves four.

Per serving: 315 calories, 22 g fat (9 g saturated), 0 cholesterol, 21 g sodium, 32 g carbohydrates, 22.6 sugars, 4 g fiber, 4 g protein

WHAT'S THE DIFF?

FOOD ALLERGY AND FOOD INTOLERANCE

When you eat a food you're allergic to, your immune system produces antibodies in reaction to the substance—leading to a rash, asthma, or other allergy symptoms. An intolerance doesn't involve the immune system. Instead your system lacks enzymes needed to digest a substance—lactose, say—leading to you getting symptoms like gas, bloating, or abdominal pain. So remember: it's not a hangover, it's an intolerance.

LOW-CAL OATMEAL COOKIES

1½	cups all-purpose flour
1	tsp ground cinnamon
1	tsp baking soda
½	tsp salt
3	cups old-fashioned or quick-cooking oats
1	cup dark or golden raisins
1	cup walnuts or pecans, finely chopped
½	cup reduced-calorie, trans fat-free margarine
¼	cup granulated sugar
¼	cup brown sugar, firmly packed
¼	cup Splenda
2	large eggs or ½ cup egg substitute
¾	cup unsweetened applesauce
1	tsp vanilla extract

1. Preheat the oven to 350°F.

2. Coat two or three heavy baking sheets with cooking spray.

3. In another large bowl, stir together the flour, cinnamon, baking soda, and salt.
Stir in the oats and then the raisins and nuts.

4. In another large bowl, with an electric mixer at medium speed, beat together the margarine, granulated and brown sugars, and Splenda until well blended. Beat in the eggs, one at a time, beating well after each (or beat in one-half of the egg substitute, followed by the other half).
Beat in the applesauce and vanilla.
With mixer at low speed, add the dry ingredients, in 2 batches, just until blended.

5. Drop the dough by heaping tablespoons onto the prepared baking sheets, spacing them 1" apart. Bake until crisp and lightly brown, 10 to 12 minutes.

6. Cool on sheet for 1 minute, then transfer cookies to racks to cool.

7. Repeat with remaining dough.

Makes four dozen cookies.

Per serving: 84.7 calories, 3.5 g fat, 0.7 g saturated), 9 mg cholesterol, 69.7 mg sodium, 11.8 g carbohydrates, 2.7 g sugars, 1 g fiber, 1.9 g protein

SERVING SIZE MADE SIMPLE:

ICE CREAM
½ cup, 143 calories

Same size as:
Tennis ball

APPLE-RAISIN CRUMB CAKE

STREUSEL

¾ cup unbleached all-purpose flour

⅔ cup brown sugar, packed

1 tsp ground cinnamon

3 Tbsp butter, cut into small pieces

CAKE

2¼ cups unbleached all-purpose flour

1 tsp baking powder

1 tsp baking soda

½ tsp salt

¼ cup butter, softened

1 cup sugar

2 eggs

1 tsp vanilla extract

8 oz sour cream

1 medium apple, peeled, cored, and finely chopped

⅓ cup golden raisins

Per serving: 355 calories, 11.8 g fat (7 g saturated), 61.1 mg cholesterol, 271 mg sodium, 58.4 g carbohydrates, 32.2 g sugars, 1.4 g fiber, 5.1 g protein

TO MAKE THE STREUSEL:

In a small bowl, combine the flour, brown sugar, and cinnamon. Add the butter and work with your fingers or a fork to form crumbs.

TO MAKE THE CAKE:

1. Preheat the oven to 350°F.

2. Grease a 9" x 9" cake pan.

3. In a medium bowl, combine the flour, baking powder, baking soda, and salt.

4. In another medium bowl, with an electric mixer on medium speed, beat the butter and sugar for 4 minutes or until creamy. Add the eggs and vanilla extract, beating until just smooth. Alternately add the flour mixture and the sour cream, beating on low speed until just blended. Stir in the apple and raisins.

5. Place the batter into the prepared pan. Top with the streusel. Bake for 40 minutes or until a wooden toothpick inserted in the center comes out clean.

6. Cool on a rack for 20 minutes and serve warm, or cool completely.

Serves twelve.

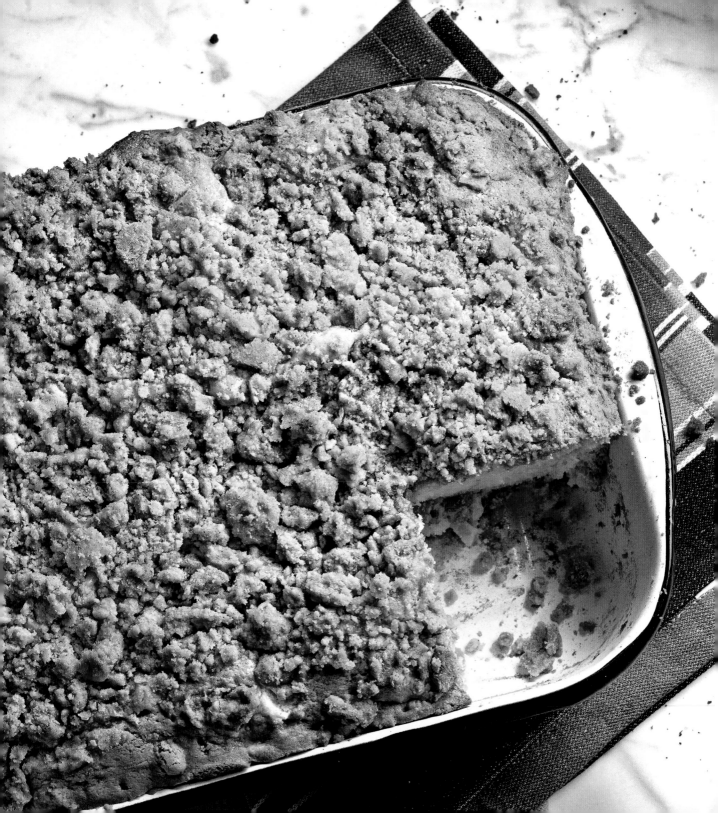

Chapter 8:
What's in Your Food?

FROM ESSENTIAL VITAMINS AND MINERALS TO
THE MOST UNPRONOUNCEABLE ARTIFICIAL ADDITIVES,
HERE'S YOUR A-TO-Z GLOSSARY OF THE GOOD, BAD,
AND UGLY STUFF FOUND IN THE FOODS YOU EAT EVERY DAY.

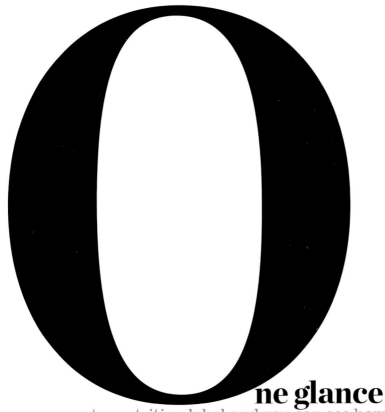

One glance

at a nutrition label and you can see how food truly is a science. You can also see how the food industry sometimes kidnaps real ingredients and replaces them with science experiments. Some substances are naturally wonderful (the B vitamin group, for example) and some are just creepy (Yellow Dye #5). But few of us know what the average food label is telling us. Yeah, we get serving size and calories. And yeah, a food with 75 percent of your recommended daily intake of vitamin D is probably a good thing. But what does vitamin D do for you? Not sure? It's crucial, and the answer is in here.

As with every chapter in this book, our goal is to educate you about what you're eating. There is good and bad in food. And frankly, not all additives are evil. Some are actually nutritious. After reading this chapter, you'll know exactly what's in the foods you eat, whether that food's as natural as a fresh fig or as artificial as a tub of icing.

The information herein is broken down into three sections: vitamins (naturally occurring good stuff in foods), minerals (naturally occurring good stuff in foods—and rocks), and food additives (unnaturally occurring stuff—good and bad—in too many foods).

For vitamins and minerals, we give you definitions, what they do for you, and which whole foods pack the biggest doses of them. And while a multivitamin may help make up for any dietary shortcomings, more and more research suggests that popping one just doesn't deliver the same health payload as vitamins and minerals in their natural state. And substituting natural sources for supplements means you're not getting the benefits of the fiber, healthy fats, and micronutrients found in fruits, vegetables, dairy, and meats. So as you read about crucial vitamins and minerals, you'll be referred back to their best natural food sources in Chapter 6 by page number so you can check them out.

We won't be referring you to any food additive sources, though. Sorry. For a lot of them, it's bad enough that they're out there at all. But after reading up on what they are and how they're used, you'll never look at an ingredients label the same way again. And that, friends, is a good thing.

Vitamins

Betaine

Betaine is best known for its power to lower homocysteine levels in the blood. Increased amounts of homocysteine, an amino acid, can cause symptoms such as extreme tiredness, osteoporosis, or blood clots. It's also linked to higher risk of major illnesses such as heart disease and stroke.
Natural Source: eggs (page 234).

Choline

Choline is the memory vitamin. Studies have shown that college students given 3 to 4 grams of choline 1 hour before taking memory tests scored higher than those who didn't receive the supplements. "We believe choline increases the release of acetylcholine, a neurotransmitter that helps your brain store and recall information," says Steven Zeisel, MD, PhD, a professor of nutrition at the University of North Carolina. Although studies have used supplements, Zeisel says that eating foods that are naturally rich in choline should do the trick just as well.
Natural Sources: eggs (page 234) and milk (page 212).

Vitamin A

A is essential for a strong immune system. USDA researchers found that an increased intake of vitamin A boosted germ-killing cells by 8 percent. Because vitamin A can build up to toxic levels in the body with too much supplementation, experts recommend avoiding vitamin A supplements and getting what you need through diet (and, at most, a simple multivitamin daily).
Natural Sources: carrots (page 80), sweet potatoes (page 78), and mangoes (page 143).

Vitamin B—Varieties

Thiamin (B₁)

The B vitamin thiamin takes a hit from a night of heavy drinking. Consuming large amounts of alcohol makes you use it faster but absorb it more slowly. The result: You end up with a deficit of a vitamin essential to normal neurological functioning. This may explain phenomena such as beer goggles and Mel Gibson's answering machine messages.
Natural Sources: beef (page 242), pork (page 246), and pasta (page 224).

THE YOLK'S ON YOU!

Ordering an egg-white-omelet to fend off heart disease? Better think twice: A USDA study found that choline—a vitamin found primarily in egg yolks—lowers levels of homocysteine in the blood by 8 precent, which improves blood flow and lowers heart disease risk.

THE FOLATE FACTOR

Many researchers and doctors now believe that folate is the nutrient that best reveals how healthy your diet is. If folate levels are low, chances are your diet needs tweaking. Cruciferous vegetables are a great source (also, see the Folate entry on this page).

Riboflavin (Vitamin B_2)

Riboflavin, or B_2, helps with oxygen absorption and the production of red blood cells. A Belgian study also found that high doses reduce the length and frequency of migraines.
Natural Sources: dairy products (page 204).

Niacin (Vitamin B_3)

At high doses, niacin, or B_3, can lower LDL (bad) cholesterol by 5 percent, cut triglycerides by 20 percent, and boost HDL (good) cholesterol by 15 percent. However, side effects include a dangerous rise in glucose levels in diabetics (so consult your doctor).
Natural Sources: poultry (page 232), fish (page 164), whole grains (page 184). Medication note: May increase some of the side effects of statins and reduce the effects of diabetes medications.

Pantothenic Acid (B_5)

Pantothenic acid helps us process proteins, carbs, and fats. It's present in most foods, though good natural sources are legumes (page 128), meats (page 242), eggs (page 234), broccoli (page 86), and avocado (page 68). Some experts recommend B_5 as an anti-stress/pro-sleep supplement. According to Ron Klatz, MD, president of the American Academy of Anti-Aging Medicine, a B_5 supplement before bed could be your antidote to too much cortisol, the stress hormone that surges in middle-age men. If that doesn't help, ask your doctor about taking some Bayer with your B;

aspirin may also help lower cortisol production.

B_6

B_6 is needed for more than 100 enzymes involved in protein metabolism. It is also essential for red blood cell metabolism—it helps the body make hemoglobin and increases the amount of oxygen carried by hemoglobin. Your nervous and immune systems also need B_6 to function efficiently.
Natural Sources: potatoes (page 76), bananas (page 137), chicken (page 234), and oatmeal (page 186).

Folate or Folic acid (B_9)

Folic acid will help keep your bloodstream streaming. A Harvard study showed that men taking the most were 30 percent less likely to suffer a stroke than those taking the least. Credit folic acid's ability to dissolve homocysteine—a compound linked to heart disease.
Natural Sources: spinach (page 92) and broccoli (page 86).

B_{12}

B_{12} is vital to the production of myelin, the fatty sheath that insulates nerve fibers, keeping electrical impulses moving through the body as they should. Because of this important function, a whole host of problems can arise when B_{12} is in short supply: memory loss, fatigue, loss of balance, decreased reflexes, impaired touch or pain perception, numbness and tingling in the arms and legs, and noise-induced hearing loss.

Researchers have discovered that a deficiency raises blood levels of homocysteine (shortages of folate and vitamin B_6 can do the same).

Unless you're vegan and avoid all animal products, it's easy to get adequate amounts of vitamin B_{12} from food sources because you need so little of it. Seafood is a terrific natural source: clams (page 178), herring (page 169), salmon (page 166), and tuna (page 164). So is ham (page 247). Vegans should look for B_{12}-fortified products or take a supplement.

Vitamin C

While vitamin C can't cure a cold, there's evidence it can shorten the sniffles by a day. The C may also stand for "calm"—University of Alabama researchers found that it may help halt the secretion of stress hormones. And scurvy? Clears it right up.
Natural Sources: citrus fruit (page 140), tomatoes (page 69), and bell peppers (page 202).

Vitamin D

Vitamin D is responsible for getting the important bone builders—calcium and phosphorus—to the places in the body where they can help bone grow in children and re-mineralize in adults. It does this first by making certain that these minerals are absorbed in the intestines, second by bringing calcium from bones into the blood, and third by helping the kidneys reabsorb the two minerals.

While your body manufactures vitamin D in response to sunlight, it's important to get plenty of it, especially as you get older. After evaluating the calcium and vitamin D status of elderly people who were entering nursing homes, researchers determined that most had low vitamin D levels and that nearly 85 percent had symptoms of osteoporosis. There is mounting evidence that vitamin D deficiency in elderly people is a silent epidemic that results in bone loss and fractures.
Natural Sources: dairy (page 204). One cup of 1 percent D-fortified milk contains 100 IU (25 percent of your daily value). Fish like herring (page 169), salmon (page 166), and sardines (page 174) are good sources. Also, spend 10 to 20 minutes in the sun every day.

Vitamin E

E is tough on cancer, especially when it's paired with selenium. Research shows that this antioxidant may reduce your risk of prostate cancer by up to 53 percent and bladder cancer by almost half.
Natural Sources: vegetable oils (page 182) and leafy green vegetables (page 92). Note: Too much E may increase the effects of blood thinners or reverse the effects of statins.

Vitamin K

Vitamin K keeps paper cuts from being fatal. It's also key for liver function. Taiwanese researchers have found that a synthetic form of vitamin K stopped the spread of liver cancer in lab tests. Your diet is likely K-sufficient—its best source is leafy green vegetables (page 92).

VITAMIN K *IS* SPECIAL

One of the keys to a long life is preserving your insulin sensitivity—meaning your body doesn't produce wild swings in blood sugar after you eat, a condition that leads to diabetes. Recent research from Tufts University found that vitamin K helps keep insulin levels in check. The researchers recommend eating five or more servings a week of cruciferous or dark leafy vegetables.

Minerals

Calcium

As the overachiever of minerals, calcium builds bones, helps with weight loss, and possibly decreases the risk of colon cancer. And a study published in the *American Journal of Medicine* found that 1,000 mg of supplemental calcium can increase HDL (good) cholesterol by 7 percent.
Natural Sources: dairy products (page 204), broccoli (page 86), and kale (page 95).

Copper

Copper is multitalented. It's an antioxidant, active in nerve function and bone growth, and also helps the body burn sugar.
Natural Sources: oysters (page 180), beans (page 128), nuts (page 120), and whole grains (page 184).

Iron

Most of the body's iron is found in hemoglobin, helping the body transport oxygen. Women may face iron deficiencies because of their menstrual cycles, but for men it's better to lift this metal than swallow too much of it. If you take a multivitamin, find one that's iron-free: There may be a link between high iron levels and heart disease. Eat meat (page 242) and you're probably iron-fortified enough.

Magnesium

A drop in magnesium can be a major headache. "Blood vessels in your brain constrict, and receptors for the feel-good chemical serotonin malfunction," says Alexander Mauskop, MD, director of the New York Headache Center. Result: a migraine. The mineral also might help regulate blood pressure and could ward off stroke and diabetes.
Natural Sources: leafy greens (page 92), whole grains (page 184), coffee (page 193), and nuts (page 120).

Manganese

Manganese is an underrated nutritional superstar. It's crucial in digestion and metabolism, helping the body process cholesterol, carbs, and protein. It's also a potent antioxident.
Natural Sources: pineapple (page 138), brown rice (page 184), spinach (page 92), beans (page 128), oatmeal (page 186), and leafy greens (page 92).

56

Percentage of the population that doesn't consume enough magnesium. In an 18-year study, French researchers determined that men with the highest blood levels of the mineral have a 40 percent lower risk of early death than those with the lowest levels. The researchers think this could be because low magnesium levels are associated with greater inflammation, which is linked to heart disease and cancer (see Magnesium entry on this page).

Phosphorus

Phosphorus is found in every cell in your body, but it's best known for helping you form bones and teeth. It also helps keep your kidneys humming and regulates heartbeat. In general, if you're eating enough protein and calcium, you're eating enough phosphorus.
Natural Sources: meat (page 242) and milk (page 212).

Potassium

Research shows that most Americans come up 1,000 mg short on daily potassium intake. The consequences: elevated blood pressure and muscle cramps. Get it from your diet—potassium supplements can build up in the body and damage the heart.
Natural Sources: almonds (page 120), bananas (page 137), spinach (page 92).

Selenium

Men need selenium to produce sperm, but it's also like kryptonite to cancer. Harvard researchers found that men with the highest levels of this mineral had a 48 percent lower risk of advanced prostate cancer. It may also ward off lung cancer. If you use a supplement, go for 200 mcg from selenium yeast daily.
Natural Sources: Brazil nuts (page 122) and meat (page 242). Note: May reduce the effectiveness of statins (talk to your doctor).

Sodium

Sodium hides in processed foods, put there by food companies to preserve products that would otherwise go bad, or to make bland or bitter food taste better, or maybe just to appeal to our craving for the stuff. Current recommended daily intake is 1,500 milligrams with an upper limit of 2,300 mg. American men generally eat more than 4,000 mg sodium a day, and it's easy to take in 7,000 without trying. You do need a little bit—about 200 mg a day—to keep fluids in balance. Excessive sodium is now linked to illnesses such as stomach cancer and kidney stones. Too much can also make the body excrete calcium, threatening bone density and strength.

We also know for certain that sodium raises blood pressure. Roughly 20 percent of American adults have higher-than-optimal BP. Reducing intake by just 300 mg (about two slices of Cheddar) drops systolic pressure (the first number) by 2 to 4 points, and diastolic by 1 to 2 points, a British study shows.

Zinc

An antioxidant, zinc improves your lipid profile and blood circulation, which for men is crucial to erectile function. It may be especially important for testosterone and sperm production, and it's vital for the functioning of proteins, enzymes, and hormones. Because heavy alcohol use depletes zinc, it's critical for those who drink regularly.
Natural Sources: oysters (page 180), king crab (page 177), lobster (page 176), meat (page 242), and poultry (page 232).

THE MUSCLE MINERAL

Researchers at the Department of Agriculture's Human Nutrition Research Center on Aging, at Tufts University, found that foods rich in potassium help preserve lean muscle mass. After studying 384 volunteers for 3 years, they found that those whose diets were rich in potassium (getting more than 3,540 milligrams a day) preserved 3.6 more pounds of lean tissue than those with half the potassium intake. That almost offsets the 4.4 pounds of lean tissue that is typically lost each decade as we age.

Food Additives

DID YOU KNOW…

The Nutrition Labeling and Education Act of 1990 absolved restaurants of all nutritional liability to the American public. Under that legislation, no fast-food or chain restaurants were required to provide calorie, fat, or sodium information for any of their menu items unless they describe the items as "low sodium" or "low fat." The health-care legislation passed in 2010, however, will require restaurant chains with 20 or more outlets to post calorie information.

Acesulfame potassium (Acesulfame-K)

A calorie-free artificial sweetener that's 200 times sweeter than sugar, it is often used with other artificial sweeteners to mask a bitter aftertaste. It's found in more than 5,000 food products worldwide, including diet soft drinks and no-sugar-added ice cream. Although the FDA has approved it for use in most foods, many health experts and food industry insiders claim that the decision was based on flawed tests. Animal studies have linked the chemical to lung and breast tumors and thyroid problems.

Alpha-tocopherol

The form of vitamin E most commonly added to foods and most readily absorbed and stored in the body. It is an essential nutrient that helps prevent oxidative damage to the cells and plays a crucial role in cell communication, skin health, and disease prevention. It's found in meats, foods with added fats, and foods that boast vitamin E health claims. Also occurs naturally in seeds, nuts, leafy vegetables, and vegetable oils. In the amount added to foods, tocopherols pose no apparent health risks, but highly concentrated supplements might bring on toxicity symptoms such as cramps, weakness, and double vision.

Artificial flavoring

Denotes any of hundreds of allowable chemicals such as butyl alcohol, isobutyric acid, and phenylacetaldehyde dimethyl acetal. The exact chemicals used in flavoring are the proprietary information of food manufacturers, which use these compounds to imitate specific fruits, butter, spices, and so on. They're in thousands of highly processed foods, such as cereals, fruit snacks, beverages, and cookies. The FDA has approved every item on the list of allowable chemicals, but because food marketers can hide their specific ingredients behind a blanket term, there is no way for consumers to pinpoint the cause of a reaction they might have had.

Ascorbic acid

The chemical name for water-soluble vitamin C. You'll find it in juices and fruit products, meat, cereals, and other foods with vitamin C health claims. Although vitamin C isn't associated with any known risks, it is often added to junk foods to make them appear healthy.

Aspartame

A near-zero-calorie artificial sweetener made by combining two amino acids with methanol. Most commonly used in diet soft drinks, aspartame is 180 times sweeter than sugar. It's in more than 6,000 grocery items, including diet sodas, yogurts, and the tabletop sweeteners NutraSweet and Equal. In the past 30 years, the FDA has received thousands of consumer complaints, mostly concerning neurological symptoms such as headaches, dizziness, memory loss, and, in rare cases, epileptic seizures. Many studies have shown aspartame to be completely harmless, while others indicate that the additive might be responsible for a range of cancers.

BHA and BHT (Butylated Hydroxyanisole and Butylated Hydroxytoluene)

These are petroleum-derived antioxidants used to preserve fats and oils. You'll find them added into products such as beer, crackers, cereals, butter, and foods with added fats. Of the two, BHA is considered the most troublesome. Studies have shown it to cause cancer in the forestomachs of rats, mice, and hamsters. The Department of Health and Human Services classifies the preservative as "reasonably anticipated to be a human carcinogen."

Blue #1 (brilliant blue) and Blue #2 (indigotine)

Synthetic dyes that can be used alone or combined with other dyes to make different colors. They're use in blue, purple, and green foods, such as beverages, cereals, candy, and icing. Both dyes have been loosely linked to cancers in animal studies, and the Center for Science in the Public Interest recommends that they be avoided.

Brown rice syrup

A natural sweetener about half as sweet as sugar. It is obtained by using enzymes to break down the starches in cooked rice. It's used in protein bars and organic and natural foods. Brown rice sugar has a lower glycemic index than table sugar, which means it provides an easier ride for your blood sugar.

867

Calories in the average entrée at a sit-down chain restaurant, compared to 522 calories in the average fast-food entrée (based on an analysis of 24 national chains).

Carrageenan

A thickener, stabilizer, and emulsifier extracted from red seaweed, it is found in jellies and jams, ice cream, yogurt, and whipped topping. Although it's technically natural, in animal studies, carrageenan has been shown to cause ulcers, colon inflammation, and digestive cancers. While these results seem limited to degraded carrageenan—a class that has been treated with heat and chemicals—a University of Iowa study concluded that even undegraded carrageenan could become degraded in the human digestive system.

Casein

A milk protein used to thicken and whiten foods. It often appears by the names "sodium caseinate" or "calcium caseinate." It is a good source of amino acids and is found in protein bars and shakes, and in sherbet, ice cream, and other frozen desserts. Although casein is a byproduct of milk, the FDA allows it and its derivatives—sodium calcium caseinates—to be used in "nondairy" and "dairy-free" creamers. Most lactose intolerants can handle casein, but those with broader milk allergies might experience reactions.

Cochineal extract (or carmine)

A pigment extracted from the dried eggs and bodies of the female Dactylopius coccus, a beetle-like insect that preys on cactus plants. It is added to food for its dark crimson color and is used in artificial crabmeat, fruit juices, frozen-fruit snacks, candy, and yogurt. Carmine is the refined coloring, while cochineal extract comprises about 90 percent insect-body fragments. Although the FDA receives fewer than one adverse-reaction report a year, some organizations are asking for a mandatory warning label to accompany cochineal-colored foods. Vegetarians, they say, should be forewarned about the insect juices.

Corn syrup

A liquid sweetener and food thickener made by allowing enzymes to break cornstarches into smaller sugars. USDA subsidies to the corn industry make it cheap and abundant, placing it among the most ubiquitous ingredients in grocery food products—including breads, soup, sauces, frozen dinners, and frozen treats. Corn syrup provides no nutritional value other than calories. In moderation, it poses no specific threat, other than an expanded waistline.

Dextrose

A corn-derived caloric sweetener. Like corn syrup, dextrose contributes to the American habit of more than 200 calories of corn sweeteners per day via bread, cookies, and crackers. As with other sugars, dextrose is safe in moderate amounts.

Erythorbic acid

A compound similar to ascorbic acid, but with no apparent nutritional

THINK ABOUT YOUR LAST MEAL

British scientists found that people who thought about their last meal before snacking ate 30 percent fewer calories that those who didn't stop to think. The theory: Remembering what you had for lunch might remind you of how satiating the food was, which then makes you less likely to binge on your afternoon snack.

value of its own. It is added to nitrite-containing meats to disrupt the formation of cancer-causing nitrosamines and is used in deli meats, hot dogs, and sausages. Erythorbic acid poses no risks, though it may improve the body's ability to absorb iron, which is not an entirely positive quality for men. They should limit their iron intake because of the mineral's link to cardiovascular problems.

Evaporated cane juice

A sweetener derived from sugarcane, the same plant used to make refined table sugar. It's also known as "crystallized cane juice," "cane juice," or "cane sugar." Because it's subject to less processing than table sugar, evaporated cane juice retains slightly more nutrients from the grassy sugar cane. You'll find it in yogurt, soy milk, protein bars, granola, cereal, chicken sausages, and other natural or organic foods. Although pristine sugars are often used to replace ordinary sugars in "healthier" foods, the actual nutritional difference between the sugars is minuscule. Both should be consumed in moderation.

Fully hydrogenated vegetable oil

Extremely hard, waxlike fat made by forcing as much hydrogen as possible onto the carbon backbone of fat molecules. (Yes, this is actually in your supermarket, being sold as an ingredient in food.) To obtain a manageable consistency, food manufacturers will often blend the hard fat with unhydrogenated liquid fats, the result of which is called interesterified fat. It's used in baked goods, doughnuts, frozen meals, and tub margarine. In theory, fully hydrogenated oils, as opposed to partially hydrogenated oils, should contain zero trans fat. In practice, however, the process of hydrogenation isn't completely perfect, which means that some trans fat will inevitably occur in small amounts, as will an increased concentration of saturated fat.

Guar gum

A thickening, emulsifying, and stabilizing agent made from ground guar beans. The legume, also known as a cluster bean, is of Indian origin, but small amounts are grown domestically. Guar gum is used in pastry fillings, ice cream, and sauces. It's a great example of a food additive that actually enhances the food's nutritional value: Guar is a good source of soluble fiber and might even improve insulin sensitivity. One Italian study suggested that partially hydrolyzed guar gum might have probiotic properties that make it useful in treating patients with irritable bowel syndrome.

High-fructose corn syrup (HFCS)

A corn-derived sweetener representing more than 40 percent of all caloric sweeteners in the supermarket. The liquid sweetener is created by a complex process that involves breaking down cornstarch with enzymes, and the result is a roughly 50/50 mix of fructose and glucose. Although about two-thirds of the HFCS consumed in the U.S. is in beverages, it can be found in every grocery aisle in products such as ice cream, chips, cookies, cereals, bread, ketchup, jam, canned fruits, yogurt, barbecue sauce, frozen dinners, and so on.

Since around 1980, the U.S. obesity rate has risen proportionately to the increase in HFCS, and Americans are now consuming at least 200 calories of the sweetener each day. Some researchers argue that the body metabolizes HFCS differently, making it easier to store as fat, but this theory has not been proved. What is known is that in some people, fructose can interfere with the body's ability to process leptin, a hormone that tells us when we're full.

Hydrogenated vegetable oil

See fully hydrogenated vegetable oil.

Hydrolyzed vegetable protein

A flavor enhancer created when heat and chemicals are used to break down a vegetable—most often soy—into its component amino acids. It allows food manufacturers to achieve stronger flavors from fewer ingredients and is used in canned soups and chili, frozen dinners, and beef- and chicken-flavored products. One effect of hydrolyzing proteins is the creation of MSG, or monosodium glutamate. When MSG in food is the result of hydrolyzed protein, the FDA does not require it to be listed on the packaging.

Interesterified fat

A semi-soft fat created by chemically blending fully hydrogenated and nonhydrogenated oils. It was developed in response to the public demand for an alternative to trans fats, because fully hydrogenated fats are supposedly free of trans fatty acids. You'll find it in pastries, pies, margarine, frozen dinners, and canned soups. Testing on these fats has not been extensive, but the early evidence doesn't look promising. A study by Malaysian researchers showed that a 4-week diet of 12 percent interesterified fats increased the ratio of LDL to HDL cholesterol. Furthermore, this study showed an increase in blood glucose levels and a decrease in insulin response.

Inulin

Naturally occurring plant fiber in fruits and vegetables that is added to foods to boost the fiber in or help the texture of low-fat foods. Most of the inulin in the food supply is extracted from chicory root or synthesized from sucrose. It's in smoothies, meal-replacement bars, and processed foods trying to gain legitimacy among healthy eaters. Like other fibers, inulin can help stabilize blood sugar, improve bowel functions, and help the body absorb nutrients such as calcium (good) and iron (not so good).

Lecithin

A naturally occurring emulsifier and antioxidant that retards the rancidity of fats. The two major sources for lecithin as an additive are egg yolks and soybeans, and it's used in pastries, ice cream, and margarine. Lecithin is an excellent source of choline and inositol—compounds that help cells and nerves communicate and play a role in breaking down fats and cholesterol.

Maltodextrin

A caloric sweetener and flavor enhancer made from rice, potatoes, or, more commonly, cornstarch. Through treatment with enzymes and acids, it can be converted into a fiber and thickening agent and you'll find it in canned fruit, instant pudding, sauces, dressings, and chocolates. Like other sugars, maltodextrin has the potential to raise blood glucose and insulin levels.

Maltose (malt sugar)

A caloric sweetener that's about a third as sweet as honey. It occurs naturally in some grains, but as an additive it is usually derived from corn. Food manufacturers like it because it prolongs shelf life and inhibits bacterial growth. It's used in cereal grains, nuts and seeds, sports beverages, deli meats, and poultry products. Maltose poses no threats other than those associated with other sugars.

Mannitol

A sugar alcohol that's 70 percent as sweet as sugar. It provides fewer calories and has a less drastic effect on blood sugar. You'll find it in sugar-free candy, low-calorie and diet foods, and chewing gum. Because sugar alcohols are not fully digested, they can cause intestinal discomfort, gas, bloating, flatulence, and diarrhea.

Modified food starch

An indefinite term describing a starch that has been manipulated in a non-specific way. The starches can be derived from corn, wheat, potato, or rice, and they are then modified to change their response to heat or cold, improve their texture, and create more efficient emulsifiers, among other reasons. You'll see modified food starch in most highly processed foods, low-calorie and diet foods, pastries, cookies, and frozen meals. The starches themselves appear safe, but the nondisclosure of the chemicals used in processing causes some nutritionists to question their effects on health, especially of infants.

Mono- and diglycerides

Fats added to foods to bind liquids with fats. They occur naturally in foods and constitute about 1 percent of normal food fats. They're in peanut butter, ice cream, margarine, baked goods, and whipped topping. Aside from being a source of fat, the glycerides themselves pose no serious health threats.

Monosodium glutamate (MSG)

The salt of the amino acid glutamic acid, used to enhance the savory quality of foods. MSG alone has little flavor, and exactly how it enhances other foods is unknown. It's used in chili, soup, and

1920s

Decade when scientists began to induce genetic mutations in crops by bombarding living cells with radiation.

WHAT ABOUT IODINE?

Your thyroid gland requires iodine to produce the hormones T3 and T4, both of which help control how efficiently you burn calories. That means insufficient iodine may cause you to gain weight and feel fatigued.

The shortfall:
Since iodized salt is an important source of the element, you might assume you're swimming in the stuff. But when University of Texas at Arlington researchers tested 88 samples of table salt, they found that half contained less than the FDA-recommended amount of iodine. And you're not making up the difference with all the salt hiding in processed foods—US manufacturers aren't required to use iodized salt. The result is that we've been sliding toward iodine deficiency since the 1970s.

Hit the mark:
Sprinkling more salt on top of an already sodium-packed diet isn't a great idea, but iodine can also be found in several nearly sodium-free sources: milk, eggs, and yogurt. Animal feed is fortified with the element, meaning it travels from cows and chickens to your breakfast table.

foods with chicken or beef flavoring. Studies have shown that MSG injected into mice causes brain-cell damage, but the FDA believes these results are not typical for humans. The FDA receives dozens of reaction complaints each year for nausea, headaches, chest pains, and weakness.

Neotame

The newest addition to the FDA-approved artificial sweeteners. It's chemically similar to aspartame and at least 8,000 times sweeter than sugar. It was approved in 2002, and its use is not yet widespread, though it's used in Clabber Girl Sugar Replacer, Domino Pure D'Lite, and Hostess 100-Calorie Packs. Neotame is the second artificial sweetener to be deemed safe by the Center for Science in the Public Interest (the first was sucralose). It's considered more stable than aspartame, and because it's 40 times sweeter, it can be used in much smaller concentrations.

Olestra

A synthetic fat created by Procter & Gamble and sold under the name Olean. It has a zero-calorie impact and is not absorbed as it passes though the digestive system. It's used in light chips and crackers. But it's hardly a perfect solution for those trying to cut calories: In even moderate doses, Olestra can cause diarrhea, intestinal cramps, and flatulence. Studies show that it impairs the body's ability to absorb fat-soluble vitamins and vital

carotenoids such as beta-carotene, lycopene, lutein, and zeaxanthin.

Oligofructose

See inulin.

Partially hydrogenated vegetable oil

A manufactured fat created by forcing hydrogen gas into vegetable fats under extremely high pressure, an unintended effect of which is the creation of trans fatty acids. Food manufacturers like this fat because of its low cost and long shelf life. It's used in margarine, pastries, frozen foods, cakes, cookies, crackers, soups, and nondairy creamers. Cardiologists, on the other hand, hate it: Trans fat has been shown to contribute to heart disease more so than saturated fats. While most health organizations recommend keeping trans fat consumption as low as possible (no more than 2 to 2.5 grams daily for an average American), a loophole in the FDA's labeling requirements allows marketers to add as much as 0.49 grams per serving and still claim zero in their nutrition facts. That means you could eat four servings of "trans-fat-free" packaged goods and still approach your daily allotment. Progressive jurisdictions such as New York City, California, and Boston have approved legislation to phase trans fat out of restaurants, and pressure from watchdog groups might eventually lead to a full ban on the dangerous oil.

Pectin

A carbohydrate that occurs naturally in many fruits and vegetables, used to thicken and stabilize foods. You'll find it in jellies and jams, sauces, pie fillings, smoothies, and shakes. Pectin is a source of dietary fiber and might help to lower cholesterol.

Polysorbates

A class of chemicals usually derived from animal fats and used primarily as emulsifiers, much like mono- and diglycerides. Polysorbates are found in cakes, icing, bread mixes, ice cream, and pickles. Polysorbates allow otherwise fat-soluble vitamins to dissolve in water, an odd trait that seems to have a benign effect.

Propyl gallate

An antioxidant used often in conjunction with BHA and BHT to retard the rancidity of fats. It's found in mayonnaise, margarine, oils, dried meats, pork sausage, and other fatty foods. Rat studies in the early 1980s linked propyl gallate to brain cancer. Although these studies don't provide sound evidence, it is advisable to avoid this chemical when possible.

Red #3 (erythrosine) and Red #40 (allura red)

Food dyes that are orange-red and cherry red, respectively. Red #40 is the most widely used food dye in America. Red dyes are used in fruit cocktail, candy, chocolate cake, cereal, beverages, pastries, maraschino cherries, and fruit snacks. The FDA has proposed a ban on Red #3 in the past, but so far the agency has been unsuccessful in implementing it. After the dye was inextricably linked to thyroid tumors in rat studies, the FDA managed to have the liquid form of the dye removed from external drugs and cosmetics.

Saccharin

An artificial sweetener that's 300 to 500 times sweeter than sugar. Discovered in 1879, it's the oldest of the five FDA-approved artificial sweeteners. It's used in diet foods, chewing gum, toothpaste, beverages, sugar-free candy, and Sweet'N Low. Rat studies in the early 1970s showed saccharin to cause bladder cancer, and the FDA, reacting to these studies, enacted a mandatory warning label to be printed on every saccharin-containing product. The label was removed after 20 years, but the question over saccharin's safety was never resolved. More recent studies show that rats on saccharin-rich diets gain more weight than those on high-sugar diets.

Sodium ascorbate

See ascorbic acid.

Sodium caseinate

See casein.

Sodium nitrite and sodium nitrate

Preservatives used to prevent bacterial growth and maintain the pinkish color of meats and fish. They're used in bacon, sausage, hot dogs, and cured, canned,

1879

The year that saccharin was discovered.

500

Number in millions of Twinkies baked each year. Number of days in a Twinkie's shelf life? 25.

and packaged meats. Under certain conditions, sodium nitrite and nitrate react with amino acids to form cancer-causing chemicals called nitrosamines.

Sorbitol

A sugar alcohol that occurs naturally in some fruits. It's about 60 percent as sweet as sugar and used to both sweeten and thicken. You'll find it added to dried fruit, chewing gum, and reduced-sugar candy. Your body digests sorbitol slower than sugars, which makes it a better choice for diabetics, but it can cause intestinal discomfort and diarrhea.

Soy lecithin

See lecithin.

Sucralose

A zero-calorie artificial sweetener made by joining chlorine particles and sugar molecules. It's 600 times sweeter than sugar and largely celebrated as the least damaging of the artificial sweeteners. It's use in sugar-free foods, pudding, beverages, some diet sodas, and Splenda. After reviewing more than 110 human and animal studies, the FDA concluded that use of sucralose does not cause cancer. The sweetener is one of only three artificial sweeteners deemed safe by the Center for Science in the Public Interest.

Tartrazine

See Yellow #5.

Vegetable shortening

See partially hydrogenated vegetable oil.

Yellow #5 (tartrazine) and Yellow #6 (sunset yellow)

The second and third most common food colorings, respectively. They're used in cereal, pudding, bread mixes, beverages, chips, cookies, and condiments. Several studies have linked both dyes to learning and concentration disorders in children. One study found that mice fed high doses of sunset yellow had trouble swimming straight and righting themselves in water. Despite these results, the FDA does not view these as serious risks to humans.

Xanthan gum

An extremely common emulsifier and thickener made from glucose in a reaction requiring a slimy bacteria called Xanthomonas campestris—the same bacterial strain that appears as black rot on cruciferous vegetables such as broccoli. It's used in whipped topping, dressings, marinades, custard, and pie filling. Xanthan gum isn't associated with any adverse effects.

Xylitol

A sugar alcohol that occurs naturally in strawberries, mushrooms, and other fruits and vegetables. It is most commonly extracted from the pulp of the birch tree and is used in sugar-free candy, yogurt, and beverages. Unlike real sugar, sugar alcohols don't encourage cavity-causing bacteria. They do have a laxative effect, though, so heavy ingestion might cause intestinal discomfort or gas.

A Final Tip of the Hat to Antioxidants

Antioxidants are our nutritional best friends. They fight free radicals, which are unstable molecules in the body that can cause DNA mutation. Any molecule that protects your cells against oxidation is technically an antioxidant—anything from certain vitamins to flavonoids and polyphenols. There are about 8,000 varieties in all, but if you eat a wide variety of fruits and vegetables, your diet is naturally rich in thousands of antioxidants. But what foods are best?

Oxygen Radical Absorbance Capacity, or ORAC, is a method of measuring antioxidant capacities of different foods. The higher the score, the more antioxidant power a food has. Here's a sampling of foods to give you an idea of how they finish—berries, legumes, and some vegetables come in high. Pure cocoa is the world champ. But other foods that are considered nutritious are low in antioxidants (see bananas and corn). That doesn't mean you shouldn't eat low-scoring foods, just don't assume you get antioxidant protection from them.

PER 100g SERVING	ORAC SCORE*
Apple, red delicious, with skin	4,275
Artichokes, raw	6,552
Bananas, raw	879
Black beans, raw	8,040
Navy beans, raw	1,520
Blueberries	6,552
Broccoli, raw	1,362
Cocoa, dry, unsweetened	80,933
Corn, raw	728
Cranberries	9,584
Elderberries	14,697
Garlic, raw	5,346
Lentils, raw	7,282
Oranges, raw	1,819
Spinach, raw	1,515

* The amount shown is the ORAC score per 100 grams, according to the USDA (see usda.gov for a comprehensive ORAC food list).

Index

Boldface page references indicate illustrations. <u>Underscored</u> references indicate tables or text in margins.